# DEVILS, DRUGS AND DOCTORS

THE STORY

*of the Science of Healing*
*from Medicine-Man to Doctor*

*By* HOWARD W. HAGGARD, M.D.

WITH MANY ILLUSTRATIONS FROM
ORIGINAL SOURCES

POCKET BOOKS, INC., ROCKEFELLER CENTER, NEW YORK

Harper edition published April, 1929

1st-7th printings . . . . . . . . . . . . . . . . . . 1929
8th-13th printings . . . . . . . . . . . . . . . . . 1930
14th-17th printings . . . . . . . . . . . . . . . . 1931
18th-20th printings . . . . . . . . . . . . . . . . 1932
21st printing . . . . . . . . . . . . . . . . . . . 1933
22nd printing . . . . . . . . . . . . . . . . . . . 1945

Blue Ribbon edition published November, 1933

1st-3rd printings . . . . . . . . . . . . . . . . . 1933
4th-7th printings . . . . . . . . . . . . . . . . . 1934
8th-9th printings . . . . . . . . . . . . . . . . . 1936
10th-11th printings . . . . . . . . . . . . . . . . 1937
12th printing . . . . . . . . . . . . . . . . . . . 1938
13th-14th printings . . . . . . . . . . . . . . . . 1940

*Pocket Book* EDITION PUBLISHED JUNE, 1946

1st printing . . . . . . . . . . . . . . . . . . . May, 1946

THIS POCKET BOOK INCLUDES EVERY WORD
CONTAINED IN THE ORIGINAL, HIGHER-
PRICED EDITION. IT IS PRINTED FROM BRAND-
NEW PLATES MADE FROM COMPLETELY
RESET, LARGE, CLEAR, EASY-TO-READ TYPE.

PRINTED IN THE U. S. A.

THIS BOOK IS DEDICATED TO
## JOSEPHINE F. HAGGARD

# CONTENTS

## Part One

# THE CONQUEST OF DEATH AT BIRTH

*Part Two*

# THE STORY OF ANESTHESIA

# CONTENTS

## *Part Three*

# THE PROGRESS OF SURGERY

## VI. MAKING AN ANATOMY

*Part Four*

# THE PASSING OF PLAGUE AND PESTILENCE

## Part Five

## THE HEALING ART

## XIII. WHITE MAGIC AND BLACK                               316

Crazy Sal—Hogarth's caricature—Andrew Still gives bone-setting
a new name—Osteopathy—Laying on of hands with impressive
force—The English opinion—Disease from dislocated spines—Faith
healing by diet—Cyril's liver—Fish and brains—Vitamins—Yeast
—Appliance cures—Dr. Perkins of Yale—The famous Dr. DuBuke
branded for stealing indigo—Perkins tractors—Cures with blue
glass—Doctors avoid faith healing—An unsympathetic attitude.

## XIV. A Drug on the Market 337

Drugs as a form of faith healing—The history of a drug told in
the definition—Potatoes as a medicament—Potable gold—The
treatment of Sir Unton—A bottle of medicine and a box of pills
—The belief in their necessity for treatment—An example by
Oliver Wendell Holmes—Carlyle and his wife's medicine—Drugs
and superstition—Egyptian mummy—A protest by Paré—Unicorn's horn—A gift from Pope Clement VII—Unicorn used by
kings of France—Its properties investigated by the Royal Society
—Governor Endicott loans Governor Winthrop a horn—The bezoar stone of Charles IX—The king and Paré experiment on a
condemned criminal—The bezoar fails as an antidote—The moss
from the skull of a criminal—A piece of the hangman's rope—
Cotton Mather prescribes sow bugs—Robert Boyle includes the
sole of an old shoe—Urine recommended as a mouth wash—
Madame de Sévigné—Richelieu's potion—The sympathetic powder
of Sir Kenelm Digby—King James tries it—Proprietary medicines
as faith cures—A fallacious test for drugs—Drugs and spices—The
drug trade—Sea supremacy and exploration—The Dutch control
the drug trade—Bloodshed for the clove—The death of King
Charles II—The medical treatment he received—An endless array
of drugs—King James I resists medical treatment—Poison lore—
Cleopatra as a medical writer—Mithridates, King of Pontus, experiments—Egyptian medicine—The universal antidote—Theriac
—Dioscorides compiles the medical drugs—Medieval Herbals—
Galen's system of treatment—Vegetable simples—Galen's life—
His medical theories—The qualities of the body—"Cool as a cu-
cumber"—Herb doctors—The apothecaries' trade at Rome—Apoth-
ecaries of Europe—The grocers sell drugs—Conserves and other
things for Sir Walter Raleigh and a physic for Mr. Edward
Nichols—"Retired for physic"—An appalling amount of unnec-
essary purging—Bleeding as a form of treatment—Dr. Sangrado—
Apothecaries that prescribed—The objections of the physicians—
Situation in France and England—The comments of Pope and
Dr. Johnson.

# CONTENTS

## Part Six

## MEDICINE THROUGH THE AGES

beginning of the nineteenth century—The scientific spirit ampli-
fied—Great advances that resulted—Anesthesia—Control of puerperal infection—Trained nurses—Aseptic surgery—Preventive medicine—The healthiest period the world has ever known—The possibilities of scientific medicine—No assurance that these possibilities will be realized—Medicine depends upon advancing civiliza-
ton—Civilization prone to regress—The dangers to civilization and
to medicine—The persistence of bigotry and obscurantism.

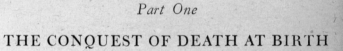

*Part One*

# THE CONQUEST OF DEATH AT BIRTH

"To overthrow superstition, to protect motherhood from pain, to free childhood from sickness, to bring health to all mankind:

"These are the ends for which, through the centuries, the scholars, heroes, prophets, saints and martyrs of medical science have worked and fought and died, as are here recounted."

—Yandell Henderson

. . .

"On either side of the river, was there the tree of life, which bare twelve manner of fruits, and yielded her fruit every month: and the leaves of the tree were for the healing of the nations."

—Revelation, xxii, 2

# CHAPTER I

## CHILDBIRTH AND CIVILIZATION

he position of woman in any civilization is an index of the advancement of that civilization; the position of woman is gauged best by the care given her at the birth of her child. Accordingly, the advances and regressions of civilization are nowhere seen more clearly than in the story of childbirth.

Child-bearing has always been accepted among primitive peoples as a natural process, and as such treated with indifference and brutality. At the height of the Egyptian civili-

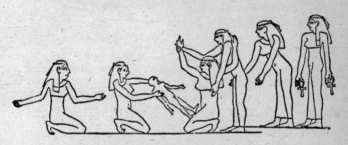

**BIRTH OF CLEOPATRA'S CHILD**

From a bas-relief on the Temple of Esneh. The amazingly large size in which the child is represented is indicative of its royal parentage. The position taken by Cleopatra is still used during childbirth by many primitive peoples.

zation and again at the height of the Greek and Roman civilizations the art of caring for the child-bearing woman was well developed. With the decline of the Greek and Roman civilizations the care of woman deteriorated; for thirteen centuries the practices developed by the Greeks were lost or disregarded in Europe. The art of caring for the child-bearing woman was not brought back to its former development until the sixteenth or seventeenth century of our era.

The medieval Christians saw in childbirth the result of a carnal sin to be expiated in pain as defined in Genesis III:16. Accordingly, the treatment given the child-bearing woman was vastly worse than the mere neglect among the primitive peoples. Her sufferings were augmented by the fact that she

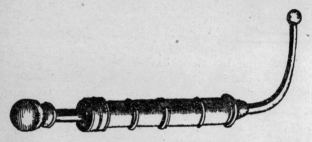

BAPTISMAL SYRINGE

For applying this rite to infants before birth in cases of difficult labor. The particular syringe shown here was designed and described by Mauriceau in the seventeenth century and Laurence Sterne, in *Tristram Shandy,* quotes the original description in full. This syringe was the "squirt" of his "Dr. Slop." In some varieties of the instrument the opening of the nozzle was made in the form of a cross to add sanctity to its use.

was no longer a primitive woman, and child-bearing had become more difficult. Urbanization, cross-breeding, and the spread of disease made child-bearing often unnatural and hazardous. During medieval times the mortality for both the child and the mother rose to a point never reached before. This rise of mortality was in part the consequence of indifference to the suffering of women. It was due also to the cultural backwardness of the civilization and the low value placed on life. It was aggravated by the increasing difficulty attending childbirth. These were the "ages of faith," a period characterized as much by the filth of the people as by the fervor and asceticism of their religion; consequently nothing was done to overcome the enormous mortality of the mother and of the child at birth. It was typical of the age that attempts were made to form intrauterine baptismal tubes, by which the child, locked by some ill chance in its mother's womb, could be baptized and its soul saved before the mother and the child were left to die together. But nothing was done to save their lives. No greater crimes were ever committed in the name of civilization, religious faith, and smug ignorance than the sacrifice of the lives of countless mothers and children in the first fifteen centuries after Christ among civilized mankind.

With the Renaissance of European civilization there came a change in the care given the child-bearing woman. This change was slower in advancing than were many of the other changes which marked this period. Material advancement was made before humanitarian advancement.

The care of the child-bearing woman is an index of the civilization of the community as a whole and not alone of the leaders of the civilization. These leaders blaze the way, they show the path to a better civilization, but that civilization comes only when the path is followed. Throughout the story of childbirth these leaders of the conquest of death at birth stand out from other men like giants in their times. These men, whose praise is unsung and whose names are unknown to most people, rank higher in the advance of our civilization and are greater men by every standard than any of the kings and statesmen whose names are taught to school children and whose works are measured by the ephemeral boundaries which they won for the countries where they fought and intrigued. The great men who were the champions in the conquest of death at birth have not fought in vain. Their glory, to the measure which the advance of civilization will allow, is in every child who lives today and in every woman who bears a child.

The modern conquest of death at birth was started in the sixteenth century. As a result of its advance, the woman of today, if she will and if the civilization of her community gives her the privilege, may look upon pregnancy not as a curse, not as the inevitable result of a "sin," but as a privilege of her sex, to be indulged in only when she chooses to do so. Hers is a pregnancy no longer darkened with the shadow of the wing of death, but illuminated with the clear light of the precise medical knowledge of her condition. She is told in advance the safety of her state and delivered of her child with a minimum of suffering never dreamed of by her primitive sister of twenty-five centuries ago, nor even by her sister of three centuries ago, as she expiated her sin in the heritage of womankind or was butchered to death by the midwife or the barber.

The conquest of death at birth has made its victories. In its means of advancement it has run ahead of the slowly moving civilization. It now waits for that lag of culture, the slow pulling of the feet out of the mire of medieval ignorance, which must end before woman can benefit to the fullest by the victories of the conquest. The neglect of the parturient woman and her child, seen in the deaths at birth and in the hazard of bearing children, is no fault of the medical profession. That profession has led in the conquest, but it can give no more than the community will accept. It cannot of itself overcome the inertia of civilization, nor say what value shall be placed on the lives of women and children.

Young civilizations are like adolescent boys: they are strong and aggressive, they take a noisy pride in the toys of their material advancement, but the very uncertainty of their unproven strength makes them ashamed to stoop to acts of kindness for fear they will be accused of weakness. They have the Utopian ideals of adolescence, but they have, too, its self-consciousness and blindness and ignorance; they reach for the stars and tread the lilies underfoot; they ignore the real problems of life and civilization. There are twenty civilized countries in the world which record the proportion of mothers and children who die at childbirth. The order of those fatalities places the civilization of a country. The United States ranks nineteenth from the top. In only one of these twenty countries, and that one in South America, is there a greater hazard for the child-bearing woman.

Child-bearing among primitive peoples is today what child-bearing was to our ancestors twenty-five centuries ago, and little different from what it was three centuries ago, except that some of the hazards were greater at the later period than at the earlier. Intuition would lead the primitive woman, as it would the animal, to bear her young, and by laceration with her teeth to sever the cord which attaches the child to its mother. The primitive woman had little difficulty with childbirth; but she had not been exposed to the evils of civilization. Distortion of the bones of her pelvis by rickets, and the consequent difficulty or impossibility of natural birth, did not affect her, for she had not yet been subjected to the diet evolved by civilization nor did she shut herself from the radiations of the sunlight by glass and clothing. Furthermore, she was not subject to that mongrelization characteristic of civilization, the cross-breeding which commerce makes possible. Her people were of one size; her baby was suited to the size of the pelvis through which it must emerge.

The native woman led a life of active work; in consequence, her child was small. By her exertions, carried on to the day of her delivery, the child was literally shaken into the normal head-down position for the easiest and safest birth. Even in urban communities today hard work and some privation have their effects in making childbirth easier. Among women who do no heavy manual work the babies are heavier at birth than among those women who do manual work; the easier births among the working class are not, as is often supposed, due to a nearer approach to natural conditions—often far from it—but, if they occur, are due to the smaller size of the children born.

The woman of native or primitive peoples was not in horror of the devastation of childbed fever. The hand of no medical student or *accoucheur* of the pre-antiseptic age brought to her the contamination from the autopsy room or from her stricken sisters. Nor did she take her place in the filthy bed of a hospital of the seventeenth, eighteenth and even early nineteenth centuries, to lie perhaps with four other patients in a bed five feet wide, as at the Hôtel Dieu at Paris, and wait, if she survived the fetid air, the pestilence of the place, and the butchery of the midwife or student, for the fever, engendered by the "weather," which killed from two to twenty of every hundred of her sisters who were forced to accept the fatal charity of such places. The primitive woman met all of these refinements of civilization later —when she met the civilized peoples. She met also other things which influenced her child-bearing; she met syphilis and tuberculosis, plague and typhus fever, gonorrhea and alcohol, and worst of all she met the crowding into cities and the shame taught by the Christian religion.

The fact that labor is a more natural process among primitive women does not imply that most civilized women cannot bear their children with little help. But a vastly higher percentage are unable to do so than was the case with the primitive women. Civilization and its blessings imposed an increasing number of penalties upon child-bearing, and for centuries, while our modern type of civilization was developing, no progress was made to counteract these penalties. Modern science has intervened at last and is able to compensate, and more than compensate, for the handicap of civilization. It can now save lives that would have been lost even under the most natural conditions. It can do more, for it can minimize for women the effects that child-bearing might have upon length of life, a consideration that did not affect the short-lived primitive peoples. The primitive woman had but one great fear in childbirth; that was that the child she carried would be in an abnormal position—as, for instance, transversely across the pelvis instead of in the normal head-down position—so that it could not be born. Such cases were fatal to both the child and the mother, but they are so no longer.

In childbirth among primitive peoples the woman usually retired from her tribe as the birth of the child became imminent. In some cases she would go alone, but more often she would be accompanied by a friend or some old woman, the prototype of the midwife. She retired either into the woods beside a stream or lake, or into a shelter set apart for child-bearing; in some instances the women retired also to these shelters for the duration of their menstrual periods. While isolation was the usual custom, it was not so always; among the natives of the Sandwich Islands the "confinement" was public and the performance was witnessed by all who happened to be about. There, contrary to the common practice, an old man usually served in the capacity of midwife and the woman was delivered sitting on his lap, while her friends gathered about to render assistance and give advice. A surgeon of the American army attended, in the middle of the last century, the wife of an Umpqua chief. He states that he found the patient in a lodge rudely constructed of driftwood, packed to suffocation with women and men. The stifling odors that arose from their sweating bodies, combined with smoke, made it impossible for him to remain in the apartment longer than a few moments at a time. The assembly was shouting and crying in the wildest manner and crowding about the unfortunate sufferer, whose misery was greatly augmented by the kindness of her friends.

Among most primitive peoples the mother bathed in cold water when the child was born, and either returned immediately to her tasks or waited for some time until she had undergone a period of isolation and sacramental purification. The purification among some peoples developed into a rite of a religious nature. Fundamentally it served the purpose of giving the woman a much-needed rest, but often the ceremonial aspects which attached to it made it more of a torture than otherwise. For instance, among the Siamese it was required that the expulsion of the child should be followed by a month of penance for the mother. It was impressed upon the female mind in Siam that the most direful consequences to both mother and child would ensue unless for thirty days after the birth of her first child—a period diminished to five days at subsequent births—she exposed her naked abdomen and back to the heat of a blazing fire, not two feet distant from her, kept up incessantly day and night.

The woman, acting as her own turnspit, exposed front and back to the excessive heat, while the husband or nurse was at hand to stir up and replenish the fire. The practice had at least one virtue—it allowed the women of that land to escape the evils that result so often among other natives from resuming household duties too soon after the birth of their children. The Siamese mother was guaranteed by this custom one month of undisturbed rest by her own fireside.

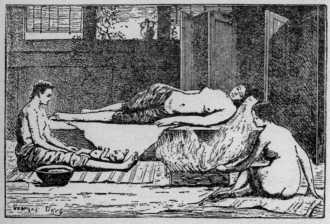

CEREMONIAL PURIFICATION AFTER CHILDBIRTH AMONG THE SIAMESE

For thirty days after the first child, and for a shorter period after each subsequent child, the mother exposed her back and abdomen to a fire kept burning day and night and at a distance scarcely two feet from her.

Most primitive peoples have held the belief, which has persisted even among some civilized peoples almost to the present time, that labor was a voluntary act upon the part of the child, due to its desire to escape from its confined quarters. The woman who assisted at the birth did all she was able to coax out the child by promises of food, and resorted to threats if the child was obdurate. The expectant mother was even starved during the last week of her pregnancy in order that the child might be more willing to emerge and obtain the milk that awaited it. The character of the labor undergone by the woman was referred to the disposition of the child; all difficulties were blamed upon its evil disposition. This belief afforded good grounds for the destruction of the child by efforts at forcing its delivery and even by instruments designed for this purpose, since a child so perverse as to refuse flatly to appear merited death, as did the mother who carried such a child.

If the labor of the primitive mother was difficult, assistance of the straightforward type might be called into play. She was picked up by the feet and shaken, head down, or rolled and bounced on a blanket, or possibly laid on the open plain in order that a horseman might ride at her with the apparent intention of treading on her, only to veer aside at the last moment, and by the fear thus inspired aid in the expulsion of the child. Again, she might be laid on her back to have her abdomen trod upon, or else be hung to a tree by a strap passed under her arms, while those assisting her bore down on a strap over her abdomen. Such practices as these last were known in Europe four hundred years ago. Music, as in singing or the beating of drums, might form a part of the accompaniment of labor, and even a volley of gun-fire has been used. Among the ancient Greeks sacred songs were sung during childbirth, and even today the lower class of Jewish women wail their accompaniment to the shrill cries of the parturient woman. In difficult labor the medicine-man of the tribe, or his successor at later periods, the priest, might be called in; the latter, perhaps, would hastily mumble a few verses of some book, for example the Koran, spit in the patient's face, and leave the rest to nature. If one doubts the efficacy of saliva, particularly fasting saliva, to aid the parturient woman, one has but to turn to Pliny's Natural History to see the multitude of diseases it cured in his time. Before we smile at Pliny's gullibility, or the natives' unsanitary practice, let us remember that Jesus cured the blind with spittle.

In even the most remote period, however crude or primitive the people, aid was given the child-bearing woman. The delivery of children and the healing of wounds are two arts that can be traced to earliest records and of necessity received attention from the most primitive people. Women

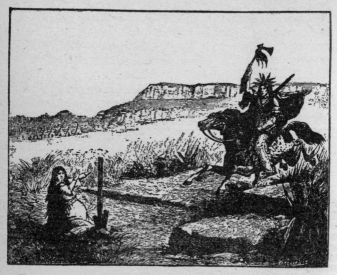

AN INDIAN BRAVE HASTENING LABOR

Formerly among some of the tribes of American Indians labor was hastened by placing the woman on the prairie and having a horseman ride at her with the apparent intention of trampling her. Although the rider turned aside at the last moment, the fear inspired in the woman was sometimes effective in shortening her labor.

who had themselves borne children and were thus taught by experience assisted their neighbors, just as warriors or hunters, exposed to injury, rendered aid to their injured fellow men. As the organization of the community advanced, some of these women who assisted at childbirth did so regularly, and later for gain. Thus arose the midwife, at first a blessing and a comfort, but later the greatest impediment to the advance of the obstetrical art. With the coming of civilization the care of the wounded soldier or hunter fell into the hands of the physician, the priest, the barber or surgeon; advance was made, although slowly, because it was held back by blind prejudice. Not so with childbirth, for the midwife held her position. The art was in the hands of women of low caste. Assistance at childbirth was looked upon as a woman's work, and because of the type of women who plied this trade progress was impossible. The aid of the priest, or man possessed of mystical power, and later the physician, was called in difficult cases only when the efforts of the midwife were ineffective. It is only at the peak of ancient civilizations and quite late in our own, that the physician personally took charge of labor in occasional cases.

The midwife is found in the very beginning of those civilizations which have contributed to our own. The progress of these civilizations and the height to which they reached are marked by the development of regulations to control the practices of the midwives and by the care given to childbearing women. Among the ancient Jews more attention was paid to the hygiene of pregnancy and childbirth than to any active assistance for the lying-in woman. Hygienic measures were, with the Jews, a part of religion, while in difficult births the women "were comforted until they died." With them delivery took place on a stool or in the lap of another woman. In the first chapter of Exodus, when Pharaoh commands the midwives to slay all Jewish infants of the male sex, mention is made of the obstetrical chair, "when you do the office of the midwife to the Hebrew women, and see them upon the stools—." It was not until the nineteenth century after Christ that the obstetrical chair ceased to be a necessary professional equipment of the midwife, which she trundled from patient to patient. Mauriceau of France in the seventeenth century started the innovation of using a bed for childbirth.

Among the Egyptians in 3000 B.C., and in India in the period of Brahmanism, 1500 B.C., the epoch of priestly aid was at its height. The priest no longer beseeched divine interference, but actually rendered effective assistance when called in by the midwife; surgical procedures were practiced, manipulation was resorted to, and instruments for removing

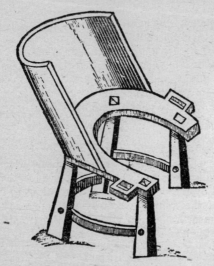

AN OBSTETRICAL CHAIR

The obstetrical chair upon which women sat during childbirth is mentioned in the Old Testament. The Greeks occasionally used a special bed or couch for this purpose, but the obstetrical chair continued in general use until the seventeenth century and was often used as late as the nineteenth century. Many different types of chairs were designed, but the one shown here was recommended by Eucharius Roslin in 1513.

the dead child began to appear. The priesthood, with a certain knowledge of anatomy and medicine, by manipulation, by internal remedies, more especially cathartic and nauseating, and by mental impressions, overcame some of the difficulties of labor. Even podalic version, to be described and discussed later, at its reappearance in the sixteenth century, was known. Religious laws dictated Cæsarean section upon the dead, and a proper care of the pregnant and especially of the unclean or infected woman. The practices used in India for difficult labor involved calling in the physician, and he made it a bloody practice, a tendency to which the Orien-

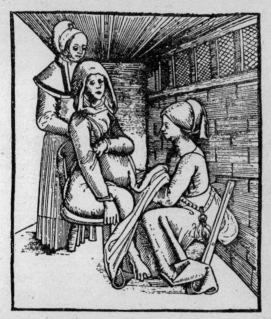

OBSTETRICAL CHAIR IN USE

A reproduction of a sixteenth-century woodcut appearing in *The Garden of Roses for Pregnant Women*, by Roslin.

tal physician was given, but from which he was restrained to some extent by religious precepts. The Indian practice involves the following directions: "When a child cannot be brought forth, the physician may employ the knife in such a way that he by no possibility cuts a living child with it; for if a child is injured, the physician may destroy both child and mother together." In the detailed description of the operation which followed this injunction of caution the only anesthesia mentioned was that embodied in the phrase, "Having cheered up the woman, . . ." Nor was there any anesthesia for such cases anywhere in the world until the nineteenth century. The same operation of piecemeal removal of the dead child after the prolonged labor in impossible delivery appears in the bloody practices of medieval Europe. In fact, its performance then was the only excuse for calling in male help, but the caution against injuring the mother was not observed at this later period.

The Susruta, a book containing the ancient system of midwifery formerly handed down by word of mouth, states that a woman should be delivered by four aged and knowing women whose *nails were well trimmed*. The law regarding midwives, as it appeared in Athens, states that the midwives must be women themselves past the age of child-bearing, but who have had a child. It was in effect as if it had been said that the requirements for a surgeon were that he had passed the age of fighting and had been wounded. In the Christian era there were no regulations for midwives until 1555, and at that time only in the city of Ratisbon.

Modern medicine comes from Greek medicine. The Greeks were organizers of culture. They assimilated all that previous civilizations had to offer and took the best from existing civilizations. They had the faculty of arranging these foreign elements and raising them to an extraordinary perfection. As the medicine of the early Greeks became organized it was in the hands of the priests of Æsculapius, whose temples of healing were located about the countryside. Æsculapius was probably a real character, but in time he was deified and woven into the Greek system of mythology. According to legends, Æsculapius suffered many vicissitudes in his early life. By one tale he was said to be the son of Coronis and Apollo, and was saved at birth only by taking him from his mother's womb as she was brought to her funeral pyre. According to another tale his mother was Ascinoe and, while there were no difficulties in the matter of his birth, he was abandoned as an infant, but was saved from starvation by a goat. Æsculapius survived his stormy childhood and lived to marry twice. By his first wife he had a daughter named Hygeia. His second wife was Lampetia, daughter of the sun-god. The name Æsculapius has passed from common usage in the language, but that of Hygeia is present in its various forms, such as hygiene, hygienic, and hygienist. The symbol of Æsculapius, the caduceus—the two snakes twined on a staff—has survived, and is still used today as a medical emblem. It is not to be wondered at that a god whose father, Apollo, was a physician and who had been so intimately concerned with a Cæsarean section, and one of the earliest examples of the artificial feeding of an infant, should turn quite naturally to the study of medicine. His instructor in the art was the centaur, Chiron, who, in spite of being half horse and half man, was the most versatile of the celestial professors. The death of Æsculapius came about as the result of an occurrence which has been attributed to no physician since his time. Pluto complained to Zeus that the prolongation of life on the earth, due to the ministrations of Æsculapius, was keeping down the population of Hades. Zeus, to restore the balance of population, slew Æsculapius with a thunderbolt,

So great, as the Greeks believed, was the power of Æsculapius over disease, so wonderful were the cures which he accomplished, and so noble and pure his character, that they not only made him a god, but erected temples in his honor. These temples were not places of barren worship, but were sanatoria, termed Æsclepieia, which in the course of time became the prototypes of our hospitals, sanatoria, and schools of medicine. The means chiefly employed for the restoration of health were sunlight, fresh air, pure water, exercise, and diet. The priests did not, however, hesitate to use drugs and even perform operations if the patient's condition seemed to warrant them, but the whole of their medical procedure was strongly tinctured with superstition and religious practices. In spite of the excellent care given to the sick by the early Greeks, two classes of people were discriminated against—

those who were moribund and women about to be confined were not allowed in the temple inclosure. The management of the latter class of cases was left entirely to the midwives. Later, as a mark of progressing civilization, the Emperor Antoninus Pius provided a special building at Epidaurus in which confinement cases and those likely to end fatally might be lodged.

Instruction in medicine was given in the Temple of Æsculapius. This instruction was oral, since there were no written medical works among the Greeks before the fifth century before Christ. At the conclusion of the medical course the pupils took an oath which embodied the tenets of the physician. This oath, often called the oath of Hippocrates, is in principle as applicable to the ethics of the physician to-day as it was 2,500 years ago. It is, in part: "I swear by Apollo, the physician, and Æsculapius and Hygeia and Panacea and all the gods and all the goddesses . . . so far as power and discernment shall be mine, I will carry out regimen for the benefit of the sick and will keep them from harm and wrong. To none will I give a deadly drug even if solicited, nor offer counsel to such an end; likewise, to no woman will I give a substance to produce abortion; but guiltless and hallowed will I keep my life and my art. I will cut no one whatever for the stone, but will give way to those who work at this practice. Into whatsoever house I shall enter I will go for the benefit of the sick, holding aloof from all voluntary wrong and corruption, including the seduction of females and males, of freemen and slaves. Whatsoever in my practice or not in my practice I shall see or hear amid the lives of men I will not divulge, as reckoning that all such things should be kept secret. . . ."

With the lapse of time the religious features of the temple fell away to give place to more and more rational medical treatment, and the priest and the physician separated. The greatest of these early Greek physicians was Hippocrates. His teachings are extant and in many respects form a basis of modern medical practices. Hippocrates the Great was born in the island of Kos in 460 B.C., thirty years after the

keep the child, she "exposed" it on a hillside or temple steps, where it might die from starvation or be taken for adoption by some passer-by. At that period infant desertion was a legitimate practice and remained so until the Christian era. The midwife likewise gave advice on the physical eligibility of those contemplating matrimony—she ran a sort of primitive matrimonial bureau—treated diseases of women and produced abortion if desired. Abortion was then common and not illegal, but under the Hippocratic oath was not ethical for physicians. With their manifold social and medical duties the Greek midwives were an institution, but their field did not extend over into that of the physician.

While the Greeks were developing their rational system of medicine their warlike neighbors, the Romans, were without any systematized medicine. The Romans had, instead, systematized superstitions. They looked for aid from their deities, of which there was one for every disease and indeed for every stage of every disease. Their medical practice is summed up in the statement that "even the itch was not without its goddess." About two hundred years before the birth of Christ a few Greek physicians wandered over into the virgin Roman field. The Romans, like any other superstitious people, were ready to embrace a new cult. They had never paid fees for having their sick helped. The votaries to the gods had been voluntary and that meant that they had probably consisted of promises of great awards while the illness lasted, but only slight compensation on the second thought after the illness was over, and, quite logically, no award if death resulted. The Greek physicians collected their fees. This fact impressed the Romans with the virtue of the treatment, on the principle of that which costs money must be worth having. As Cato phrases it, "a profession which they exercise for lucre, in order that they may win our confidence."

The early experiences of the Romans with Greek physicians were discouraging. Some of the physicians who came first to Rome were the dregs of the profession; they took advantage of the gullible Romans and badly misbehaved themselves. Cato, that irritable misanthrope of the second century B.C., as would be expected, had a condemning word to say of Greek physicians. Cato was a Roman Cotton Mather and had a good opinion only of Cato, for in his words he "owed less to the people of Rome than the people of Rome owed to him." Cato it was who concluded his speeches in the Senate by croaking out: "Carthage must be destroyed," to urge Rome on to the second Punic war. Of Greek physicians he says among other things: "They [the Greeks] are a most iniquitous and intractable race, and you may take my word as the word of a prophet when I tell you, that whenever that nation shall bestow its literature upon Rome it will mar everything; and that all the sooner if it sends its physicians among us. They have conspired among themselves to murder all barbarians with their medicine. . . . They are in the common habit, too, of calling us barbarians. . . . I forbid you to have anything to do with physicians." The Romans had then "got on for six hundred years without physicians," and as subsequent events showed, Cato's warning was not without its merits. Some of his ire, however, may have arisen from jealousy, for he is said to have had a famous book of recipes by aid of which he treated the maladies of his sons, his servants, and also, Pliny says, his friends, although, knowing Cato's character, that seems dubious.

The Romans at first had no laws to punish malpractice, poisoning, and the manipulation of wills by hired physicians. Pliny mentions some of the abuses which resulted from the inadequacy of legal protection. He says: "It is at the expense of our perils that they learn, and they experimentalize by putting us to death, a physician being the only person that can kill another with sovereign impunity. Nay, even more than this, all the blame is thrown upon the sick man only; he is accused of disobedience forthwith, and it is the person who is dead and gone that is put upon trial." Pliny lived in the first century after Christ and was active in the practice of law at Rome and was a politician. By having a secretary to take down his dictation, at any hour of the day or night, he managed in his spare time to turn out 108 large books, covering biography, political history, and natural history, but containing very little that was original or even critically considered. His most famous work is his *Natural History,* in thirty-seven volumes, which covers almost every conceivable subject which might be classified

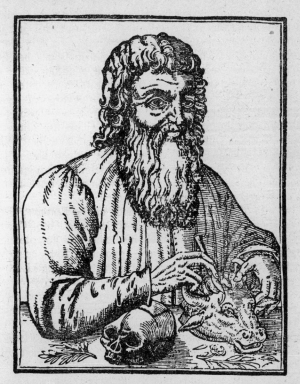

"HIPPOCRATES OF COOS, THE PRINCE OF PHYSICIANS"

From a woodcut in the *Surgery* of Ambroise Paré, sixteenth century. Hippocrates was the father of modern medicine; he lived in the fifth century before Christ, but the principles he set forth for medicine were not developed fully until the nineteenth century.

under this title. He had great respect for the opinions of Cato, but was somewhat more just in regard to physicians, for he says: "These [malpractices and ignorance] are faults, however, which must be imputed to individuals only; and it is not my intention to waste reproof upon the dregs of the medical profession, or call attention to the ignorance displayed by that crew."

As Pliny points out, the predictions of Cato were realized, particularly in the unprofessional philanderings of Drs. Eudemus and Vectius Valens, early medical arrivals in Rome. Eudemus had an intrigue with Livia and poisoned her husband, Drusus Cæsar; and Valens had an affair with the notorious Messalina, who in turn had Livia executed and was herself murdered. Livia was the daughter of Agrippina, who, with the aid of the physician Xenophon of Kos, poisoned her husband, the Emperor Claudius. Pliny exclaimed over the misconduct of Eudemus and Valens: "What adulteries have been committed in the very houses of our princes, even!" If the Romans were unfamiliar with malpractice, they at least had a familiarity with adultery. Eudemus was tortured and Valens was executed.

In spite of the unfriendly attitude of the Romans, Greek medicine migrated to Rome after the destruction of Corinth in 146 B.C. Eventually Greek medicine was accepted and city and court physicians were appointed. Nero employed the latter to treat the bruises he contracted during his nightly revels incognito in the streets of the city.

Greek medicine continued to develop at Rome and culminated in the ancient practice of midwifery as told in the writings of Soranus of Ephesus, second century after Christ. Soranus lived in Rome in the time of Trajan and Hadrian. His work on midwifery and the diseases of women set a standard beyond which there was no further advance for fourteen centuries and indeed much regression. His contempt for the Roman system of medical deities is complete in his blunt statement that "the midwife should be no believer in spirits." He had considerable knowledge of the anatomy of the female reproductive tract, but it was far from exact in its details, for the Greek religion would not tolerate human dissection, and for such anatomy as was not visible he was forced to base his knowledge on dissection of animals. His teachings brought the child-bearing woman a kindness of treatment she had never before received. He disapproved of the reckless employment of medicines for hastening labor or applying force to the woman for this purpose. He taught sensible, rational care and assistance

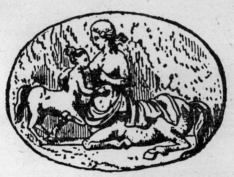

A CENTAURESS NURSING HER CHILD
From an ancient cameo

based on knowledge and not on superstition. He reintroduced podalic version. This procedure of turning and extracting the child, instead of employing instruments to destroy it, marks the peaks of ancient midwifery. Its revival in the sixteenth century after Christ marks the point where medieval midwifery was finally raised to a par with that of the ancients. Soranus himself practiced midwifery, a custom that two centuries later passed from the Western civilization, to be not only ignored by the physician, but actually prohibited by custom and law until only a little over three centuries ago, when a king of France progressed far enough in his civilization to have a regard for his mistress, if not for his wife, such that he was moved to again call in the physician as a midwife.

The following extract from the book of Soranus shows something of the character of this great physician of antiquity, the greater because he devoted his services to the sufferings of motherhood: "There is a disagreement; for some reject destructive practices, calling to witness Hippocrates, who says: 'I will give nothing whatever destructive; and deeming it the special province of medicine to guard and preserve what nature generates.' Another party maintains the same view but makes this distinction, namely, that the fruit of conception is not to be destroyed at will because of adultery or of care for beauty, but is to be destroyed to avert danger appending to birth, if the womb be small and cannot subserve perfection of the fruit, or have hard swellings and cracks at its mouth, or if some similar condition prevail."

# CHAPTER II

## SAIREY GAMPS AND THE MIDMEN

ivilizations, like human beings, grow old, become decrepit, and die. But also like human beings their influence is sometimes felt long after they have died. The Roman Empire declined, and Greek medicine deteriorated. The Christian religion was in ascendancy, and under the influence of its theology attention was turned from the physical aspects of life to the spiritual. Revelation replaced reason; the cause of disease became possessions by devils, and the cure of disease was attempted by exorcism or miracles. Rational medicine was replaced by superstition. The teachings of such Greek physicians as Hippocrates and Soranus were lost to the practices of the Western world. Yet these teachings were preserved in the manuscripts collected in the monasteries of Christian Europe. They were buried there, to be resurrected, rediscovered, centuries later. While they waited, the struggle for medical knowledge was crushed by the power of the Church; the clergy zealously retained the gathered learning within the monasteries as a scepter to sway the masses, who were kept in ignorance. The teachings of able men were laid aside to be replaced by ridiculous theories and methods which originated in fanaticism and grew upon the ignorance of the people.

The Middle Ages were the most unfortunate period in the history of womankind. Complete ignorance prevailed, without the intuitive skill of the primitive period and without the knowledge of previous civilizations. Women were deprived of the aid, however poor, of the male physician, and at the same time the penalties of urban civilization were making childbirth more and more hazardous. The practices of the Middle Ages present the accumulated evils of previous periods aggravated by ignorance and barbarism. Womankind had indeed fallen into evil days in that Christian era. She paid for the mythical fall of man, under her temptation of him, in the coin of pain and blood and death.

Primitive woman had resorted to abortion when she thought the birth of her child might be difficult or when she

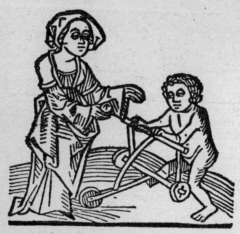

FIFTEENTH-CENTURY KIDDY-CAR

This woodcut, with variations, was used in the past in many books dealing with the care of children. It originally appeared in "Versehung des Leibs," a poem on the care of children written by a monk of the fifteenth century.

was nursing another child. From the quotations from Soranus given at the end of the last chapter it is evident that whatever the attitude of the midwives might have been, the Greek physicians themselves looked upon abortion in much the same light as do physicians today, to be performed not lightly, but only when the life or health of the mother was in danger. The Roman Church of medieval times put a bar to even this mode of escape for the tortured women of that period; the penalty of eternal damnation was threatened for the operation of abortion, and Cæsarean section was advocated to replace the accursed procedure. The opening of the abdomen and uterus to remove the child was then an operation to be performed without anesthesia, with no knowledge of antiseptics, and with a crudity of procedure equal to that of the most barbaric people. The physician of the Middle Ages did not perform surgical operations; such things were below his professional dignity and belonged to the executioner or to the barber, who was the forerunner of our surgeons, or to whoever cared to undertake them, regardless of his qualification to do so. In the middle of the thirteenth century Bishop Paulus of Meirada, in Spain, is said to have performed a Cæsarean operation on a living woman, though it is doubtful if he did; the next to practice the art was a hog-gelder, who, two centuries later, performed the operation on his own wife.

Sex concepts have always been mingled with religion; thus we find today venereal disease defended by a quasi-religious attitude as a punishment of sin; and the prevention of conception, which is an economic measure, similarly contested. In the medieval times religion took over the supervision of the prostitutes and the oversight of the practices of the midwives. Thus the Dominican monk, Albertus Magnus (Albert von Bollstädt, 1193-1280), wrote a book for the guidance of midwives, and the Church councils passed edicts on their practices. These instructions and edicts were not, however, for the better care of the child-bearing woman, for the relief of her suffering or the prevention of her death. They were designed to save the child's life for a sufficient time to allow it to be baptized. Thus the Council of Cologne in 1280 decreed that on the sudden death of a woman in labor her mouth was to be kept open with a gag so that her child would not suffocate while it was being removed by operation. The intention involved was better than the physiology.

There is little actual knowledge of the practices of the midwives in medieval times, but their degradation can be judged by those at the beginning of the Renaissance. Even in a normal delivery the woman often died from infection or eclampsia. In difficult labor she was left to die or butchered to death if her midwife was of the type of Dickens's Sairey Gamp, or if a vagabond "surgeon" or hog-gelder could be found to assist at the slaughter. As a rule the matter was left entirely in the hands of the midwife, and in 1580 a law was passed in Germany to prevent shepherds and herdsmen from attending obstetrical cases—an indication both of the advance of civilization and what it had advanced from.

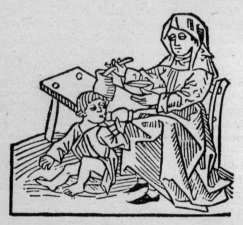

FIFTEENTH-CENTURY NURSE AND CHILD

From "Versehung des Leibs." Accompanying this picture were the following directions for selecting a nurse (translation is from Ruhrah, *Pediatrics of the Past*).

"At times it happens that from various causes the Mother cannot suckle the child herself. In such a case one must choose a nurse for the child. Her qualifications should be as follows. The nurse must be of shapely stature, not too young and not too old. She must at all times be free from illness of eyes or body. Moreover, her nature must be such that there is no defect in her body. Mark also, that she must be neither too slim, nor too plump. If there should be any defect in her, the child would incline towards it. She must have a good character, modest, chaste and clean. Her food should be in conformity with the following directions, so that the milk may remain fully nourishing. I

The state of affairs that existed in the medieval period and early Renaissance is not to be wondered at, for this was a time when public, domestic, and personal hygiene was at its lowest ebb. The walled cities were for the most part densely crowded and had no drainage. Filth accumulated in the unpaved streets. The dwelling-houses were described by Erasmus as containing open cesspools, their floors were strewn with refuse, and in them was a pestilence of flies and vermin. They were indeed sinks of filth and infection. Ancient Rome had paved streets; Paris had none until the eleventh century. Handkerchiefs, nightgowns, and table forks did not come into use until centuries later. London had its first paved streets in the sixteenth century. In that same century Frankfort-on-the-Main started the innovation of requiring each house to have a privy and ordered that the pigpens of the city should be cleaned.

Fifteen centuries of the Christian era culminated in the production of one book, worthy of the name, for the direction of midwives, who throughout this time had been left literally to their own discretion. Eucharius Roslin, of Worms, in response to the wishes of Catherine, the Duchess of Brunswick, wrote a manual from which the ignorant and careless old women who made up the midwives might learn to conduct their work in a safer and more efficient manner. This book was published in Worms in 1513 and contained

---

prescribe her to eat white bread and good meat, also rice and lettuce every day. Almonds as well as hazelnuts she should not do without. Her beverage must be a pure wine; and moderation must be used in bathing. Nor must she do much labor. In case her milk should give out, she must not forget to eat peas frequently and in quantity, also beans, and in addition gruel which should be boiled in milk beforehand. She must also rest and sleep a good deal so that the child may thrive on the milk. Moreover, she must carefully avoid onions and garlic; as well as any bitter or sour food and any dish containing pepper. She must eat no over-salted food, nor anything prepared with vinegar. Love's intercourse she must also avoid or go in for it very moderately. For in case she should become pregnant, her milk would be harmful to the child. In order that the child may not be harmed in such a case, one must wean it from the milk."

nothing that was new, but did bring to light the work of the
Greeks; it was, however, marked with the superstition of
medieval medicine, fumigation with dove's dung, and similar
practices, and with the horrible doctrine of medieval surgical
midwifery. The prejudices which at that time existed in the
minds of the people, particularly in cities, against the slightest participation of males in the practice of midwifery, were
so great that Roslin, who had probably never seen a child
born, may have felt something of the humor of his position,
for the title of his book was *The Garden of Roses for
Pregnant Women and for Midwives*. The book, nevertheless,
accomplished much good; it was extensively plagiarized by
later authors and was translated into Latin, French, Dutch,
and English, in which last country the title became *The
Byrthe of Mankynde*. The exclusion of men from the study
of the child-bearing woman rose in some instances to fanatical heights. Dr. Wertt, of Hamburg, in 1522, put on the
dress of a woman to attend and study a case of labor. As a
punishment for his impiety he was burned to death.

In the sixteenth century can be detected the first stir that
presaged the sweeping advances to be made in the care given
the child-bearing woman and her child. The *Rose Garden* of
Roslin was the first indication that this gentler influence was
making itself felt in civilization, and after that came attention, not to the woman, but to the child, and in this Ambroise
Paré was the prominent figure.

Ambroise Paré, of France, typified the highest type of
medical mind of his time and he was a character of which
any generation might be proud. Paré was a man of gentleness, and as Soranus, from the greatness of his character,
had given attention to the child-bearing woman, so Paré gave
attention to the child to be born. Paré came to Paris in 1529
during the reign of Francis I. He was then a rustic barber's
apprentice, nineteen years of age. He received his early surgical training as a dresser at the Hôtel Dieu. This institution,
typical of the hospitals throughout the world at that time,
deserves mention, that one, having in mind the modern hospital, may have also some conception of the conditions under

which Paré got his training and so appreciate his work the
more. The Hôtel Dieu is said to have been founded between

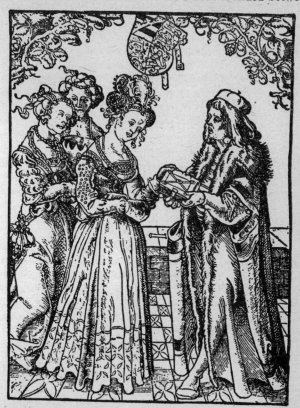

**EUCHARIUS ROSLIN PRESENTING HIS BOOK TO THE
DUCHESS OF BRUNSWICK**

An illustration from *The Garden of Roses,* 1513, showing the author
presenting his book on obstetrics to his patroness. This was the first
book on midwifery in Europe for nearly fourteen centuries. It was
translated into many languages and was extensively plagiarized. The
English edition appeared in 1555 under the title *The Byrthe of Mankynde.*

the years 641 and 649 by Saint Landry, Bishop of Paris, but the first mention made of it in the records is in 829. Upon it Dr. J. S. Billings made this comment: "When the

The fyrſt booke.        fol. v.

⸿ In this fyrſt chapiter is bryefly declaryd the contentes of the fyrſte booke.

Lthough that many thynges entreatyd of in this fyrſte booke, ſhall ſeme vnto ſum not very neceſſary to the vnderſtandynge of the ſeconde booke: yet them contrary do I enſure and certifye (as I haue ſufficiently ſaid in the prologue that the ignorant in the fyrſte, ſhalbe full blynde in the ſeconde: to the which the fyrſt is as a key, openyng and clearyng the matters to be entreated of in the ſeconde.

⸿ In this fyrſt booke then ſhalbe declaryd the forme, maner, and ſytuation of thinwarde partes of a woman: ſuche as are in them. by nature

D.iii.

*(marginal notes:)* Thuclite of the fyrſt oooke.

The contentes of this booke.

A PAGE FROM *THE BYRTHE OF MANKYNDE*

William Raynalde's English translation of Roslin's book on midwifery.

medieval priest established in each great city of France a Hôtel Dieu, a place for God's hospitality, it was in the interest of charity, as he understood it, including both the helping of the sick poor and the affording to those who were neither sick nor poor an opportunity and a stimulus to help their fellowmen; and doubtless the cause of humanity and religion was advanced more by the effects on the givers than on the receivers." The truth of the last statement is amply

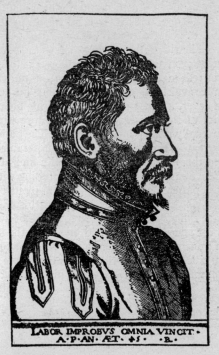

LABOR IMPROBVS OMNIA VINCIT
A·P·AN·ÆT·45·B·

AMBROISE PARÉ AT THE AGE OF FORTY-FIVE

This famous French surgeon of the sixteenth century was then the chief surgeon of King Henry II.

proven by Tenon in his memoirs of the hospitals of Paris. In the Hôtel Dieu there were 1,200 beds, of which 486 were for single patients; from three to six patients occupied each of the remaining beds, which were five feet wide. The large halls, unlighted and unventilated, held 800 or more patients crowded together and often lying about on heaps of straw which were in a vile condition.

Max Nordau has said of the hospital: "In one bed of moderate width lay four, five, or six persons beside each other, the feet of one to the head of another; children beside gray-haired old men; indeed, incredible but true, men and women intermingled together. In the same bed lay individuals affected with infectious diseases beside others only slightly unwell; on the same couch, body against body, a woman groaned in the pangs of labor, a nursing infant writhed in convulsions, a typhus patient burned in the delirium of fever, a consumptive coughed his hollow cough, and a victim of some disease of the skin tore with furious nails his infernally itching integument. . . . The patients often lacked the greatest necessities. The most miserable food was doled out to them in insufficient quantities and at irregular intervals. The nuns were in the habit of feeding with confectionery those patients who seemed to them pious enough, or at least those who reeled off their rosaries with sufficient zeal, but the body exhausted by disease required not sweets, but cried for meat and wine. Such food, however, the sick never received in profusion, save when it was brought to them by the wealthy citizens from the city. For this purpose the doors of the hospital stood open day and night. Anyone could enter; anyone bring whatever he wished; and while the sick on one day might be starved, on another day they might very likely get immoderately drunk and kill themselves by overloading their stomachs. The whole building fairly swarmed with the most horrible vermin, and the air of a morning was so vile in the sick wards that the attendants did not venture to enter them without a sponge saturated with vinegar held before their faces. The bodies of the dead ordinarily lay twenty-four hours, and often longer, upon the deathbed before they were removed, and the sick during this time were compelled to share the bed with the rigid corpse, which in this infernal atmosphere soon began to stink, and over which the green carrion-flies swarmed. . . ."

In this hospital there were beds for children; in fact, eight such beds, which accommodated a total of 200 infants and young children, of whom the majority necessarily succumbed to the charity extended to them. About one-fifth of the patients in the Hôtel Dieu died. Recovery from any surgical operation was in the nature of a rarity. The attention given to surgery in such hospitals may be judged from a description of one in Lyons in 1619. In that hospital, accommodat-

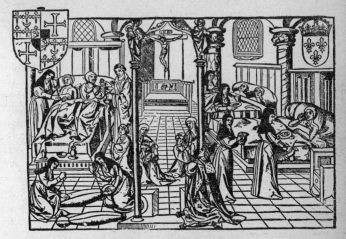

A ROOM IN THE HÔTEL DIEU

From a woodcut of the sixteenth century. The beds shown were intended for two patients, but frequently five or six, regardless of sex or disease, were crowded into each one. Less fortunate patients found refuge on heaps of straw in the dark hallways. This hospital was indescribably filthy, as were all others at this period.

ing 549 patients, there was only one medical man whose duty it was to look after the surgical cases; he resided outside of the building. When this surgeon required assistance in the dressing of wounds or in performing surgical operations, he was authorized to make use of the "apothecary boy." No doubt Paré gave the equivalent of assistance in the hospital of Paris. The stock of surgical instruments possessed by the hospital consisted of just five, which included a trephine for opening the skull and a mouth plug for keeping the jaws separated. In considering the barrenness of the provisions for surgery it must be borne in mind that this art had not yet been rendered "respectable" by the edict of Charles V, although Emperor Wenzel had made it so in Germany in 1404; but the German army surgeons' duty included the shaving of the officers as late as the eighteenth

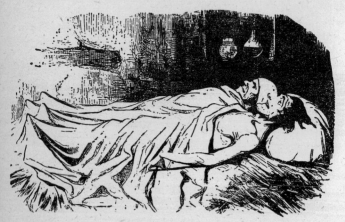

HOSPITAL PATIENT IN BED WITH A CORPSE

A common occurrence in charity hospitals of two or three centuries ago. An etching by Daumier.

century. In the memoranda relating to the duties of the medical staff in the civil hospital of Padua (1569) there is the statement: "And a barber who is competent to do, for the women as well as the men, all the other things that a good surgeon usually does." The "all other things" included every surgical procedure practiced except the applying of ointments to sores and wounds, that being the more "respectable" office of the surgeon himself.

In spite of the gross neglect of the sick and lack of organization, the Hôtel Dieu of Paris was not free from the managerial difficulties which are sometimes encountered by hospitals even today. It was under ecclesiastical supervision, with the care of the sick in the hands of lay brothers and sisters; but in 1505 the parliament of Paris nominated a commission of eight citizens to manage the temporal affairs of the hospital. Whatever the shortcomings in medical practice may have been, there was at least a healthy directness in handling administrative difficulties; the monks and nuns who objected to the changes that were made were dismissed, and the physicians who sided with them were committed to prison.

After three years of training in the Hôtel Dieu, Paré became a lowly army surgeon under Anne de Montmorenci, lieutenant-general in the army of Francis I. France was at this time embroiled in the wars with Emperor Charles V which had resulted from the attempted conquest of Italy. Paré saw his first service at the battle of Turin in 1537, and of it he says:

"In the year 1536 the great King François sent a great army to Turin to recover the cities and castles which had been taken by the Marquis de Guast, lieutenant-general of the emperor: where Monsieur the Constable [Anne de Montmorenci], then grandmaster, was lieutenant-general of the army, and Monsieur de Montegan was colonel-general to the infantry of which I was the surgeon. A great part of the army having arrived at the Pass of Suze, we found the enemy holding the passage. . . . Captain Le Rat climbed with many soldiers from his company on a little hill, whence they fired directly on the enemy. He received a shot from an arquebus in the ankle of his right foot, wherewith he suddenly fell to the ground and then said, 'Now the Rat is taken.' *I dressed his wounds and God healed him.*

"We thronged into the city and passed over the dead bodies and some that were not yet dead, hearing them cry under the feet of our horses, which made a great pity in my heart, and truly I repented that I had gone forth from Paris to see so pitiful a spectacle. Being in the city, I entered a stable, thinking to lodge my horse and that of my man, where I found four dead soldiers and three who were propped against the wall, their faces wholly disfigured, and they neither saw, nor heard, nor spoke, and their clothes yet flaming from the gunpowder, which had burnt them. Beholding them with pity there came an old soldier who asked me if there was any means of curing them. I told him no. At once he approached them and cut their throats gently and without anger. Seeing this great cruelty I said to him that he was an evil man. He answered me that he prayed God that when he should be in such a case, he might find some one who would do the same for him, to the end that he might not languish miserably."

Ten years after this battle, which gave Paré his first experience with military surgery, Francis I died, and his son, Henry II, came to the throne of France. He brought with him a woman to whom his affections were given, the former mistress of his father, Madam de Breze, better known as Diane de Poitiers. She was nineteen years his senior and a widow with two children. He also brought with him to the throne a wife who was embittered by the loss of her husband's affection and by the treatment she had received from the French because of her sterility during the first ten years of her marriage to the Dauphin. Although she subsequently had ten children in thirteen years, her rancor persisted. This wife later was to leave a mark of blood and ruin on the history of France. She was the Italian Catherine de' Medici. The excellency of Paré's work brought him to the attention of the king and he was made his chief surgeon. What was even more important, he became the friend of Catherine de' Medici. When, during a tournament in 1559 the lance of the ill-fated Montgomery accidentally pierced the helmet of the king and entered his brain, Paré attended him. His patient died, and with him passed the supremacy of Diane de Poitiers. Catherine de' Medici was free to vent her malignance on the French through her sons, Francis II, Charles IX, and Henry III. To each of these in turn Paré was chief surgeon, and with Henry III he received the additional title of "counselor to his majesty." After the brief reign of Francis II, husband of Mary Queen of Scotland, Catherine de' Medici ruled during the minority of her son Charles IX. She introduced then that intrigue, corruption, and financial disorganization which Rabelais, the doctor and priest, attacked with gross allegory. She was instrumental, too, in the persecution of the Protestants which through the activity of the family of Guises rose to its peak in the massacre of St. Bartholomew's night. Paré is said to have been the only Protestant for whom there was royal edict to spare his life on that night, but it is also said that there was some question as to the fervor of his religious affiliations.

One of Paré's greatest claims to distinction was his breaking away from the pseudo-Hippocratic and pseudo-Galenic tenets that bound the medical profession of his time; it took a man of courage to depart from a course rigidly prescribed for centuries. His first advance in this direction was in the treatment of gunshot wounds, and although its bearing is greater on the work of surgery to be given in a later chapter, it is used here to illustrate Paré's character for a quotation cannot be given from his work on podalic version. He did not write extensively of that method, but taught it to his assistants, one of whom saved the life of Paré's daughter by its application.

Gunshot wounds were a new feature of the Renaissance surgery; and according to the precept that "disease not curable by iron was curable by fire," they were treated with boiling hot oil. The story of Paré's gentler innovation, so typical of the man, is best told from his own writings, which were sprinkled often with the phrase at once so modest and so true, "I dressed his wounds, and God healed him." In speaking of his experiences with the army in Turin in 1537, from which a quotation has already been given, Paré says:

"Now all the soldiers at the Chateau, seeing our men coming with a great fury, did all they could to defend themselves and killed and wounded a great number of our soldiers with pikes, arquebuses, and stones, where the surgeons had much work cut out for them. Now I was at that time an untried soldier; I had not yet seen wounds made by gunshot at the first dressing. It is true that I had read in Jean di Vigo, first book, *Of Wounds in General,* chapter eight, that wounds made by firearms were poisoned wounds, because of the powder, and for their cure he commands to cauterize them with oil of elder, scalding hot, in which should be mixed a little theriac; and in order not to err before using the said oil, knowing that such a thing would bring great pain to the patient, I wished to know first, how the other surgeons did for the first dressing, which was to apply said oil as hot as possible, into the wounds, of whom I took courage to do as they did. At last my oil lacked and I was constrained to apply in its place a digestive made of the yolks of eggs, oil of roses, and turpentine. That night I could not sleep at my ease, fearing by lack of cauterization that I should find the wounded on whom I had failed to put the said oil dead or empoisoned, which made me rise early to visit them, where beyond my hope I found those upon whom I had put the digestive medicament feeling little pain, and their wounds without inflammation or swelling, having rested fairly well throughout the night; the others to whom I had applied the said boiling oil, I found feverish, with great pain and swelling about their wounds. Then I resolved with myself never more to burn thus cruelly poor men wounded with gunshot."

Paré's medical writings were in the vernacular; he was not a scholar; the medical writings of all other prominent medical men of the time were in Latin. The organized physicians of Paris found therein an excuse for attacking the works of Paré and attempting to prevent their publication: they cited not only his ignorance, "a man very impudent and without any learning," but also that in his teachings he departed from the established practices of the ancients. In reply, among many other things, Paré states: "In outward dislocation of the vertebræ Hippocrates commands to bind the man straight on a ladder, the arms and legs tied and bound, then after having raised the ladder to the top of a tower or ridge of a house, with a great cable in a pulley, let the patient fall like lead on the firm pavement, which Hippocrates said was done in his time. But I do not teach any such way of giving the strappado to men, but I show to the surgeon in my works, the method of reducing them safely and without great pain."

Sufficient of the life of Paré is given here to make clear the character of this man who brought back to civilization and described fully a procedure, podalic version, which was for the child what the discovery of the infectious nature of childbed fever, three centuries later, was for the mother. Podalic version, as described by Paré, was to be used in those cases where the child was not in the normal position to be born. It consisted in inserting the hand into the uterus, grasping one or both feet (hence podalic) of the unborn child, and turning it (*i.e.*, version) into such a position that it could be born. The child was usually extracted, pulled out, at the same time. In the few words which suffice to describe podalic version it seems like an obvious procedure, one that would have occurred even to the medieval midwives. But its application waited centuries for a man who had at heart the kindly interest of humanity and who had the humility to stoop, in that age, to such lowly things as the woman and her child. Paré had many attributes in his character which are seen in those of the founders of great religions, but not always seen in the zealous followers of such religions.

The importance of podalic version for the child-bearing woman can be understood best from a comparison with the conditions existing before its development. As stated in the previous chapter, the primitive woman had but one great fear at childbirth—that her child might be in such a position, as, for instance, transversely across her pelvis instead of in the normal head-down position, that it could not be born. Such cases were fatal for both the child and the mother, but fortunately were rare because of the active life led by the primitive woman. With the coming of civilization a means was found for possibly saving the mother's life at the sacrifice of that of the child; the child, in an increasing number of cases, was killed and removed piecemeal with instruments that the pagan priest and later the physician devised for this purpose. Indeed, until the time of Paré the performance of this act was the only reason for calling in the physician or barber to see the child-bearing woman.

There was one other procedure which gave an alternative

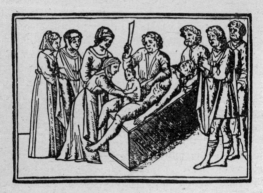

THE BIRTH OF CÆSAR FROM THE 1506 EDITION OF SEUTONIUS

This illustrates the popular belief that Julius Cæsar was born by the so-called Cæsarean operation. In his time the operation was not performed on living women, but only after death as a religious measure. Cæsar's mother lived for several years after he was born. The operation obtained its name from the fact that the Roman law required this procedure in case of the mother's death; the laws under the emperors became Cæsarean laws, and the operation the Cæsarean operation.

to that above; a means was also found of possibly saving the life of the child at the expense of the mother, a procedure advocated by the Roman Church—Cæsarean section. This operation, far different in its effects then than in its frequent performance today, consists in removing the child through a cut made in the front of the abdomen. The name Cæsarean attached to it has given rise to the belief that Julius Cæsar was brought into the world by this means, but at the time when Cæsar lived the operation is not known to have been performed on the living woman, and his mother, Julia, lived many years after his birth, as is proven by his letters to her. The probable explanation for the name is as follows: In 715 B.C. the king, Numa Pompilius, codified the Roman law, and in the *lex regia*, as it was called, it was ordered that the child should be removed from every woman who died when far advanced in pregnancy, even in cases where there was no chance of survival for the child, so that the mother and child might be buried separately. The *lex regia* became the *lex Cesare* under the rule of the emperors, and the operation became known as the Cæsarean operation, or section. Few such operations had been performed on living women at the time of Ambroise Paré, and, for even centuries after, the suffering it entailed and the high mortality that resulted from it made the operation one of last resort.

Paré opposed Cæsarean section, and his opinion checked its further advance for more than a century; in its stead he suggested podalic version. This procedure cannot replace either Cæsarean section or the destroying of the child in all cases, for it is not applicable to women who have abnormally small pelvises, but Paré did not have a sufficient knowledge of anatomy to know this; he believed, as had the Greeks, that the pelvis separated in the middle and opened out during the birth of the child and that the pains of childbirth were due to this separation of the bones. Podalic version was at the time a tremendous advance in the saving of the lives of infants and the suffering of women.

The development of podalic version constituted the first step since the fall of the Roman Empire in the emancipation of the child-bearing woman from the exclusive hands of the ignorant midwives. It was something with which the physician could assist the woman in difficult labor without killing her or mutilating the child; it took the operative assistance of the child-bearing woman from the hands of the surgeon and laid the foundation for an independent art of medicine —obstetrics.

In Paré's time a school for midwives was opened at the

Hôtel Dieu at Paris. The position occupied by the child-bearing woman in civilization was rising; after centuries of neglect she received the consideration of the physician. The women graduated from the school of midwifery were of a type vastly superior to the bedraggled hags who had formerly trundled their obstetrical chairs from house to house. Louise Bourgeois, "sworn midwife" of the city of Paris, was

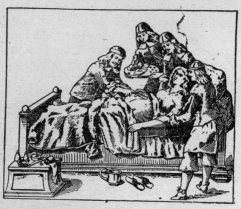

A CÆSAREAN OPERATION IN THE SEVENTEENTH
CENTURY

Very few such operations were performed at that time, for there was no anesthesia, asepsis, or adequate means of controlling hemorrhage. The woodcut shown here appeared in the works of Johann Schultes, a surgeon of the seventeenth century.

among the first of the graduates; in 1601 she officiated at the birth of the Dauphin (later Louis XIII), and afterward at the birth of the other children of Marie de' Medici.

The customs of the time were changing; trained and supervised midwives were a step toward the betterment of the child-bearing woman, and the next step was the participation of the physician himself in midwifery. Boucher was called in to attend La Vallière, mistress of Louis XIV, and the king is said to have evidenced his interest in this reinstatement of male midwifery by watching the procedure from the concealment offered by some curtains. In 1670 Julian Clement attended Madame de Montespan at the birth of the Duc de Main, and in 1682 he delivered the Dauphin. Clement received the title of *accoucheur,* to replace the somewhat derisive appellation of man midwife, or mid-man. Soon male midwifery became the fashion among the ladies of the court. The princesses of the period hastened to place themselves under the care of *accoucheurs.* Clement went three times to attend the wife of Philip V of Spain.

THE AUTOGRAPH OF
AMBROISE PARÉ

## CHAPTER III

## "THE COMPASSION OF PETER CHAMBERLEN"

n the sixteenth century civilization had progressed far enough so that Paré could reintroduce podalic version, and thus bring midwifery back to the level it had reached among the ancients and open the way for the participation of the physician in midwifery. Paré reintroduced also the ligature in surgery, changed the method of treating wounds, founded orthopedics, and introduced massage and artificial eyes. In that same century Magellan circumnavigated the world, Charles V sacked Rome and declared surgery "respectable," and Cortez entered Mexico; Copernicus described the revolution of the planets about the sun, Galileo demonstrated the law of falling bodies, Paracelsus founded chemicotherapy, Vesalius laid the foundation of human anatomy, and Fracastoro named the new plague syphilis. The Reformation took place, the black death, influenza, and the sweating sickness swept Europe, and Catherine de' Medici, from behind the French throne which held her dissolute son, declared war on the Huguenots, and ordered the massacre of Saint Bartholomew's night in 1571. Paré survived the massacre; he was a friend of Catherine de' Medici's and so was spared, but to avoid it another Huguenot physician, Chambellan, fled from France to England.

This Chambellan came to England at a time when Henry VIII had concluded his matrimonial experiments; the year of the king's death was coincident with the founding of an insane asylum at St. Mary's of Bethlehem, London, which was to enrich the language with a corruption of its name, "bedlam." By the time the Chambellan family had settled and changed its name to Chamberlaine, Queen Elizabeth had

been on the throne ten years, Shakespeare was six and
Francis Bacon ten years old, and witchcraft had been made
a capital offense. By the time the name Chambellan had
gone through its final evolution of adoption to England and
become Chamberlen, William Harvey was born, Timothy
Bright had invented shorthand, and the Spanish Armada
had been destroyed. These events bring us up to the year
1588, and the two sons of Chamberlen, Peter the younger

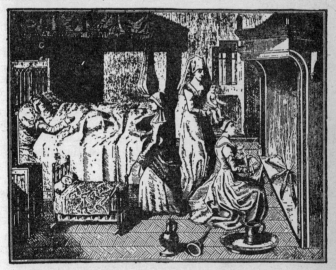

A FIFTEENTH-CENTURY LYING-IN ROOM

and Peter the older, were devoting their attention to midwifery and had invented the obstetrical forceps.

The Chamberlen brothers kept the secret of their invention and attempted to control the instruction of midwives.
In justification of their pretensions they claimed that they
could deliver patients when all others had failed. They
passed along their jealously guarded secret to the next
generation of Chamberlens, which was represented by

another Peter, son of the younger of the two brothers. He was a man of considerable ability, but his character united at the same time some of the virtue of a religious enthusiast and many of the devious qualities of a quack. Like his father and uncle, he attempted to monopolize the control of the midwives. When refused this privilege, he set forth his own views in a pamphlet entitled *A Voice in Ramah, or the Cry of Women and Children as Echoed Forth in the Compassion of Peter Chamberlen*. Ambroise Paré had said of his patients, simply, "I dressed his wounds, and God healed him."

The secret which was Peter Chamberlen's was that of the obstetrical forceps which had been handed on to him by his father and uncle. This in turn he handed on to his sons, of whom Hugh, 1630-1706, was the most important. The secret was kept in the family, and in the words of Hugh Chamberlen, "My father, brother, and myself (though none else in Europe as I know) have by God's blessing and our own industry attained to and long practiced a way of delivering women in this case without prejudice to them or their infants." He still kept the secret.

At the time Hugh Chamberlen, following the family custom, was attempting to control the instruction of midwives in England, physicians were making very slow advancement into the field of obstetrical practice. Paré had given impetus to the movement, and the title of *accoucheur* conferred on Clement had supplied a dignified name for the profession; but the attempts of the physicians to practice obstetrics were met with opposition. Except in the case of royalty the male-physician encountered prudery which rose to amazing heights. Sometimes he was forced to tie one end of a sheet to his neck and the other end to his patient's neck; while the view of both parties was unobstructed above this guard, the physician could not see beneath it. He made his manipulations blindly, but he spared his patient's blushes. The title of *accoucheur* was not at first generally accepted and contemptuous names were often used to belittle physicians who practiced obstetrics. Thus when Dr. William Smellie,

in the eighteenth century, established a school in London
for teaching midwifery, he was christened by his competitor,

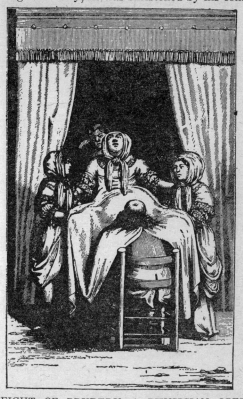

**THE HEIGHT OF PRUDERY—A PHYSICIAN OPERATING
UNDER THE SHEET**

For thirteen centuries the physicians of Europe were not allowed to
attend normal cases of delivery, but in the seventeenth century they
began to participate to some extent. Except among royalty they met
with amazing prudery and were often forced to carry out their manipulations blindly, as shown here, in order to spare the blushes of their
modest patients. A woodcut from the works of a Dutch physician,
Samuel Janson, 1681.

Mrs. Nihell, the Hay Market midwife, "a great-horse-god-mother of a he-midwife." Smellie is remembered in medical history because he made and published the first exact measurements of the pelvis, but he has his place, too, in literature. He is in Laurence Sterne's *Tristram Shandy* under the alias of "Andrianus Smelvgot." He got into that delightful book by mistaking the words *Lithopædii Seno-nensis Icon* for the name of an author, whereas they were in reality the heading of a drawing of a petrified fetus. The error was pointed out by Dr. John Burton, of York, the original of the "Dr. Slop" who competed with a midwife to deliver Tristram.

The opposition to the participation of physicians in obstetrics did not cease altogether until nearly the present century. As late as the 'forties of the nineteenth century John Stevens, of London, denounced and exposed in his pamphlets "the dangers and immorality" of employing "men in mid-wifery." He dedicated his efforts to the Society for the Suppression of Vice. The obstetrician of today is no longer exposed to condemnation and open derision. Nevertheless, in those countries which are backward in their cultural development there still exists a remnant of the earlier atti-tude; it is shown in a certain evident, if unspoken, belittle-ment of the physician who assists the child-bearing woman. He is felt by some people to be of lower caste than physicians in other branches of the medical profession—the surgeon, for instance. This attitude is reflected in the inefficiency of the instruction in obstetrics given in medical schools, and some-times in the inferior type of men who choose this branch of the profession. It is always reflected in the statistics of mortality at childbirth.

In the time of Hugh Chamberlen the opposition to male midwifery was at its height and he gained no popularity from the choice of his specialty; moreover, he dabbled in politics. The politics of England in the latter half of the seventeenth century were two-edged and Hugh Chamberlen found them so by his contact with them. In consequence he retired to

Paris for the quieter atmosphere of Louis XIV's reign. While there he attempted to sell his precious family secret and was directed to Mauriceau, who was then the leading obstetrician of France.

Mauriceau had at that time just made the bold innovation of having his patients delivered in bed and had dispensed with the obstetrical chair, whose antiquity was greater than that of the Bible; in spite of the innovation, the obstetrical chair held its supremacy and the brides of Holland continued to provide them with their trousseaus until the nineteenth century. Chamberlen boasted to Mauriceau that by means of his secret he could deliver the most difficult case in a few moments. Mauriceau promptly placed at his disposal a woman deformed and dwarfed by rickets for whom every effort at assistance to deliver her child had failed. Hugh Chamberlen with a great display of confidence undertook the case, but after working for three hours admitted that he was having some difficulties—the woman died from the injuries she received from his manipulations. "To complete the story," says Mauriceau, "it should be remembered that six months before the occurrence of these events, this physician had come to Paris from England and boasted that he possessed a secret method by means of which he could, even in the most difficult case, promptly effect the delivery of the child, and had told the king's physician-in-ordinary that he would sell the knowledge of this secret for the sum of 10,000 Thalers" (about $7,500).

From the standpoint of medical ethics alone, not to mention humanitarian aspects, the behavior of the members of the Chamberlen family in keeping secret a method by which suffering might be alleviated and lives saved was most reprehensible. A man may invent a mechanical device for the comfort, profit, or pleasure of mankind, manufacture and sell it to his financial betterment, with his process secret or protected by patents. He can do all this honorably, he may even become rich, and no one looks at him askance, indeed quite the opposite. Such is not the case in medicine, for the

tenets handed down from the time of the priests of
Æsculapius, and supported by that intangible thing called
ethics, the respect and recognition of fellow-physicians,
forbid such practices. A physician who seeks and finds a
means of alleviating human suffering or prolonging lives
makes his discoveries public, that all of his profession may
see and profit, with no financial recompense to him who
has made the discovery. Such a procedure is followed in no
other branch of human learning practiced for a livelihood.
The obligation to humanity, which the physician uncom-
plainingly accepts and himself enforces, is looked upon as
a natural course by all those people who accept, as equally
natural, quite the opposite course from all other members
of society. Medicine arose from religion; fortunately, it has
retained in its principles some of the religious virtue of
sacrificing self to the suffering of others, a course that must
seem most impracticable to many men of commerce. In all
ages, in ancient times as well as today, there have been,
and are, physicians who profit through secret methods which
are of either real or imaginary virtue. The Chamberlens were
men of this type, and there were others at that time also—
many others.

England, at about the time in which Hugh Chamberlen
exploited the obstetrical forceps, was particularly prolific in
famous charlatans. The four most prominent, besides Chamberlen, were Sir William Reed, Dr. Grant, Chevalier Taylor,
and "Spot" Ward. Reed and Grant depended for their fame
upon the fact that Queen Anne suffered from weak eyes.
There were no scientific ophthalmologists in her time and
she fell a victim to quacks. Her favorite was William Reed,
a tailor who, "having failed as a mender of garments, set
up as a mender of eyes." He was an illiterate impostor, but
through the queen's favor was made a prominent practitioner
and a knight. Dr. Grant, another oculist to Queen Anne,
started life as a tinker, tried preaching, and drifted into his
medical specialty after failing in these two ventures. His
original occupation is alluded to in an epigram of the time:

Her majesty sure was in a surprise
Or else was very shortsighted,
When a tinker was sworn to look after her eyes
And the Mountebank Reed was knighted.

Chevalier Taylor was an apothecary's assistant who became a self-made specialist of eye diseases. He is the prototype of all modern advertising medical fakers, and, as the result of his efforts became one of the most widely known men in the eighteenth century. He was even dignified by notice from Samuel Johnson, who said he "was the most ignorant man he had ever met." Taylor was appointed oculist to King George II and had among his patients Gibbon and Handel. He himself finally went blind and died in a convent hospital at Prague. He was admitted there, although in his "medical talks" he had often slyly hinted that, tautologically speaking, he had been in almost every "female nunnery in all Europe and could write volumes on the adventures of these religious beauties."

Joshua Ward, known as "Spot" because of a birthmark on his face, took up medicine when he failed in business as a dry-salter. He invented a "Pill" containing antimony, and by administering this remedy and at the same time practicing faith healing with the "laying on of hands," he developed a great reputation and became popular in the courts of King George II. Literary men in particular seem inclined to quacks, and Ward treated both Gibbon and Fielding. Gibbon, in his autobiography, mentions Ward among those "successively summoned to torture or relieve" him. Fielding had, like Molière, a very low view of the regular medical practitioners, but he was grateful to Ward for his treatments. Lord Chesterfield also took Ward's medicine and gave a testimonial for it.

Reed, Grant, Taylor, and Ward were quacks made famous by the favors they received from the English royalty. The French court under Louis XIV likewise was a hotbed of quacks, whose foibles are set forth in the amusing satires of Molière. The memory of these quacks merely shows the gullibility of prominent people and the fact that less prominent people employed the quacks because the kings, queens, statesmen, and famous writers of the day did so. Even today the medical opinion of prominent but non-medical people is sometimes looked upon with respect by the public, even though the men offering the opinion are not qualified to do so.

None of the charlatans described above had anything of value for treating disease. The Chamberlens, on the other hand, held a valuable secret, and even in their time they were censured for their unethical procedure. There is no uncertainty in the words of de La Motte, obstetrician of Volgens, as he comments on the secrecy which has surrounded the discovery of the obstetrical forceps: "He who keeps secret so beneficial an instrument as the harmless obstetrical forceps deserves to have a worm devour his vitals for all eternity. . . ."

Hugh Chamberlen was less successful than many of the contemporary English charlatans. His political views got him into trouble and he was forced to flee to France. There, because of the intervention of Mauriceau, he failed to sell his secret. He returned to England, but in 1699 he was forced to flee again.

This time he went to Holland There he sold his secret, but it continued to spread, perhaps from association, a blot on the fragile medical ethics of that time. The Medico-Pharmaceutical College of Amsterdam had the sole privilege of licensing physicians to practice in Holland, and it also had Hugh Chamberlen's secret. To each of its licensees it sold the secret for a large sum. This disreputable practice continued until a group of generous-spirited men purchased the secret and made it public. It was then found that Chamberlen—possibly it was the college—had perpetrated a grim joke and had swindled the purchasers. The device they had purchased consisted of only a half, and a quite useless half, of the forceps. The final chapter in the story of the Chamberlen family comes from the son of Hugh, Hugh Junior, an intimate friend of the Duke of Buckingham and a prominent physician in England. During the later years of his life he allowed his family secret to leak out, and the instrument soon came into general use.

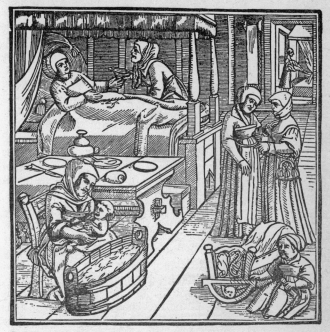

SIXTEENTH-CENTURY LYING-IN ROOM, SWITZERLAND

After a woodcut appearing in the works of Jacob Rueff, a Swiss physician of that period. In nearly all of the old pictures of the lying-in room the nurse is shown washing the child. Frequently she has her feet immersed in the water to test its temperature. The human foot is a much more sensitive "thermometer" than the hand.

The ideas of ethics are so strongly inculcated in the profession of medicine that the credit for the discovery of the obstetrical forceps is not always given to the Chamberlens, but instead to a Belgian, Jean Palfyne, who developed an instrument which he presented freely to the Paris Academy in 1721.

The forceps in their early form were crude, but rapid development in their design followed after their general adoption. Something of the crudity of the early forceps, particularly in the lock that held the blades together, is suggested by Laurence Sterne in *Tristram Shandy*. He says: "Dr. Slop had lost his teeth—his favorite instrument [the obstetrical forceps]—by some misapplication of it, unfortunately slipping, he formerly, in a hard labour, knocked out three of the best of them with the handle of it. . . ."

The purpose of the forceps is to assist in the extraction of the child when the propulsive forces of the mother are lacking, or when, by reason of her condition, or of that of the child, it is advisable to terminate labor rapidly. The forceps did not take the place of the podalic version of Ambroise Paré. Each of the three procedures of assisting at the birth of the child—podalic version, the use of forceps, and the operation of Cæsarean section—has its particular province. Podalic version makes it possible to correct the position of the child and to extract it by its feet, but to apply podalic version the child must still be in the uterus and freely movable there. If labor has advanced with the child in the normal position, the head is forced into the inelastic ring formed by the pelvic bones. From this position it cannot be disengaged and pushed back into the uterus. It is then impossible to hasten its birth by pulling on its feet, as in podalic version, for its feet can no longer be reached. If the strength of the mother failed at this point an impasse was reached for the earlier practitioners of midwifery, for they had no satisfactory way of drawing the child from its position. Even in births which progressed normally several hours might elapse after the time the child's head became engaged in the pelvis but before it was delivered. If, during this time, the child's life became endangered, the earlier practitioners could not at once go to its assistance and extract it. They were forced to wait until it was born in the usual manner, and it was then often too late to save its life.

The obstetrical forceps overcomes these difficulties. It was applicable when podalic version could no longer be used.

The forceps consists of two wide flat blades curved to fit gently over the child's head. The blades are inserted and brought into position separately, and are then locked together, firmly gripping the head. By turning and gently pulling the child is extracted. Any opening through which its head will pass will readily allow the passage of the remainder of its body, for the baby's head is of larger diameter than is its trunk or hips or shoulders.

The invention of the forceps brought another aid to the child-bearing woman which was to play its part in the saving of the lives of children and the suffering of women, but, like all things of which the limitations have not been defined, the use of the forceps was abused in the early stages of its development. Neither the application of forceps nor podalic version will aid birth when the ring made by the bones of the pelvis is too small to admit the head of the child. The efforts of Hugh Chamberlen with the deformed woman whom Mauriceau gave him as a patient were an instance of this kind. The only procedure which could have been applied to save her life and that of the child was Cæsarean section, but Cæsarean section was then far from the relatively safe and painless operation that it is today. Mauriceau refused to undertake it.

Although it was clearly recognized, by those who dealt with midwifery in the sixteenth century, that the child must pass through the ring formed by the pelvic bones, they did not know the exact structure or relation of these bones. Paré, in fact, believed, as did most other physicians, that the pelvis separated in the front and spread, as might a broken hoop, to make room for the child's head to pass. It was Andreas Vesalius (see Chapter VI) who, in his book of anatomy, in 1543, first showed, although crudely, the true relation of the bones of the pelvis. Three bones in all make the ring through which the child must pass. The flaring hip bones form the sides of the pelvis. In the rear they are joined by ligaments to opposite sides of the spinal column, at that part where the vertebræ are fused to form the sacrum, which is shaped like a blunt arrow head. In front, stout projections from the hip bones circle the bottom of the abdomen. They are united by ligaments at the mid-line, and act as braces to hold the shape of the pelvis against the thrust of the legs. The sacrum locks the pelvis in the rear like a keystone in an arch, but this keystone is an inverted one and when pushed outward by the forces at birth it locks tighter and no expansion is given to the pelvic ring.

Anatomical study, as begun by Vesalius, gradually showed the fallacy of the separation of the pelvic bones during childbirth. An extract from a book on midwifery published in 1682 indicates both the passing of this fallacy and also the means for the study of anatomy used by men as eminent as Paré. This book is entitled, *The English Midwife, Enlarged, Containing Directions to Midwives; . . . the Whole Fitted for the Meanest Capacities.* It was published in London, where it was "Printed for Rowland Reynolds, next door to the Golden Bottle in the Strand, at the middle *Exchange* door." The book was a plagiarism of Wolveridge's *Speculum Matricis Hibernicum,* a standard text of its time, but now the rarest British book of its kind. The quotation in question, written a century after the time of Vesalius and Paré, is as follows: ". . . Ambroise Paré, a most famous Chirurgion in his time at Paris (quoting many witnesses to the thing), gives us an History of a Woman in whom (having been hang'd 14 days after she was delivered in Child-birth,) he found (as he saith) the share bone separated in the middle the breadth of half a finger, and the flanck-bones themselves disjointed from the hoop-bone. But we will not in this matter accuse him of an imposture as having too much respect, and a better opinion of so worthy a person, and believing him to be too sincere as to commit such a crime; but do indeed believe the good man might be mistaken in this separation; for we cannot probably conceive that being so at the time of her labor it would remain so a fortnight after, the breadth of half a finger; for then they would have been forc'd to carry this Woman to execution;

(for they are executed at *Paris* within the City or Suburbs,) because she would not have been able to have supported

---

THE

## English Midwife

ENLARGED,

Containing

## Directions to Midwives;

Wherein is laid down whatever is most requisite for the safe Practising her Art

ALSO

Instructions for Women in their Conceiving, Bearing and Nursing of Children.

With two new Treatises, one of the Cure of Diseases and Symptoms happening to Women before and after Child-birth.

And another of the Diseases, &c. of little Children, and the conditions necessary to be considered in the choice of their Nurses and Milk.

The whole fitted for the meanest Capacities.

---

Illustrated with near 40 Copper-Cuts.

---

*London*, Printed for *Rowland Reynolds*, next door to the *Golden Bottle* in the *Strand*, at the middle *Exchange* door. 1682.

---

TITLE PAGE OF *THE ENGLISH MIDWIFE, ENLARGED*

Published in 1682. The text of this book is presented as a dialogue between the doctor and the midwife, and much sound practical advice is given. The book not only covers obstetrics, but also the diseases of children and the diseases peculiar to women; the limited knowledge on these subjects is shown by the fact that they are covered in 300 pages. The type of women undertaking midwifery and the care of women and children is indicated by the statement on the title page, "The whole fitted for the meanest capacities."

her self, or climbe the ladder of the Gibbet; and keep her
self on her Legs according to the custome of other Malefac-
tors; because the body is only supported by the stability of

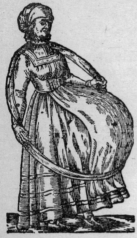

LIB.25.    *Of Monsters and Prodigies.*    655

*The picture of Dorothie, great with childe with manie children.*

*Martin Cromerus* the autor of the Polish histo-  The ninth
rie, writeth that one *Margaret*, a woman  Book of the
sprung from a noble and ancient familie neer  Polish Histo-
*Cracovia*, and wife to Count *Virboslaus*,  rie.
brought forth at one birth thirtie five live
children, upon the twentieth daie of *Jan.*
in the year 1296. *Franciscus Picus Mirandula*
writeth that one *Dorothie* an Italian had
twentie children at two births; at the first
nine, and at the second eleven, and that shee
was so big, that shee was forced to bear up
her bellie, which laie upon her knees, with
a broad and large scarf tied about her neck, as
you may see by this figure.

## "DOROTHIE, GREAT WITH CHILDE WITH MANIE CHILDREN"

One of the many marvels that Ambroise Paré figured in his *Surgery*.
Paré was skeptical for his times, but he accepted on very slight evidence many occurrences of which he was not a witness. The story of
Dorothie, however, was conservative in comparison with that of the
Countess Hagenan, who was said to have been delivered of three hundred and sixty-five children at a single birth; one hundred and eighty-
two of them were reputed to be female, a like number males, and the
odd one bisexual. Pepys in his *Diary* mentions that he saw the basin
in which these children were baptized.

these bones; wherefore we must believe, as most probable,
that such a disjunction and separation were caused either
from the falling of this Woman's body from the high Gibbet

to the ground after execution or from some blow on that place from some hard thing."

As this book indicates, the pelvis cannot spread apart. The head of a child, when larger than the pelvic ring, therefore, cannot pass through it. This disproportion does not, as a rule, result from the abnormal size of the child's head, but rather from the small size or distorted shape of the pelvis. Such abnormality of the pelvis occurs particularly as a consequence of the disease rickets. Rickets is essentially a disease of civilization. It is due to lack of sunlight and is greatly influenced by improper diet. The actinic, or chemically active, light of the sun acting through the skin influences the growth and development of bones. The disease rickets occurs in children; the growing bones do not harden normally and become distorted. The actinic light from the sun which prevents the disease is in excessive quantities harmful. It is the cause of sunburn. The natives of tropical or semitropical countries, where the actinic rays of the sun are particularly strong, are protected from the injurious effects of the rays by pigment in their skin. A dark skin does not keep out heat any better than a white skin, but it affords a partial protection against the actinic rays of the sun. Even people of the blond races tan and freckle when exposed excessively to the sun's rays, and thus, so to speak, develop their own physiological sunshade. The dark-skinned people of the tropical and subtropical regions do not lose their pigment when they migrate to the cities of the temperate zone; consequently they remain too strongly protected against the feebler sunlight. To add to their trouble, the smoke pall which covers cities, of itself and from the fog that it causes, further cuts off the sunlight. The cold weather of winter drives children indoors, where the sunlight is filtered through glass, which stops the few remaining rays of chemically active light. For the children so placed a special diet rich in such substance as cod-liver oil is necessary to prevent rickets. In consequence of the ignorance or disregard of this requirement the disease is particularly prevalent among the dark-skinned people in the dingy slums of modern cities.

A well-developed case of rickets presents an unmistakable picture. The head is large and flat on top. The ribs are roughened and feel like beads to the touch—the so-called "rachitic rosary." The legs, and to a less extent the arms, are bowed. In older children pronounced bowleggedness is the most evi-

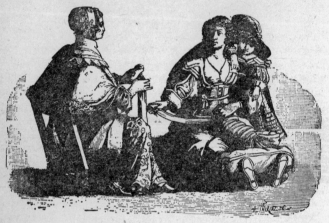

NURSES SWADDLING A CHILD

In the seventeenth century, the period of this woodcut, the baby, at birth, was first bathed and then salted all over (in accord with the teachings of Galen), and its head tightly bandaged to shape it. Next it was bound round and round in swaddling bandages until it was unable to make the slightest movement. These bandages were usually taken off only once a day, when the child was allowed a few minutes of exercise. The swaddling continued for several months. About half of the children so treated died during the first year of life. Even in the United States today a fifth of all deaths are in the first year of life—a very high mortality in comparison with other civilized countries.

dent feature left by the disease, and with it goes distortion of the pelvis. A walk through the slums of any large city in the temperate zone, where there is a fair proportion of the dark Mediterranean peoples or negroes, will show, even to the casual observer, many cases in which rickets has left its mark.

In one of our large cities a series of measurements was made of the pelves of women who were pregnant; among the white women, 8.5 per cent were below the normal size; among the black women the percentage was 32.6. The difference is in

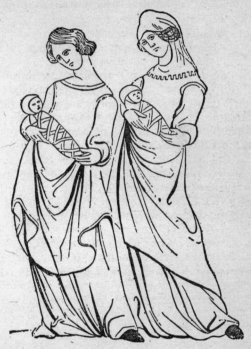

THIRTEENTH-CENTURY NURSES WITH SWADDLED
CHILDREN

This old woodcut shows the bandaging which babies had to endure for the first few months of life.

part compensated by the smaller size of the children borne by the negro women.

Measurement of the pelvic opening can be made readily by the physician. He does so by determining the distance between certain bony prominences about the pelvis or by X-ray examination. Such measurements are a regular part of the proper care of pregnant women of the present day and are made early in pregnancy. If any serious abnormality is found, provision can be made for it in time to avoid danger to life of the child and mother.

Prior to the time of anesthesia and asepsis—that is, before the beginning of modern surgery in the last part of the nineteenth century—the woman with a deformed pelvis met serious difficulties at the time of her delivery. Cæsarean section with its then high mortality for the mother might be attempted, or the pelvic bones might be cut apart at their joint at the front of the body, or the resort of earlier times might be used and the child destroyed, but in serious deformity even this last procedure was far from successful. The induction of abortion, or later of premature labor, offered a solution to this difficulty. Abortion had been practiced by primitive peoples when there was any reason for not wanting the child to be born. With the development of the Greek and Roman culture the practice of inducing abortion was continued, and indeed used extensively by the midwives for any and all reasons. The more conservative position taken by the better class of physicians is clearly outlined in the quotation given from Soranus: ". . . The fruit of conception is not to be destroyed at will because of adultery or of care for beauty, but is to be destroyed to avert danger appending to birth. . . ." With the supremacy of the Catholic Church in Europe the practice of abortion was forbidden under penalty of eternal damnation.

It was in England in the eighteenth century that the practice of the primitive peoples and of the ancients was revived as a means of avoiding, in part at least, the tragic consequences of birth with contracted pelvis. The means of measuring the size of the pelvis were sufficiently established then, so that the physician could recognize the abnormality. In such cases the pregnancy was brought to an end late in the seventh month or during the early part of the eighth month, and thus before the child had reached its full development. The smaller size of the child made its birth possible through a pelvis much narrower than the normal. With good care the child thus prematurely born could be raised. It is of interest to note that the old Hippocratic belief that

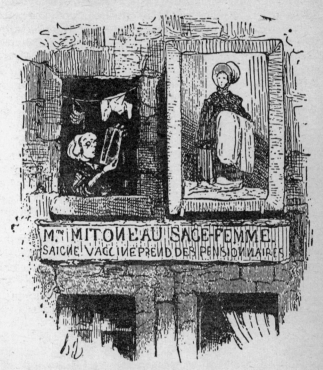

**SAGE-FEMME**

An etching by Daumier showing the midwife and her sign.

there was a better chance for raising the child born during the seventh than one born during the eighth month was passing with the medical profession at this early date. This fallacious idea persists today as a popular superstition. By inducing premature labor it was possible to secure a living child in cases in which the destruction of the child had been necessary in previous deliveries at full term.

The French physicians did not follow the example of the English physicians, and in failing to do so were probably acting under the influence of the Catholic Church in France. In spite of the attitude taken by the medical profession of that country and in spite of civil and ecclesiastical decrees and proclamations, abortion was extensively practiced and had been for many years, but its practice was not for medical reasons. The great ladies of the day made light of the earthly and spiritual terrors held up to them and resorted to the crime to hide the consequences of their sexual irregularities. Bayles, indeed, uses this fact to support the theory that fear of worldly shame is a stronger sentiment than that of religion. The conditions existing in Paris at this time, seventeenth and early eighteenth centuries, can be gathered from a letter of Guy Patin, at one time dean of the Faculté de Médicine. Patin was a man of satirical humor and of keen observation, as may be judged from the fact that as early as 1657 he made the statement: "As to our publishers—I can hope for nothing from them. They print nothing at their own expense but *novela utrisque*" (sex novels). The complaint has persisted! At the time Patin wrote there was a large class of men and women who made a business of producing abortion; the women in this trade were chiefly from the midwives. Patin's letter, written in 1660, comments on the case of Mademoiselle de Guerchi, who had been seduced by the Duc de Vitry and who had died from infection resulting from an induced abortion:

"They make a great clamor here about the death of Mademoiselle de Guerchi. They had imprisoned the midwife at the Chatelet, but she had been taken from there to the *conciergerie* by order of the court. The curé of Saint Eustache has refused sepulture to the body of the lady. They say that it was carried to the hôtel de Condé, and was there put in quicklime in order to consume it soon, so that it could not be identified if anyone came to see it. The midwife had defended herself well up to now. . . . But I believe the question [torture] will be put to her. The vicars-general and the plenipotentiaries went to complain to the Premier President that in a year six hundred women, by actual count, have confessed to killing and destroying their fruit."

The midwife was later found guilty and hanged at Croix de Trahoir, as Patin says, "in good company."

At the time the English physicians revived the practice of inducing premature birth as a means of avoiding difficult labor, midwifery had not been separated from surgery. In

*VOVS estes priez d'assister au Convoy, Service & Enterrement de deffunt noble homme M<sup>e</sup> Guy Patin, Conseiller Medecin, Lecteur, & Professeur du Roy au College Royal de France, & Docteur Regent en la Faculté de Medecine à Paris, decedé en sa maison rüe du Chevalier du Guet: Qui se fera V endredy premier iour d'Avril 1672 à vnze heures precises du matin, en l'Eglise Saint Germain Lauxerrois sa paroisse, où il sera inhumé. Les Dames s'y trouveront s'il leur plaist.*

*Vn De profundis.*

INVITATION TO GUY PATIN'S FUNERAL

earlier times the only reason for calling in the physician at the time of childbirth was because of the necessity for performing some destructive surgical procedure. The revival of podalic version and the invention of the forceps reduced the number of cases in which it was necessary to destroy the child. The practice of obstetrics nevertheless remained in the hands of the surgeons. They quite naturally had a tendency to make child-bearing a surgical operation and to use instruments whenever possible. The general use of the obstetrical forceps gave even a wider play to this habit of "meddlesome midwifery." It was said at that time of one prominent German obstetrician that he employed instruments twenty-nine times in sixty-one births, and of another that he "began to cut and slash" as soon as everything was not precisely normal, and in this way had a mortality of twenty per cent. The surgeons, moreover, could not resist carrying with them into the obstetrical field their practice of blood-letting, and the parturient woman was bled for prophylaxis if everything seemed normal, and for treatment if anything seemed abnormal.

The revival of the practice of inducing premature labor to avoid the necessity of surgery at childbirth was a reaction on the part of the English physicians against the participation of the surgeon in obstetrics. It was, in fact, a definite move in the direction of separating these two branches of medical practice. Like most reactions, it was carried to an extreme. Even beneficial surgical and instrumental procedures at childbirth were discarded for a time. Thus in the middle of the eighteenth century William Hunter, to emphasize his views of interfering with childbirth, was in the habit of showing his obstetrical forceps covered with rust, as evidence of the fact that he never used it. William Hunter was trained in the University of Glasgow, an institution destined to be associated with the names of many men of medical fame, and he was the leading consultant in midwifery in London. His views had a strong influence on the physicians in England. The practice of avoiding the use of instruments and trusting in the powers of nature went so far that in 1819 Sir Richard Croft, obstetrician to Princess Charlotte, upon whose life depended the hope of the dynasty, permitted the princess to remain in labor for fifty-two hours. The child was born dead and the mother died six hours later. Croft shot himself in remorse over what he realized was his mismanagement. The reaction against operative interference gradually extended to France and the rest of the Continent. There the reaction was less extreme and the only violent manifestation of the new order of midwifery was in the frenzied activities of a Parisian fanatic, Sacomb, who, about the time of the French Revolution, opened an anti-Cæsarean school in Paris and fought the Cæsarean operation, and in fact all other operative interference, with all the weapons of the charlatan. While Sacomb's hysterical activities made no great impression at the time, it is of interest to note that there is no record of a Cæsarean operation having been performed in Paris for a period of ninety years after his short-lived efforts. The mortality for the women undergoing Cæsarean section was at that time about 80 per cent.

The reaction against operative interference in childbirth served its purpose. The obstetrical art was no longer taught as a branch of surgery. In the nineteenth century obstetrics became a recognized part of medical education and practice. The rational use of forceps and other operative procedures returned, but no longer as primary instruments of delivery, merely as necessary aids in difficult cases.

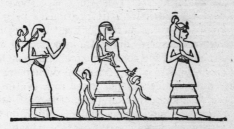

EGYPTIAN WOMEN CARRYING THEIR
CHILDREN

# CHAPTER IV

## "A GENTLEMAN WITH CLEAN HANDS MAY CARRY THE DISEASE"

y the nineteenth century obstetrics was well developed from the mechanical side. Great progress had been made in the art of assisting the child-bearing woman during the three hundred years which had passed since Paré had opened the way for the return of the physician to the lying-in room. But some of the advantages derived from the development of obstetrics and the extensive participation of physicians in the art were offset by the increasing prevalence of a disease known as child-bed fever, or puerperal infection. This disease, which struck only at women who bore children, had been known from antiquity as an occasional occurrence. During the seventeenth, eighteenth, and nineteenth centuries, however, it became a pestilence. Between the years 1652 and 1862 there were two hundred epidemics of this disease, which was then attributed largely to the state of the weather. In 1773 a great epidemic of puerperal fever more than decimated the lying-in hospitals of Europe, and after raging for three years culminated in Lombardy, where it is said that for a year not one woman lived after bearing a child.

The ravages of puerperal infection were greatest in the lying-in hospitals of Europe. This was particularly unfortunate, for there is no institution which in principle seems more humane than the lying-in hospital, where destitute women can receive aid during the birth of their children. But from the seventeenth to nearly the twentieth century these hospitals, which had been built for and dedicated to the care of child-bearing women, were humane in spirit only. In reality most of them were deadly for the women who entered them. These hospitals were the centers in which puerperal infection flourished. At one time the deaths from the disease rose to such heights in the old Maternité of Paris and in the lying-in hospital of Vienna, that 10 to 20 per cent of all women who entered them died there. The attention of the public at large was finally attracted and the abolition of these

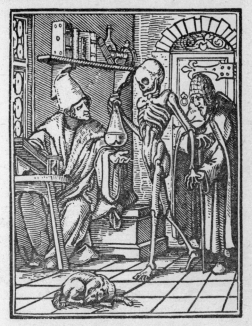

DEATH AND THE PHYSICIAN
A woodcut by Hans Holbein.

institutions as menaces to public health was considered. They would have been abolished if any other means could have been found of caring for the destitute women who had no other place to go to bear their children or who went to the hospitals in spite of the dangers because the state would then accept their children as orphans even if the mother survived. A means of controlling puerperal infection was developed in the nineteenth century; before that time childbirth ranked in mortality with some of the serious infectious diseases.

Puerperal fever starts within a few hours to a few days after the birth of the child. There is high fever and all the symptoms which are known today to accompany infection of the kind popularly called blood-poisoning. But such things as blood-poisoning or wound infection were unrecognized until half of the nineteenth century had passed and Lister had applied to surgery the work of Pasteur. Even as late as the nineteenth century the formation of pus in wounds was considered, as it had been since the beginning of the Christian era, as a normal part of the healing process; it was called "laudable pus." The enormous mortality from surgical operation and the prevalence of wound infection in hospitals before the time of Lister are dealt with at length in Chapter VI.

Brief extracts from the record of a case of puerperal fever described by a physician practicing during an epidemic at Aberdeen, 1789 to 1792, give some insight into the course of the disease and also into the medical practice of the time: "In the afternoon of the 19th of August, 1790, John Low, miller of Justice-mills, came to my house, requesting me to go immediately to his wife, who, he said, '. . . was in great danger.' I accordingly went, and found her in a dangerous situation; she complained of an acute pain in the lower part of the abdomen, attended with a very great degree of fever, the velocity of the pulse being at the rate of 140 strokes in a minute.

"The disorder commenced with a violent rigor at six o'clock in the morning, being about thirty-six hours after delivery. . . . I accordingly ordered bleeding to the quantity of sixteen ounces."

The physician also ordered a physic and raised a blister on the patient's abdomen, gave her opiates to relieve the pain in that location, and concludes, " . . . the scene was soon closed." With his patient dead he philosophizes at length on the ingratitude of the patient's friends in particular and on the hardships of medical practice in general!

". . . On this, as well as many other occasions, I found that scientific practice and popular opinion very seldom correspond.

"According to a vulgar custom in this country, the women came from all quarters to see the patient, and to offer their advice. Several ladies likewise joined the crowd; and though they neither knew the nature, nor even the name of the disease, yet they gave their advice with great freedom! Some said it was wrong to bleed, others that it was improper to purge a patient in such a situation; some prescribed heating, and others astringent medicines; and seemingly actuated by other motives than the good of the patient, they proposed different practitioners. . . ."

The first definite statement, although unheeded, as to the cause of childbed fever, came from the United States. The narrative of the conquest of death at birth turns for the first time to this country.

In Colonial days obstetrics did not receive the attention in this country that it did abroad; and with the conditions of life here at that time there is no reason to expect that it should. Childbirth in those early days of American civilization was considered a simple physiological function, to be carried out in secrecy with a friend or a midwife. The wife of Dr. Samuel Fuller, who landed from the *Mayflower,* was the first midwife of the Colony. The next was Mrs. Hutchinson of Boston, who was banished for her political heresy. She was succeeded by Ruth Barnaby, who lived to be one hundred and one. The first person to be executed in the Colony of Massachusetts Bay was Margaret Jones, female physician; she was accused of witchcraft. Incidentally, she is the only physician whose name was in any way associated—and her association was involuntary—with the scandalous persecutions which were guided by those zealots, Cotton Mather and Samuel Parris.

The efforts of the Chamberlens to control midwifery in England and Mauriceau's innovation of conducting childbirth in bed did not influence the activities of the Colonies, but other things from Europe did. Syphilis entered Boston in 1646, ten years after Harvard College was founded. The appearance of diphtheria in Roxbury, Massachusetts, was timed closely with Louis XIV's ascension to the throne. While Hugh Chamberlen was trying to sell his obstetrical forceps in Paris, New York was busy with an epidemic of yellow fever, and Boston, soon after, with one of its numerous epidemics of smallpox. Forty-six years after Clement delivered the Dauphin of France and made male midwifery popular among the ladies of the court, New York City passed the first ordinance in America to control the activities of the midwives. In 1716 the professional ability of anyone and everyone in this country to officiate at childbirth was still, nearly a hundred years after the landing of the *Mayflower*, taken for granted, but apparently the civil activities of those participating in this art needed some regulation, for the ordinance reads:

"It is ordained that no woman within this corporation shall exercise the employment of midwifery until she has taken oath before the mayor, recorder or an alderman . . . to the following effect: That she will be diligent and ready to help any woman in labor, whether poor or rich; that in time of necessity she will not forsake the poor woman and go to the rich; that she will not cause or suffer any woman to name or put any other father to the child, but only him which is the very true father thereof; indeed, according to the utmost of her powers; that she will not suffer any woman to pretend to be delivered of a child who is not indeed, neither to claim any other woman's child for her own; that she will not suffer any woman's child to be murdered or hurt; and as often as she shall see any peril or jeopardy, either in the mother or child, she will call in other midwives for council; that she will not administer any medicine to produce miscarriage; that she will not enforce a woman to give more for her service than is right; that she will not collude to keep secret the birth of a child; will be of good behavior; will not conceal the birth of bastards. . . ."

In 1739 a special department for instruction in obstetrics

was created in the University of Glasgow, while in America it was six years after that date that there was the first record of a "man midwife." The *New York Weekly Post Boy* of July 22, 1745, states: "Last night died in the Prime of Life, to the almost universal Regret and Sorrow of this City, Mr. John Dupuy, M.D., Man Midwife; in which last Character, it may be truly said here, as David did of Goliath's Sword, there is none like him." Later there is mentioned Dr. Attwood of the same city, who "is remembered as the first doctor who had the hardihood to proclaim himself a man midwife; it was deemed scandal to some delicate ears, and Mrs. Granny Brown, with her fees of two dollars or three dollars, was still deemed the choice of all who thought that women should be modest."

In 1762, the same year that New York was maintaining its modesty and its preference for Granny Brown of the two dollar or three dollar fees, Dr. William Shippen, Jr., was opening a school for midwifery in the less modest but more progressive city of Philadelphia. Dr. Shippen had returned from abroad, where, after studying with John Hunter and his brother William Hunter, he of the rusty forceps, he had completed his medical studies at the University of Glasgow. Shippen brought back with him the advanced ideas of European obstetrics and at once opened a school to impart them to his less enlightened brothers and sisters in midwifery. His class started with an enrollment of twelve students. Dr. Shippen provided "convenient lodgings" for the accommodation of poor women during their confinement, and may thus be said to have established the first lying-in hospital in America. The following advertisement, inserted by Shippen, appears in the *Pennsylvania Gazette* of January 1, 1765:

"Dr. Shippen, Jr., having lately been called to the assistance of a number of women in the country in difficult labors, most of which was made so by the unskilled old women about them; the poor women having suffered extremely, and their innocent little ones being entirely destroyed, whose lives might have been easily saved by proper management; and being informed of several desperate cases in the different neighborhoods which have proved fatal to the mothers as well as to their infants, and were attended with the most painful circumstances, too dismal to be related. He thought it his duty immediately to begin his intended Course in Midwifery, and has prepared a proper apparatus for that purpose, in order to instruct those women who have virtue enough to own their ignorance and apply for instruction; as well as those young gentlemen now engaged in the study of that useful and necessary branch of surgery, who are taking pains to qualify themselves to practice in different parts of the country with safety and advantage to their fellow citizens."

So far as is known, no women had "virtue enough to own their ignorance and apply for instruction." It is of interest that, although a disciple of the English school of moderation in midwifery, Shippen, nevertheless, called his art a "branch of surgery." Three years after he established his private school he joined with Dr. John Morgan of Philadelphia in organizing the medical department of the College of Philadelphia, later the University of Pennsylvania, and there taught anatomy, surgery, and obstetrics.

The College of Philadelphia gave the first regular medical degree in America, conferring the Bachelor of Medicine on ten men in 1768. The following year King's College of New York, later Columbia University, graduated two men in medicine, having overcome in the meantime its regard for Granny Brown to the extent of giving instruction in obstetrics. The term "regular medical degree" is used here because prior to those given by the two American Medical schools there had been two irregular degrees conferred. One of these was in 1663, by order of the court of Rhode Island, to Captain John Cranston to "administer physicke and practice chirurgerie . . . and by this court styled Doctor of Physicke and chirurgerie by the authority of this the general assembly of the colony." The other degree was given by Yale College. Although the Yale Medical School was not established until 1810, the Academic College in 1720 conferred the honorary degree of M.D. on Daniel Turner in acknowledgment of books that he had presented to the institution. It was said facetiously that

Yale's degree of M.D. in this case signified *multum donavit*. "Doctor" Turner's writings dealt largely with venereal disease; he effected improvements in the methods for contraception and was a staunch supporter of "prenatal influence." Some of the books which Turner presented to Yale have been used as sources of material for this book.

The American Revolution interrupted the teaching of obstetrics at the newly founded medical school of Pennsylvania. In 1775 Congress appointed Dr. Morgan "director-general and physician in chief" of the American army. He was unjustly dismissed in 1777 and his place was taken by Shippen. Under Shippen the famous physician Benjamin Rush served for some time as a surgeon-general. He was one of the signers of the Declaration of Independence, but at Valley Forge he deserted Washington to join the Conway Cabal. Dr. Rush, although probably the ablest practitioner of his time, was somewhat of a theorist and a propagandist given to extravagant statements. It is of one such statement, "Medicine is my wife and Science my mistress," that Oliver Wendell Holmes made the caustic comment, "I do not think that the breach of the Seventh Commandment can be shown to have been an advantage to the legitimate owner of his affections."

This same Oliver Wendell Holmes, just one hundred years after Mr. John Dupuy, M.D., man midwife of New York, "died to almost universal regret," read before the Boston Society for Medical Improvement a paper entitled, "The Contagiousness of Puerperal Fever." In this paper he showed clearly that the disease which ravaged the women in the lying-in hospitals of Europe, and which in America also took its toll of lives, was an infectious disease, and that the infection was carried by the physician or midwife from one patient to another through lack of cleanliness. This paper, setting forth the essentials of the greatest discovery ever made in the care of the child-bearing woman, was received with indifference in Boston, and with heated condemnation in Philadelphia by Dr. Meigs, who had succeeded Shippen in the chair of obstetrics at the university. Dr. Holmes replied to the attack with a paper, "Puerperal Fever as a Private Pestilence," and in it stated that one "Senderein" had lessened the mortality from the disease by scrubbing his hands with chloride of lime. The "Senderein" was Semmelweis, of whom much more will be said presently. Holmes's papers were not even heard of in Europe until resurrected as historical curi-

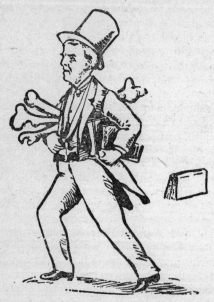

OLIVER WENDELL HOLMES AS DRAWN BY HIMSELF
From a pencil sketch.

osities over fifty years later. Holmes became professor of anatomy at the Harvard School of Medicine two years after the publication of his paper on puerperal infection, and, probably being engrossed in his new duties, he did not push further the discovery which he had tried to show to the obstetricians of America. The credit for one of the greatest boons that medicine has given to humanity goes instead to Semmelweis.

Oliver Wendell Holmes is not known to most people as a physician. His fame comes from his literary work in quite another field than medicine, but his *Medical Essays* are as fascinating to the layman as to the physician, for his literary talents shone as brightly in these as in any of his other writings. They are perhaps more brilliant in places, for he was urged by the ardor of the reformer. A passage picked at random, somewhat broad in its satire, but suited to the fight he fought against the overdosing of the defenseless sick with medicine and pertinent here because of the treatment that was inflicted on the sufferer from puerperal fever, is given here:

"How could a people which has a revolution once in four years, which has contrived the Bowie knife and the revolver, which has chewed the juice out of all the superlatives in the language in Fourth of July orations, and so used up its epithets in the rhetoric of abuse that it takes two great quarto dictionaries to supply the demand; which insists in sending out yachts and horses and boys to outsail, outrun, outfight, and checkmate all the rest of creation; how could such a people be content with any but 'heroic' practice? What wonder that the Stars and Stripes wave over doses of ninety grains of quinine and that the American eagle screams with delight to see three drachms (180 grains) of calomel given at a single mouthful?"

Nor did the rhetoric of Holmes fail him when he dealt with puerperal infection. The most virulent opposition of Holmes's theory of the transmission of the disease through the agency of the physician's hands came from Dr. Meigs of Philadelphia, a most estimable physician but a chronic obstructionist. He was incensed by Holmes's imputation that the physician's hands were not clean; and he quoted a number of cases of infection which had occurred in the practice of the great Dr. Simpson of Edinburgh, an "eminent gentleman," according to Dr. Meigs. Holmes replied by first defining his position in the argument with Meigs as, "I take no offense, and attempt no retort. No man can quarrel with me over the counterpane that covers a mother with her newborn infant at her breast." He goes on to say in regard to Simpson: "Dr. Simpson attended the dissection of two of Dr. Sidney's cases (puerperal fever), and freely handled the diseased parts. His next four childbed patients were affected with puerperal fever, and it was the first time he had seen it in his practice. As Dr. Simpson is *a gentleman* (Dr. Meigs as above), and as a gentleman's hands are clean (Dr. Meigs as above), it follows that a gentleman with clean hands may carry the disease."

Carlyle has said: "Consider how the beginning of all Thought worth the name is Love: and the wise head never yet was, without first the generous heart." How well this describes Soranus, Paré, and Holmes; each championed the cause of the child-bearing woman. In the character of each there must have been much of the generous heart and humility which, though centuries apart, made them giants in the world. To these three must be added a fourth, the greatest of them all, Ludwig Ignaz Philipp Semmelweis.

Semmelweis, unsung in the history of the world, little known even though an international statue to him was unveiled in Budapest in 1906, has the mute testimony of his greatness in every child that is born and in every mother that bears a child in the civilized world. Holmes was not an obstetrician, but as a man of gentleness he was shocked by the deaths from puerperal fever and he pointed out to his fellow physicians what he reasoned out to be its cause. His passing words were unheeded. Semmelweis labored through a lifetime of oppression and persecution in the vile wards of the great charity lying-in hospitals of Europe. He found the cause of puerperal fever. He controlled it in the hospitals where he worked. He gave a practical method for its eradication. He died of its infection.

To obtain the setting for Semmelweis's work the narrative must return to Europe, to the Vienna of the eighteenth century. There Maria Theresa was ruling Austria first through her husband, Francis I, and after his death in 1765, through her son, Joseph II. There is a lull in the Austrian wars; the Turks have been driven from the walls of Vienna; Frederick the Great is on the throne of Prussia, and Maria Theresa's daughter, Marie Antoinette, is married to the Dauphin of France, later Louis XVI. In this time of general peace Maria Theresa turned her attention to the cultural development of her country. The fruits of her endeavors were the Viennese school of music with Haydn and Mozart at its head, and the founding of the old school of Viennese medicine, which is of importance because it laid the foundation for the brilliant new school of Vienna which came with the nineteenth century. For the re-establishment of medicine Maria Theresa turned quite naturally to Dr. Gerhard van Swieten. When the Archduchess Maria Anna had suffered an abortion, van Swieten had attended her with such satisfaction that she had recommended him to her sister, the empress, who up to that time had been barren. Following the advice given by van Swieten, Maria Theresa had sixteen pregnancies and assured the succession of her family. Van Swieten was in Leyden, where his position was that of a physician and private teacher, for, being a Catholic, he could not hold a public professorship there at that time. Maria Theresa brought him to Vienna and made him president of the General Medical Department of Austria. She also made him a baron and appointed him censor; in the latter capacity he incurred the animosity of the Jesuits and of Voltaire and Haller, who accused him of applying his "damnature" to their works.

Van Swieten made an official systematization of medical practice and instruction in Austria, which had the weakness of allowing inefficient men in high positions for no other reason than that of official favoritism. A more beneficial aspect of this organization is seen in the handling of the charlatan Mesmer. He established his séances of mesmerism in Vienna, was immediately investigated, and ordered to leave within twenty-four hours. It so happened, however, that this hasty departure worked no hardship on the exponent of animal magnetism, for he went to Paris, and there, under the protection of Marie Antoinette, acquired with his séances a fortune from broken-down *roués* and amorously inclined ladies.

In van Swieten's time the city hospital of Vienna consisted of twelve beds, six for women and six for men. As a result of the reorganization of medical affairs the "Allgemeines Krankenhaus," the great general hospital, was built in 1784. This institution included a lying-in hospital which was the largest in the world. Dr. Boer, who was to be the director of the new lying-in hospital, was sent by Emperor Joseph II to France and England to learn the practices of midwifery used there. On his return he introduced the conservative English methods; he practiced forbearance and trusted nature, interfering only when it was absolutely necessary to do so.

Two years after Boer undertook his work Joseph II died, and, during the political reaction that followed, Boer struggled on under serious discouragements. In spite of official persecution his work was extremely successful. In the last and thirty-fourth year of his service, 3,066 women were delivered in the wards of his hospital and of these only 26 died—that is 8.4 deaths in 1,000 births, a low rate in those days and one which does not compare unfavorably with that in the United States today.

Four years before Boer retired, in 1818, Semmelweis was born in Budapest, the capital of Hungary. He was the fourth son among eight children of a prosperous shopkeeper. The educational standards in Hungary were at that time at a low level and Semmelweis received a deficient elementary training which shows in places in the style of his later writings. As he himself said, he developed in his youth "an innate aversion to everything that can be called writing." If Semmelweis had wielded the pen of Oliver Wendell Holmes his great discovery would have been adopted throughout Europe in the first twelve months after it was made; instead, he died too soon to see the general application of the principles which he set forth.

When nineteen years old Semmelweis undertook the study of law at the University of Vienna, but, disappointed with that, turned to medicine. He completed his medical studies, and, after signing a declaration that he did not intend to remain in Vienna, received his doctor's degree in 1844, and later the same year the degree of master of midwifery. He at once applied for a position as assistant in the lying-in hospital and, at the hands of Klein, the successor of Boer, received the first of the official injustices which were to be his lot. His application, at first granted, was later rejected, and the term of the assistant then in office was extended for two years. As Semmelweis says, that was contrary to the custom prevailing in the Obstetrical Clinic, and "Dr. Breit was the first to whom this favor was granted." Dr. Klein, to whom Semmelweis, after two years of waiting, became assistant, lacked the qualities of his predecessor, Boer; from first to last his career depended upon official favoritism. Boer had refused to teach midwifery to the students through the use of a dead body, and that had been given as one of the excuses for his dismissal. Klein consented to do so. His first year as director resulted in the loss of 237 lives from the 3,036 women delivered in the hospital, a mortality of 78 in 1,000 births.

While Semmelweis waited for his appointment as assistant he obtained the friendship of two of the medical leaders who were to make the Vienna school of the nineteenth century a great center of medical learning. These two were Skoda and Hebra. Skoda was the first physician at Vienna to adopt a "specialty." He devoted his attention to diseases of the chest and developed the method of diagnosis by percussion—that is, tapping on the chest with the finger to obtain, from the sound elicited, a conception of the state of the structures of the interior—a procedure familiar to anyone who has undergone a physical examination. At Skoda's time the practice "annoyed" the patients, and as it was considered a foolish procedure he was put in charge of the insane patients. He triumphed, however, over this act of official pettiness and was rewarded in time with a whole division of the hospital devoted to diseases of the chest. Hebra, without suffering the reverses of Skoda, developed his specialty in diseases of the skin and laid the foundation for the modern study of that subject. Both Skoda and Hebra remained firm friends of Semmelweis's. They defended him as best they could and even wrote papers setting forth his discovery when he found himself unable to do so.

An appreciation of the task to which Semmelweis set himself in trying to rid the lying-in hospital of childbed fever can be had from a brief description of the conditions existing in these hospitals throughout Europe. England and the Scandinavian countries had at this time, the middle of the nineteenth century, some ideas of cleanliness in hospitals, but the rest of Europe was untroubled with any scruples in this direction. In England childbed fever came as an occasional epidemic; in the hospitals on the Continent it was a perennial epidemic. Speaking of these epidemics, and still bound to the idea of "miasma"—that is, noxious air as a cause of contagion—Oliver Wendell Holmes said, "Now add to all this [transmission of the disease by contact] the undisputed fact that within the walls of lying-in hospitals there is often generated a miasma, palpable as the chlorine used to destroy it, tenacious so as in some cases almost to defy extirpation, deadly in some institutions as the plague; which has killed women in an Old World hospital so fast that they were buried two in a coffin to conceal its horrors." The miasma in these cases was filth.

Bearing in mind that childbed fever is wound infection caused by the contamination of the raw surface left in the uterus after the birth of the child, consider the state of cleanliness in the Maternité of Paris as described by La Forte after his visit there in 1864, only thirty-six years before the present century:

"The principal ward contained a large number of beds placed in alcoves like English horse-stalls along each side. Ventilation was almost impossible. Floors and partitions were washed once a month . . . the ceilings showed that they had not been whitewashed for many years. Lying-in women who became ill were transferred to an isolation room regardless of the nature of their illness—puerperal fever cases and patients affected with diarrhea, bronchitis, measles, or any other eruptive fever. Midwife pupils attended normal lying-in patients and fever cases alike, and performed all the necessary manipulations for every class of case."

La Forte speaks of the apparent aversion to water at the hospital, of the clouds of dust raised by dry sweeping the unwashed floors, and concludes: "It is not astonishing that the Maternité of Paris has furnished a mortality without example in any European country. From 1861 to 1864 the patients numbered 9,886 of whom 1,226 died; equal to a mortality of 124 in 1,000 births." This is not a hospital of medieval times mentioned here, but a hospital in a center of culture and in years from which many of the children born must be living today.

In 1858 Semmelweis, while advocating chemical treatment of the hands as a prevention of the spread of puerperal fever, received a letter from one of his students describing the conditions at Gratz: "Infection of all sorts occurs at the Gratz lying-in hospital. . . . The dissection-room is the only place where the students can meet and pass the time when waiting for their midwifery cases, and they often devote their attention to dissecting or studying and manipulating preparations." (Be it noted parenthetically that the cadavers of the dissecting-room at that time were not embalmed in antiseptics as they are today, and in Germany, where an autopsy occurred invariably after each death in the hospital, the body, afflicted with whatever disease, furnished material for the medical student.) "When they [the students] are summoned to the lying-in hospital, which is just across the street, they do not make any pretense at disinfection; some of them do not even wash their hands. . . . The patients might as well be delivered in the dissecting-room. As it is, the students cross the street with hands wet and bloody from dissecting; they dry their hands in the air, and stick them a few times into their pockets, and at once proceed to make examinations. It is no longer a riddle to me why, after a clinical meeting, the medical officer of Gratz exclaimed: 'The lying-in hospitals are really nothing but murder institutions!' "

Of the lying-in hospital of Budapest in 1850, it is said that the patients' view from the window was the burying-ground, varied on the other side by glimpses of the dissecting-room, with underneath the privies and an open sewer. In 1860 the hospital was moved to a new building, and of this the following is written in a publication of that time:

"While it is not to be denied that the institutions have obtained the advantages of more room, it must be admitted also that the internal fittings (furniture, beds, etc.) are in the old wretched condition; the broken tables and the ragged and worn-out bed clothes, all brought from the old hospitals. Especially the lying-in clinic is in an indescribably pitiable condition; there poor lying-in women are to be found, some of them partly on straw spread on the floor, some of them on wooden benches, others crouching in any corner of the room, weary and worn out; only to a few is it vouchsafed to find a regular bed on which to stretch their weary limbs. Everywhere you find dirty bed linen, with bedclothes old and worn and almost in rags."

With this quotation in mind, think of a modern charity hospital. There are two classes of patients in this country today who have superlative medical attention—the very rich and the very poor who go to the charity hospitals. Both classes are served by the same physicians.

The bed linen referred to in the quotation above as being almost in rags suffered also from other difficulties. In 1860 graft was known in hospital administration and Semmelweis encountered and ended, for his wards, one of the most loathsome varieties. The mortality among his patients remained high in spite of his efforts, and he examined the instruments, the utensils, and the beddings. He made a shocking discovery. He found that patients in labor were laid upon filthy sheets which actually stank of decomposed blood and uterine discharge. These had been received and accepted as clean by the head nurse from the laundry contractor, who had accepted the contract at a specially low rate. All the circumstances pointed to dishonesty which extended all the way from the superintendent to the pupil-midwives. With his whole heart and soul filled to overflowing with desire to save from suffering and death the poor creatures consigned to his care, Semmelweis bundled together the evil-smelling "wash" and went straight to the chief official. His vehement gesture shook the linen in the face of that gentleman and demonstrated at close range to his eyes and nose the urgent call for improvement. He obtained promptly all that he demanded for the care and comfort of his patients, and obtained, besides, the dislike and hostility of the director.

It must not be thought that the conditions in the charity hospitals or the frightful loss of lives among the lying-in patients in these institutions applied likewise to the private practice of physicians among the well-to-do classes. Childbed fever occurred in occasional cases, and sometimes in epidemics, but, as Holmes particularly noticed, it was apt to run in a few consecutive cases of some one physician and then die out for a time. The lesser rate of puerperal infection outside of the hospitals, be it noted, was not due to any precaution of the physician, but rather to the ideal conditions for the spread of the disease which existed in the hospitals. Today, in the era of asepsis, the conditions are reversed; it is vastly safer for a woman to be confined in a modern hospital than at her home. Such cases of puerperal infection as are seen in hospitals originate on the outside and are brought to the hospital for treatment. Infection in the hospital has been reduced to almost the vanishing point as, for instance, one case in eight or ten thousand births.

With a picture in mind of the conditions existing in the maternity hospitals of the middle of the last century, we turn again to Semmelweis and his problem. The maternity hospital of Vienna, where Semmelweis started his work, was in two divisions; in one the medical students were instructed and in the other the women who were to become midwives were trained. In the First Division, that of the medical students, there were from 68 to 158 deaths in each 1,000 births, with an average, over a period of six years, of 99. In the Second Division, that of the midwives, the average for the same period was 33 deaths in 1,000 births. The difference in these figures started the active mind of Semmelweis to puzzling over the reason; he passed in review all the possible causes which had been suggested.

Some physicians had confidently attributed the frightful devastation wrought by childbirth fever in the First Division to epidemic influences, which in those days signified some not exactly defined state of the weather which often spread over whole districts of the country and caused fever in women bearing children. But Semmelweis dismissed this theory on the ground that the same atmospheric conditions existed in both divisions of the hospital. He recognized that the cause of the disease lay within the hospital. He said: "A very common and successful method of diminishing the ravages of a puerperal-fever epidemic is to close the lying-in hospital. The hospital is not closed in the expectation that the patients will die somewhere else, but because of the belief that if they remain in the hospital they will die, owing to the epidemic influences at work within the hospital; whereas if they are confined outside, away from the hospital, they will remain well."

Semmelweis makes point after point in tracing the course by which he established to his own satisfaction that the disease arose from some unknown cause within the hospital. It may be added that only a dreadful dilemma saved the lying-in hospitals from destruction. The patients were charity cases and most of the children born were retained under the care of the state. Due to the hospitals, many women in the bloom of life were carried off by fever. Without the hospitals a large number of women would remain well, but because of the anxiety over the maintenance of themselves and their infants they would resort to the crimes of abortion, child exposure, desertion, and murder. The hospitals were tolerated as the lesser of the two evils.

Semmelweis demonstrated that crowding could make little difference in the distribution of deaths between the two divisions of this hospital, because each was crowded. Fear was declared by some physicians to be the cause of the fever, for the dread of going to the First Division was very great; so great, indeed, that it was thought the women sickened and died for that reason. In this connection Semmelweis says: "That they were afraid of the First Division there was abundant evidence. Many heartrending scenes occurred when patients found out that they had entered the First Division by mistake. They knelt down, wrung their hands, and begged that they might be discharged. Lying-in patients with uncountable pulse, meteoric abdomen, and dry tongue, only a few hours before their death would protest that they were quite well in order to avoid medical treatment, for they believed that the doctor's interference was always the precursor of death." Semmelweis dismissed this theory that fear was the cause of the difference in mortality, because this difference in mortality would of necessity have to exist before the fear could develop.

Certain religious observances were also accused of increasing the mortality. The chapel of the lying-in hospital was so situated that the priests, bearing the last sacrament to the dying, could, in the Second Division, reach the ward where the patient lay without passing through the other wards, but in the First Division they must pass through five wards before reaching the sick-room beyond. It was usual for the priests, arrayed in their robes, with an attendant marching before them ringing a bell according to Catholic ritual, to proceed to the sick woman to administer the sacrament. According to ordinary arrangement this should be done only once in twenty-four hours, but in childbed fever twenty-four hours is a long time, and the priests had to be sent for occasionally in a few hours after their regular visit. It is easy to imagine the impression which the fateful tolling of the bell would produce upon the lying-in women. "Even to me myself," says Semmelweis, "it had a strange effect upon my nerves when I heard the bell hurried past my door; a sigh would escape my heart for the victim that once more was claimed by an unknown power. This bell was a painful exhortation to me to search for this unknown cause with all my might. During my first term of office I appealed to the sense of humanity of the servant of God, and without difficulty it was arranged that for the future the priests would take a roundabout route, without ringing the bell, so as to reach the sick-chamber in silence and unobserved. The two divisions were made similar in this respect, but the difference in their mortality still remained."

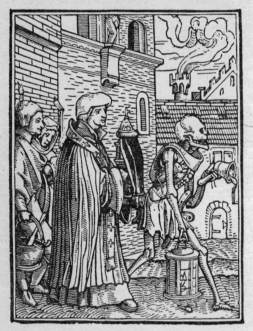

DEATH AND THE PRIEST

A woodcut by Hans Holbein. The priest is carrying the sacrament to some dying man or woman; attendants follow with tapers and holy water, and death leads the way with a lantern and a bell to announce the coming of the priest. It was the sound of this bell which distressed Semmelweis.

Other and even more absurd reasons were given for the difference in mortality. "It was alleged that the reason for the great mortality was because patients were unmarried women of the most hopeless class of the community, accustomed to earn their bread in want and misery and amid conditions which produced great and constant depression of spirits. If this had been the cause of the mortality it would have been as great in the Second Division, for to it exactly the same class of patients were admitted. The higher mortality of the First Division was ascribed to the wounded modesty of the poor women going through the process of parturition in the presence of men. Most of the patients in the First Division certainly suffered from fear, but not many were troubled with a sense of shame. Truly it shows with what want of thought the whole question of the etiology of puerperal fever has been discussed when the persons who at times are depicted as the most abandoned of the population, have attributed to them in the next sentence a tenderness of modesty such as the upper and highest classes of the community do not claim. Among the upper and even the highest ranks of society labor is conducted by physicians, and their patients do not die of puerperal fever in consequence of wounded modesty in the same proportion as is alleged of the inmates of the lying-in hospitals who, for the sake of argument, are often depicted as the most loose and abandoned of the community."

Semmelweis goes on step by step to eliminate ventilation, dirty laundry, and improper diet on the grounds that these things were the same in the two divisions. Yet as he eliminated these possible causes he knew that the real cause lay undiscovered before him in the hospital. This fact was proven by the observation that women who were overtaken with labor on the street while making their way to the hospital were not affected with childbed fever in the hospital, even though they might be taken into the First Division.

The restless energy of Semmelweis in his work in the hospital, his sympathy with suffering women, and his constant criticism of the old orthodox opinions on the causation of childbed fever, probably reached the ears of the director, Kline, in exaggerated form. Semmelweis was demoted from his position of assistant in charge of the First Division, to that of provisional assistant; another physician was put in his place. After some six months of depressing inactivity Semmelweis resumed his former position. At the same time the death of Dr. Kolletschka occurred at the hospital under circumstances which greatly impressed Semmelweis. Kolletschka, while performing a post-mortem examination, received a puncture wound on the finger from the knife of one of his pupils. In consequence of this slight wound he sickened and died. The general symptoms of his malady were those of childbed fever. Of this occurrence Semmelweis says: "In the excited condition which I then was, it rushed into my mind with irresistible clearness that the disease from which Kolletschka had died was identical with that from which I had seen so many hundreds of lying-in women die.

"Day and night the vision of Kolletschka's malady haunted me, and with ever-increasing conviction I recognized the identity of the disease from which Kolletschka died with the malady which I had observed to carry off so many lying-in women."

Semmelweis was on the verge of his great discovery that childbed fever was wound infection, blood-poisoning, which was transmitted to women by the unclean hands of the physicians and medical students who examined them during their childbirth.

"In the case of Kolletschka the cause of the disease was cadaveric material carried into the vascular system; I must, therefore, put this question to myself: Did, then, the individuals whom I had seen die from an identical disease also have cadaveric matter carried into the vascular system? To this question I must answer, Yes!"

All of the physicians and students attending the First Division of the hospital had frequent occasion to come in contact with and work upon the bodies of those who had died at the hospital. According to the usual method of washing the hands, merely with soap and water, particles adhering to the hands were never completely removed, a fact demonstrated by the odor which the hands retained. In the examination of the women in the wards, any of the students were entitled to make internal examination for their instruction; the raw surfaces left at delivery were infected; childbed fever followed. Moreover, when one woman was infected the hands of the examiner, unwashed between examinations, carried the infection to the next woman examined.

With his discovery made, Semmelweis at once required each student to wash his hands in a solution of chloride of lime before making examinations. At that time in his division there were 120 deaths in 1,000 births; in the next seven months the deaths fell to 12 in 1,000, and for the first time in the history of the hospital were below that of the Second Division. In that year also there were two months in which not one single death occurred among the patients of the First Division.

At this point in the career of Semmelweis the antipathies which his enthusiasm had aroused rose in turn to suppress him. Distracted by the petty acts of official injustice, he left Vienna abruptly and returned to Budapest. There he wrote his book setting forth his discoveries and rose to be head of the small lying-in hospital of the city. There, too, he faced hostility and official injustice. He returned but once to Vienna. In 1865 his mental state aroused the anxiety of his wife and friends and he was taken to Vienna for the examination of a specialist in mental diseases. This examination disclosed an injury to a finger which had probably occurred during one of his last operations. He was infected with the disease, blood-poisoning, whose identity with puerperal fever he was the first to recognize. He died August 13, 1865, a victim of the infection which he had devoted a lifetime to eradicate from the wards of the maternity hospitals. Thus ends a chapter in the conquest of death at birth, a chapter which gave, but not in Semmelweis's time, the modern lying-in hospital its supreme virtue—cleanliness. The work of Lister in the same decade completed what Semmelweis had started.

Today puerperal infection no longer ravages the lying-in hospitals. The infection is no longer carried there by the attendants, as Holmes says, "from bed to bed as rat-killers carry their poison from one household to another." Puerperal infection is a disease that is preventable. It will be prevented when civilization rises to that level where it will demand the prevention. It will be then, as Holmes declared it should be: ". . . if there is any voluntary blindness, any interested oversight, any culpable neglect, even, in such a matter, and the fact shall reach the public ear, the pestilence-carrier of the lying-in chamber must look to God for pardon, for man will never forgive him." All women do not go to hospitals; they have only the kind of medical care which the civilization of their community makes available for them. In the United States 6.8 women die in every 1,000 births, and of these, 40 per cent die of childbed fever. Every year in the United States more than 7,000 women die from this preventable disease and the public ear is still deaf to their deaths.

Nor are these 7,000 deaths the only consequences of the disease; for each woman who dies of it, three or more survive. Thus each year 20,000 or more women suffer from the disease and live, but many of them are left with some degree of invalidism.

The prevalence of puerperal infection is not alone the cause of the high mortality among women bearing children in the United States. Deaths from other causes account for a mortality of 4 in every 1,000 births. The death rate, even when thus modified by deducting the deaths from puerperal fever, remains higher than the general rate in some other countries. In Sweden, for instance, the death rate for mothers is 2.3 in every 1,000 births. In the care of the child-bearing woman in Sweden and the United States a striking difference lies in the fact that in Sweden 80 per cent of the deliveries are conducted by midwives, while in this country 80 per cent of the deliveries are conducted by physicians. There are physicians in this country who specialize in obstetrics and whose skill is as great as that of any obstetricians in the world. The service of these men is given to all classes in the hospitals, but outside of hospitals it is available only to those women who can pay for the best service. The vast majority of cases of childbirth do not come into their hands, but go, instead, to men who practice obstetrics as a side line to their general medical practice, or else they go to untrained and ignorant midwives.

The attitude of indifference toward the child-bearing woman in this country—evident in our disgraceful mortality —is seen particularly in the kind of training and·supervision the midwives receive. In the United States there are at least 28,000 licensed and 18,000 unlicensed midwives. They have no standing. In some states they are tolerated by law; in other states they are ignored. Their work is supervised only in the most casual manner, and with one exception there is no place where they can be trained. Nevertheless they are annually intrusted with the lives of over 500,000 women bearing children. In Sweden, on the other hand, the midwives are chosen from a class of women comparable to the better grade of trained nurses. They are thoroughly educated in the art of practical midwifery, are allowed to practice only under close medical supervision, and are required to call in a trained obstetrician in any difficult labor. The difference between the midwives in Sweden and the midwives in the United States is as great as the difference between the specialists in obstetrics and the common run of doctors into whose indifferent hands the lives of most of the child-bearing women of the United States are entrusted. These doctors are not so well trained in obstetrics as are the midwives of Sweden. Moreover, the demands of their general practice and the necessity of earning a living leave them neither the necessary time nor the patience to deal properly with their poorly paid obstetrical cases. The persisting high mortality for mothers in the United States is not a matter fundamental to the economic condition of this country; it is merely an expression of indifference.

## Part Two

# THE STORY OF ANESTHESIA

## CHAPTER V

## "IN SORROW THOU SHALT BRING FORTH CHILDREN"

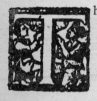he use of anesthetics to alleviate the pain of surgical operations and of childbirth was unknown before the middle of the nineteenth century. Prior to that time operations were performed only from the direst necessity; the fully conscious victim of the operation was tied with ropes to prevent his escaping from beneath the surgeon's knife, and he bore his suffering with such fortitude as he could command. This barbarous state of affairs, formerly accepted as inevitable, shows by contrast with present conditions the humane aspect of the discovery of anesthesia. No greater boon has ever come to mankind than the power thus granted to induce a temporary but complete insensibility to pain. So far as surgery is now concerned, the means of inducing anesthesia are highly developed and extremely effective. Such, however, is not the case in childbirth. Although anesthesia was early applied to relieve the pains of childbirth, and with much benefit, certain conditions, partly physiological and partly sociological, have prevented this use of anesthesia from being developed and applied to the extent that has been attained for surgery. These difficulties are dealt with in this chapter; and as they are described it will be seen that behind them lies the old indifference to the suffering of women in this case, exacerbated by religious opposition to the use of anesthesia for

relieving the pains of childbirth. All of these difficulties are being slowly overcome. A time will unquestionably arrive when the general conditions now existing in regard to anesthesia at childbirth will be looked back upon and considered as barbarous as were the conditions in surgery in the pre-anesthetic days.

The discovery of anesthesia for surgical operations was first demonstrated with the use of ether in 1846. It depended not so much upon the employment of a new drug as upon a new method of administering drugs. The anesthetics are inhaled and therein lies their especial feature. The action of a drug which is swallowed cannot be controlled once the drug has passed into the body; its effects diminish only as the drug is slowly eliminated during hours or even days. On the other hand, the action of the vapors of gases which are used as anesthetics continues fully only as long as these substances are inhaled. When the inhalation ceases they are rapidly exhaled and their action can thus be accurately controlled. The narcotic action of such drugs as opium, hemp, and mandrake has been known from antiquity, as will be seen later, but these drugs cannot be used satisfactorily as anesthetics. They deaden pain, but they also exert a depressing influence upon the action of the heart and upon respiration, which, if the dose of the drug is large, may result fatally. Moreover, pain partially counteracts the action of the narcotic drugs. Thus when they are given in the large amounts necessary to relieve the pain of an operation, they may prove poisonous when the operation is over and their effects are no longer neutralized by the pain. In the past such drugs were sometimes administered for surgical operations, but in the amounts that could be given safely they served merely to allay the sharpest agonies of the operation. The narcotic drugs did not furnish true anesthesia, and they were used in the past as they are used today—to relieve in part the suffering from wounds or painful diseases and thus to allow the sufferer to rest.

This deadening of pain by soporific potions was known even to some primitive peoples as well as those of the earliest civilizations. Helen cast "nepenthe" into the wine of Ulysses, and the Talmud of the Jews speaks of a narcotic called "samme de shinta"; there is the "bhang" of the *Arabian Nights* and the "drowsy syrups" of Shakespeare's time. Opium and Indian hemp, "hashish," were probably known

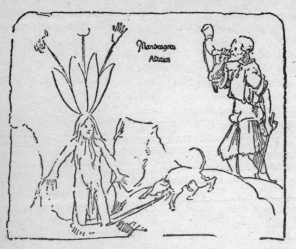

GATHERING A MANDRAKE

According to popular superstition the mandrake shrieked when pulled from the earth and anyone hearing the shriek went mad. The man shown here has tied his dog to the plant and the dog in seeking to escape is pulling out the root. As a further precaution the man is blowing on his horn to drown out the shriek. The supposedly human shape of the mandrake is evident from this old picture.

to the Egyptians and Greeks, and the mandrake to the Babylonians and Hebrews. This mandrake is the European plant, not the May apple, or mandrake, of America. Besides having narcotic properties, mandrake was said to have the power of arousing the sexual passions; Rachel sought mandrakes of Leah (Gen. xxx: 14-16), but it is uncertain for which purpose she used them. Mandrake wine was used in surgical operations by Dioscorides, an army surgeon in the service of Nero; the plant has played a part in early English and German folklore. There are tales of the human shape of its roots and the shriek of agony that it gave when it was uprooted. This shriek was supposed to cause madness in those who heard it. Shakespeare has Juliet say (Act IV, Scene 3), "And shrieks like mandrakes' torn out of the earth,—That living mortals hearing them run mad." In order to avoid the danger of hearing the shriek the plant was drawn from the ground by a dog. "Therefore they did tye some dogge or other living beast unto the roote thereof with a corde . . . and in the mean tyme stopped their own ears for fear of the terrible shriek and cry of the mandrake. In whych cry it doth not only dye itselfe but the feare thereof killeth the dogge. . . ."

Mandrake was the most popular substitute for an anesthetic during the Middle Ages. It held its vogue up to the sixteenth century and is referred to by Elizabethan poets. It was an inefficient anesthetic and ceased to be employed. Its inefficiency is evident from the fact that Paré did not use it, and he was a compassionate surgeon who did not believe in torturing "poor wounded men." Paré used no anesthesia; he simply tied his patients so that their struggles would not interfere with his work.

The surgeons of the eighteenth and nineteenth centuries sometimes intoxicated their patients with alcohol or occasionally drugged them with opium when the procedures of the operation necessitated freedom from struggling. But the surgeons of these pre-anesthetic days depended largely upon speed; an operation verged on being a sleight-of-hand affair designed to shorten to the minimum the suffering of the surgeon's victim. Thus one reads of Langenbeck, surgeon-general of the Hanoverian army in the time of Napoleon, amputating a shoulder while one might take a pinch of snuff.

In all of this nothing is said of the child-bearing woman. Soporific potions may have been used in ancient times, but no one then troubled about the pains of women. Indeed, the efforts to avoid the pangs of child-bearing sometimes called forth punishment. The Greek goddess Actemia, terrified by her mother's suffering at her own birth, besought from Zeus the favor of eternal virginity. Subsequently she seduced Endymion and was punished for her early prudery by a truly god-like superfecundation; she became the mother of fifty daughters all at one time. One of the reasons that soporific potions were not used to relieve the pain of childbirth was because the nature of the substances available—opium, for instance—precluded their employment in effective doses. They arrest the progress of the birth or are injurious to the child. There are, however, some recorded instances of painless childbirth during profound intoxication which was not induced for this purpose. One such case occurred in a woman brought into the Hôtel Dieu of Paris in 1818. There is also the celebrated case of the Countess de St.-Geran, who was rendered insensible by a draught given to her by the midwife; she was delivered and her child was abducted before she regained consciousness.

There is a prescription for relieving painful childbirth set forth in a manuscript of Zerobabel Endicott of Salem. Zerobabel was a son of Governor Endicott by his second wife, but the records provide little information as to his career other than that he was a physician, that he served on an occasional jury, and was fined, in 1659, by the Quarterly Court for excessive drinking. Endicott's prescription is given here in full: "For Sharpe & Dificult Travel in Women with child Take a Lock of Vergins haire on any Part of ye head, of half the Age of ye Woman in travill. Cut it very smale to fine Powder then take 12 Ants Eggs dried in an oven after ye bread is drawne or other wise make them dry & make them to powder with the haire, give this with a quarter of a pint of Red Cows milk or for want of it give it in stronge ale wort."

The alternative of ale for milk, as the vehicle for the ant eggs and human hair, was a wise provision; milk was exceedingly scarce in America in those days, but ale was both plentiful and cheap. While this concoction had no effect except on the imagination, it was at least less disgusting than were many of the medicaments used at that time.

The pain of child-bearing has always been woman's heritage. The pain and the fortitude with which she has met it are not new with modern civilization. It is said of the parturient in Biblical times (Jer. IV:31), "For I have heard a voice as of a woman in travail, the anguish as of her that bringeth forth her first child, the voice of a daughter of Zion, that gaspeth for breath, that spreadeth her hands, saying, 'Woe is me now! for my soul fainteth before the murderers!' " As for the fortitude of women there can be quoted (Jer. XLVIII:41, XLIX:22), "and the heart of the mighty men of Moab at that day shalt be as the heart of a woman in her pangs."

Biblical quotations are not amiss in a chapter dealing with the use of anesthesia, for Biblical quotation and Biblical interpretation formed the basis for the opposition to the use of anesthesia. The introduction of anesthesia to alleviate the pains of child-bearing and for surgical operations aroused a violent controversy. It was science *versus* theology and progress *versus* stagnation, and would seem amusing now if it were not for the human suffering involved. Similar controversies, no doubt equally amusing long after they are over, still arise and probably always will arise so long as human nature remains what it is.

The events leading up to the controversy over anesthesia started in 1800, when Sir Humphrey Davy in England experimented upon himself with nitrous oxide. He states that, "As nitrous oxide in its extensive operation appears capable of destroying physical pain, it may probably be used with advantage in surgical operations in which no great effusion of blood takes place." Forty-four years later Horace Wells of Hartford, Connecticut, began to use nitrous oxide in dentistry and thus was the first man to make a practical application of anesthesia. Wells was led to use the gas as the result of an observation made while attending a lecture given on nitrous oxide in New Haven, Connecticut. The lecturer allowed members of his audience to inhale the gas, and Wells noticed that those under its influence did not appear to be sensible to slight injuries caused by falling or by staggering against the furniture on the stage. Some years later a death resulted from an anesthesia which he gave, and this caused Wells to withdraw from practice. He eventually became depressed over what he regarded as his failure and put an end to his own life.

Wells reported the progress of his work to William Morton of Charlton, Massachusetts, a friend and former partner. Both were keenly interested in any method which promised relief from the pain caused by the extraction of teeth. They had perfected a plate to hold false teeth, but its use necessitated the removal of all old roots left in the jaw from broken teeth. Many patients refused to submit to this prerequisite, and had their dental plates formed on the broken teeth still in their jaws, because of the pain involved in extraction without an anesthetic. Cocaine for local anesthesia was not in use until 1879. Wells and Morton realized that the introduction of their method necessitated an anesthetic of some kind and, after the failure of Wells with nitrous oxide, Morton was on the lookout for some substance which would be safe and reliable.

Morton practiced dentistry in Boston and undertook at the same time the study of medicine at the Harvard Medical School. His work there brought him into contact with Dr. Charles Jackson, and from him Morton learned of the anesthetic properties of ether. Jackson had obtained this knowledge through an observation similar to that made by Wells at the lecture on nitrous oxide. Ether was sometimes inhaled by medical students at so-called "ether frolics," indulged in for amusement and for the mild intoxication of "ether jag" which the vapor produced. Jackson had noticed that when the students were thus under the influence of ether they appeared to be insensible to pain caused by falling over furniture. Jackson had never taken advantage of his knowledge to use ether for the purpose of obtaining relief from pain; but Morton, searching for an anesthetic to be used in his dental practice, at once saw the possibilities presented by ether. He accordingly experimented with ether at his home, first using the family dog as a subject, and finally anesthetizing himself. His next step was to use it in his dental practice and an opportunity to do so was soon presented in the person of one Eben Frost. The following description of his first attempt (1846) to etherize a patient is taken from an article in *McClure's Magazine* for September, 1896: "At this moment the door bell rang and he [Morton] admitted a man named Eben Frost, whose face was bandaged and who was in that stage of mingled hope and consternation so familiar to all dental surgeons. He asked if it were not possible to mesmerise him, and readily consented to inhale ether when assured that it was superior to mesmerism. To the joy of the operator and the astonishment of the patient the attempt was perfectly successful." This event occurred in the last part of September, 1846.

Morton, as stated above, was a medical student as well as a dentist, and, after his success with his patient, Eben Frost, his mind quite naturally turned to the possibility of using ether to lessen the frightful suffering from surgical operations which were then performed with nothing to relieve it. After two weeks of preparation he called on Dr. Warren, who was senior surgeon of the Massachusetts General Hospital at Boston. Morton told him of his use of ether and of his success in relieving pain, and asked for an opportunity to give a demonstration of his method on a patient undergoing a surgical operation. Dr. Warren consented and the date of the demonstration was set for October 16, 1846. On the appointed day a considerable number of spectators gathered in the operating-room. The patient was brought in. Dr. Warren, his assistant, and the guards whose duty it was to hold the struggling and shrieking patient, stood about and waited for Morton, who had not arrived. Finally Dr. Warren remarked, "As Dr. Morton has not arrived, I presume he is otherwise engaged." He picked up one of his instruments, turned to the patient, and was about to proceed with the operation. At this moment Morton entered; he had been delayed in the completion of the apparatus which he used to administer the ether. On Morton's entry Dr. Warren stepped back, indicated the man on the operating-table, and said, "Well, sir, your patient is ready." Amid the silence of the spectators, surrounded by unsympathetic and even derisive faces,

Morton proceeded to administer ether. In a few minutes he
looked up and said, "Dr. Warren, *your* patient is ready."
The incredulous audience watched in silence as the incision

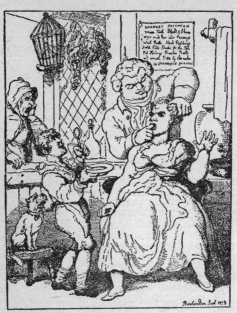

TOOTHACHE, OR TORMENT AND TORTURE, A CARICATURE
BY ROWLANDSON

In 1823, when this drawing was made, there was no anesthesia for
dentistry and in fact very little dentistry except the extraction of
teeth. Much of this extraction was conducted by itinerant quacks or
jacks-of-all-trades, who did it as a side line to their business. Joseph
Grego, who collected and annotated Rowlandson's works, says of this
sketch: "Although the rustic practitioner does not display his diploma
from the college of surgeons, his license to kill by authority, he has
made up a certificate with which, it is probable, he is equally satisfied:
'*Barnaby Factotum:* Draws Teeth, Bleeds and Shaves: Wigs made
here; also sausages. Wash Balls, Black Pudding, Scotch Pills, Powders
of the Itch, Red Herrings, Breeches Balls and Small Beer by the
maker. *In utrumque Paratus.*'"

was made through the skin. The patient neither struggled nor cried out. The operation was continued and a tumor removed. Still the patient gave no sign of pain. With the completion of the operation Dr. Warren turned to the audience and said, "Gentlemen, this is no humbug."

The word anesthesia is used here in describing Morton's work, but the word was not in use in the language when Morton gave his demonstration at the hospital. The fact that a word to define the condition was not in use is striking evidence that a state of insensibility to pain was something wholly new, for man names promptly all the phenomena which come under his observation. Nor was this new phenomenon an exception to the rule, for hardly was the hospital demonstration over before the scholar and physician, Oliver Wendell Holmes, was asked to suggest a name. He replied with the word "anesthetic" to define the substance used to produce insensibility, and the word "anesthesia" for the state of insensibility.

Twenty-one years after this demonstration at the Massachusetts General Hospital, Morton, at the age of forty-nine, died of apoplexy while driving with his wife through Central Park, New York City. His death was no doubt hastened by the controversy in which he had engaged to establish his priority to the use of ether as an anesthetic.

Soon after his demonstration of the possibilities of ether as an anesthetic Morton had joined with Dr. Jackson in an attempt to patent ether under the name of "letheon." Their intention was to control the use of letheon by issuing permits to physicians. The fees to be charged were to depend upon the size of the town in which the physician practiced, and ranged from $37 to $200 for a period of seven years. The name "letheon" could not, however, disguise the well-known odor of ether and considerable indignation was aroused among the members of the medical and dental professions at the unethical procedure of Morton and Jackson. As one journal expressed it: "The surgeons of the Massachusetts General Hospital, together with a few initiated, became astonishingly fervent in their praise of an 'innovation' which requires the combined efforts of scientific attainments and mechanical skill to develop. Classical erudition comes to their aid, and, for a season, good old 'sulphuric ether' was made to succumb to the name of 'letheon.' "

Morton and Jackson soon separated their interests. Jackson attempted to show that he alone was the "inventor" of the anesthetic. Morton, under the advice of the lawyers Rufus Choate and Caleb Cushing, applied for a patent on his application of the use of ether. At the same time Horace Wells, who had used nitrous oxide, came forward to take his part in the three-sided controversy to establish the real discoverer of anesthesia. In 1849 Morton petitioned Congress for a reward for his discovery. He was opposed by Jackson and the friends of Wells, who was then dead. The celebrated controversy, thus begun, occupied the attention of Congress for several years and was characterized by violent animosity between the former friends, Morton and Jackson. At one time it was facetiously suggested that, as a solution, statues should be erected of both Morton and Jackson and on the common pedestal the word "e(i)ther" inscribed. In 1854 a bill proposing to appropriate $100,000 to the real discoverer of anesthesia was up for its final reading before the Senate. At this stage Senator Dawson arose and stated that it had been brought to his attention that ether had been used by Dr. Long in Georgia for a surgical operation four years before Morton's demonstration at the Massachusetts General Hospital. In consequence of this declaration the appropriation was allowed to die.

Dr. Long of Athens, Georgia, was a country practitioner known only to those of the locality where he practiced. One French writer, with characteristic disregard of the geography of any country except France, called him the "Greek physician of Athens." Like Jackson, Dr. Long had observed the insensibility to pain produced by ether during "ether frolics," and he was led to try it as a means of abolishing pain during a surgical operation. The bill for that first operation under ether, made out to James Venable, the first patient, is still preserved. The charges, including anesthesia, were $2.00. Dr.

Long continued to use ether in his limited country practice, but he neither published an account of his experiences nor exercised any influence in bringing ether into general use in surgery. The controversy between Morton and Jackson had been brought to his attention through the nation-wide interest it aroused. His communication to Senator Dawson setting forth his prior claim to the use of ether was not motivated by a desire for reward, but was made simply that another might not be recognized by Congress as the discoverer of anesthesia.

The use of anesthesia in surgical operations has now become commonplace. So rapid are the advances in the application of science to the comfort of man that the conditions existing in surgical operations within the memory of men living seem barbarous. In 1896, fifty years after the introduction of anesthesia, Hayden wrote a description of two operations, one before and one after the use of ether.

### THEN

"With a meek, imploring look, and the startled air of a fawn, as her modest gaze meets the bold eyes fixed upon her, she is brought into the amphitheater crowded with men, anxious to see the shedding of her blood, and laid upon the table. With a knowledge of merciful regard as to the intensity of the agony which she is to suffer, opiates and stimulants have been freely given her, which, perhaps at this last stage, are again repeated. She is cheered by kind words and the information that it will soon be over and she freed forever from what now afflicts her; she is enjoined to be calm, and to keep quiet and still, and, with assistance at hand to hold her struggling form, the operation is commenced.

"But of what avail are all her attempts at fortitude? At the first clear, crisp cut of the scalpel, agonizing screams burst from her, and, with convulsive struggles, she endeavors to leap from the table. But force is nigh. Strong men throw themselves upon her and pinion her limbs. Shriek upon shriek make their horrible way into the stillness of the room, until the heart of the boldest sinks in his bosom, like a lump of lead.

"At length it is finished, and, prostrate with pain, weak from her exertions, and bruised by the violence used, she is borne finally from the amphitheater to her bed in the wards, to recover from the shock by slow degrees."

### NOW

"How would the same case be now? With a sweet, calm smile playing around her mouth—an evidence of pleasant dreams—her eyes fast closed as in a gentle sleep; her body extended languidly and listless as in the repose of childhood, surrounded by no ill-favored men whose powerful aid will be needed; with no crowd of medical men to guard against unforeseen accidents. The surgeon and his two assistants to pass the necessary implements, or to assist in stanching the blood, are all who are required. At his leisure—not hurried by the demands of pain to complete as soon as possible—he can coolly prosecute his work, varying it to suit any exigency of the occasion, and ready to profit by any favorable contingency which its course may present.

"When finished, and all is in the proper condition which will demand no fresh interference for some time, the patient is awakened from her slumber and receives the glad information that it is all over.

"The one grateful look which answers this news can have no value placed upon it. Alone, it is worth a lifetime of exertion and trouble."

If Hayden's description of the after-effects of a surgical operation under anesthesia seems too gentle to one who has undergone an operation, it is equally true that his description of the horrors of a surgical operation of the pre-anesthetic days also falls short of the reality.

Dr. Warren, who had performed the operation on the day of Morton's demonstration at the Massachusetts General Hospital, was a man of high standing in his profession.

He was favorably impressed by the use of ether and his opinion did much to bring about its general acceptance. Among the first in Europe to use ether was Dr. James Y. Simpson, professor of obstetrics at the University of Glasgow. He administered it to a few of his patients to alleviate the pain of childbirth, but he found difficulties in its use, particularly on account of its odor and irritating action. He was convinced, however, that other substances must possess also the property of inducing anesthesia. With his colleagues, Keith and Duncan, he examined a great variety of chemicals in the hope of finding a substitute for ether, and adopted chloroform as the most promising possibility. As a test the three friends gathered in the dining-room of Simpson's home; in front of each on the table was a tumbler of chloroform, and each inhaled the vapors which rose from the fluid. They became exhilarated, the liveliest conversation ensued, and then the three suddenly fell insensible. After their recovery they repeated the experiment, and Simpson's niece was inclined to try also. Folding her arms across her breast, she inhaled the vapor, and to the amusement of the guests she fell asleep, crying: "I'm an angel! Oh, I'm an angel!"

Soon after the experiment at the dinner table Simpson used chloroform to relieve the sufferings of a woman during childbirth. He was so struck with the blessing conferred that he at once published his results. That was in 1847. Of the first case in which chloroform was tried he writes:

"The lady to whom it was first exhibited during parturition had been previously delivered in the country by perforation of the head of the infant, after a labor of three days' duration. In this, her second confinement, pains supervened a fortnight before the full time. Three hours and a half after they commenced, and ere the first stage of the labor was complete, I placed her under the influence of chloroform . . . The child was expelled in about twenty-five minutes after the inhalation was begun. . . . The squall of the child did not, as usual, rouse her; and some minutes elapsed . . . after the child was removed by the nurse into another room before the patient awoke. She then turned around and observed to me that she had 'enjoyed' a very comfortable sleep, and indeed required it, as she was so tired, but could now be more able for the work before her. (In consequence of extreme anxiety at the unfortunate result of her previous confinement, she had slept little or none for one or two nights.) In a little time she again remarked that she was afraid her 'sleep had stopped the pains.' Shortly afterward her infant was brought in by the nurse from the adjoining room, and it was a matter of no small difficulty to convince the astonished mother that the labor was entirely over and that the child presented to her was really her 'own living baby.'"

Simpson, almost within the week, published a report of his success with chloroform. The immediate result was not an acceptance of this means of relief from suffering which he offered to women; instead, his work precipitated a violent controversy over the propriety of abolishing the pains of childbirth. A lesser man than Simpson would have been crushed by the intense opposition he encountered; but as it was, no man could have been found better suited than Simpson to enter the lists in favor of woman. He enjoyed a fight in a good cause.

In the course of the events above narrated leading up to the conquest of death at birth, a striking difference is to be noted in the character of the men particularly concerned. There was Paré, simple and direct, equally at home in the rough military camps of his time and in the treacherous intrigues of court. He survived four Catholic kings of France and was the medical adviser and councilor of each in succession, although he was a Protestant. What greater testimonial could be written on the sterling qualities of any man? The Chamberlens, half charlatans, half fanatics, held secret for nearly a century a treatment of inestimable benefit to the human race; they were, in consequence, disdained by their medical contemporaries and have been censured or ignored by historians. Holmes, a scholar and a man of the finest quality; certainly not wholly a dilettante in medicine, but certainly equally lacking in not forcing, either with the

life of sacrifice of Semmelweis or the belligerent persistence
of Simpson, the things which his keen intelligence showed
him a generation before other men saw them as clearly as he
did. Jackson and Morton were not directly concerned with
the story of childbirth, but were responsible in leading up
to one of its greatest advances. They present a mixture of
selfish interest and personal controversy which obscures the
conception of their work; many of the benefits that they
should have reaped were lost in their squabbles and went to
James Simpson. In Sir James Y. Simpson there is the character of a reformer without the dour pessimism and tragic
readiness of martyrdom common among reformers; he was
a reformer, but he was one with both feet set solidly on a
foundation of common sense, one with a genial love of his
fellow-men and a healthy disposition to argument. Rarest
of all, he was a reformer with a sense of humor.

Scotland has a legend regarding anesthesia: Thenu, the
mother of St. Kentigern, or St. Mungo, of Glasgow was
impregnated without her knowledge under the influence of
some soporific potion. In consequence, as a punishment, she
was cast down from the top of a high hill, but, wonderful
to say, she was not hurt. Not satisfied with this evidence of
divine intervention, her judges then sentenced her to be set
adrift in a small boat on the Firth of Forth, whereupon she
floated across to Fife and was received by St. Servanus. In
due time she was safely delivered of a son, who became afterward the famous St. Kentigern. Having a saint whose history
recorded an anesthesia so closely connected with childbirth
may have given the clergy some sensitiveness on the subject.
At any rate, it is a historical fact that in 1591 a lady of
rank, Eufame Macalyane, sought the assistance of Agnes
Sampson for the relief of pain at the time of the birth of
her two sons. Agnes Sampson was tried before King James,
for her heresy, was condemned as a witch, and was burned
alive on the Castle Hill of Edinburgh. Again in the nineteenth century the Scottish clergy rose, if not to burn
Simpson with fire, at least to consume his practices with their
fiery condemnations. Simpson, less submissive than the lady

of the sixteenth century, turned, and with their own weapon
of religious interpretation silenced the clergy and cleared
the way for the more serious controversy with the men of
his own profession.

Simpson and his use of chloroform in childbirth were
denounced from the pulpit and by pamphlets. Many otherwise sensible people were thus led by their religious
scruples to doubt the propriety of inhaling chloroform. The
arguments used by the clergy against anesthesia varied, but
all centered around the theme that pain, particularly the
pain of childbirth, was the ordained lot of mankind; to
prevent it was a sacrilege. As one clergyman expressed it,
"chloroform is a decoy of Satan, apparently offering itself
to bless women; but in the end it will harden society and
rob God of the deep, earnest cries which arise in time of
trouble for help." Another pointed out that chloroform, like
alcohol, produces intoxication and unconsciousness, and on
this slender foundation rose to rhetorical heights. He drew
a picture of the lying-in room with its former quiet dignity,
now giving way under the influence of chloroform to a
scene of drunken debauch during which a child was brought
into the world.

The authority claimed for these ecclesiastical attacks lay
in the Biblical curse placed upon mankind (Gen. III:16):
"Unto the woman he said, I will greatly multiply thy sorrow and thy conception; in sorrow thou shalt bring forth
children; and thy desire shall be to thy husband, and he
shall rule over thee." It was the portion, "in sorrow thou
shalt bring forth children," which was the crux of the
matter. According to the prevailing interpretation pain (sorrow) was ordained in childbirth, and the prevention of pain
during childbirth "was contrary to religion and the express
comand of Scripture."

Simpson replied to these accusations in a series of papers
which for their theological skill and sound logic left little
to be said against the use of chloroform. Simpson was a busy
practitioner. His writing was done in snatches, even at the
bedsides of the women whom he cared for in their confine-

ments. One can visualize the staunch Scotchman writing some of his passages with a sympathy and a conviction that arose from the groans of his patients. At other times a twinkle must have lit his eyes and his tongue must have pressed into his cheek as he wrote some of his religious and physiological interpretations. His smile, if it existed, did not once appear as open derision in the simple logic of his words.

Simpson's paper, "Answers to the Religious Objection Against the Employment of Anesthetic Agents in Midwifery and Surgery," 1847, is a masterpiece of its kind. First he presents the justice of his own stand by analogies in other occupations, and uses in support quotations from Genesis. He demonstrates that, if literal translation is adhered to, the farmer, in pulling up "the thorn and thistle" which the earth is doomed to bear, and in avoiding shedding "the sweat of his face" in tilling the ground through the use of horses and agricultural machinery, is also going against the express command of Scripture. He shows likewise that the physician, on the basis of too literal a translation, would be represented as wrong in attempting to save life, for it was ordained that man should be subject to death—"dust thou art, and unto dust shalt thou return." "If," said Simpson, "it be justifiable in the physician to try to counteract the effects of one part of the curse, and justifiable in the agriculturalist to try to counteract the effects of another part, it is surely equally justifiable in the *accoucheur* to try to counteract the effects of a third part of it. . . . Are those who maintain the uncanonical character of using human means to contravene the pains of childbirth ready, then, to maintain that we shall not use human means to contravene the tendency to death, or to increase the fertility and produce of the ground except by personal labor and the actual 'sweat of the brow'?"

His next step was to cast doubt upon the validity of the word "sorrow" as used in connection with child-bearing. I am no judge of Simpson's philology, but to his own satisfaction at least he translates the Hebrew word to mean toil or labor rather than "sorrow." He then goes on to demonstrate at length that childbirth among the human species,

because of the erect posture, is a more "laborious" procedure
than among quadrupeds. The Biblical word, according to
his interpretation, amounts merely to an early recognition
of this physiological fact.

Simpson next explains that opposition, particularly on
theological grounds, had been presented against every
humane innovation in the past. He cites as an instance the
opposition to the introduction of vaccination against smallpox. Those opposed to its introduction had argued against
it on religious grounds. "Smallpox," they had said, "is a
visitation from God, and originates in man: but the cowpox [vaccination] is produced by presumptuous, impious
man. The former Heaven ordained; the latter is a daring
and profane violation of our holy religion." A more practical
opponent told of the effects of this "profane violation" in
the case of "a lady who complained that since her daughter
was inoculated she coughs like a cow and has grown hair
all over her body." Another pointed out that vaccination
was discontinued in one part of the country "because those
who had been inoculated in that manner bellow like bulls"!

Simpson carried his illustration further and told of the
attempted frustration of advancement in the field of agri-
culture. There had been strong opposition to the introduction
of the winnowing machine which separates chaff from grain.
This process had been carried out formerly by throwing
grain into the air and allowing the wind to carry the chaff
away. "Winds," it was argued by those opposed to the
innovation of farm machinery, "were raised by God alone,
and it was irreligious in man to attempt to raise wind for
the aforesaid purpose for himself, and by the efforts of his
own." One clergyman had debarred from communion such
of his flock as used the winnowing machine. Simpson carries
his examples even further and says: "Some day a canal will,
in all probability, be made through the Isthmus of Panama.
It has, as you are well aware, long been proposed to cut one;
and there and thus unite the Atlantic and Pacific Oceans."
But when this proposal was made in the sixteenth century
a priest by the name of Acosta brought forward the follow-

ing reason against it: "I am of opinion that human power should not be allowed to cut through the strong and impenetrable bounds which God has put between two oceans, of mountains and iron rocks, which can stand the fury of the raging seas. And, if it were possible, it would appear to me very just that we should fear the vengeance of Heaven for attempting to improve that which the Creator in His almighty will and providence has ordained from the creation of the world." The arguments advanced in the nineteenth century against the use of anesthesia at childbirth varied in form not at all from the arguments brought against the proposal for a Panama Canal in the sixteenth century, and the winnowing machine in the eighteenth century.

Simpson completed his paper with a piece of almost irrefutable logic, and certainly one of the most amazing. He more than meets his opponents, for he takes their weapons for his own use. He says: "Besides, those who urge, on a kind of religious ground, that an artificial or anesthetic state of unconsciousness should not be induced merely to save frail humanity from the misery and tortures of bodily pain, forget that we have the greatest of all examples set before us for following out this very principle of practice. I allude to that most singular description of the preliminaries and details of the first surgical operation ever performed on man which is contained in Gen. 11:21: 'And the Lord God caused a deep sleep to fall upon Adam, and he slept: and he took one of his ribs, and closed up the flesh instead thereof.' In this remarkable verse the whole process of a surgical operation is briefly detailed. But the passage is principally striking as affording evidence of our Creator himself using means to save poor human nature from unnecessary endurance of physical pain." The first surgical operation was thus shown to have been performed with the patient under anesthesia.

Completing his religious controversy to his satisfaction, Simpson turned to vanquish equally effectively the more serious opposition raised by some of the physicians themselves. The most outspoken opponent of the use of anesthesia in childbirth was Dr. Meigs of Philadelphia, the same Dr. Meigs in whom the observations of Holmes on puerperal

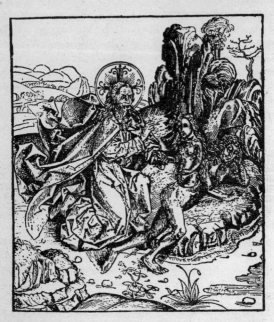

### THE BIRTH OF EVE—THE FIRST ANESTHESIA

A representation of the "first surgical operation," the incident used by Sir James Simpson to allay the opposition to the use of anesthesia. The deep sleep—anesthesia, according to Simpson—into which Adam was cast is quite evident in this woodcut from a history by Hartmann Schedel written in 1493. Vesalius in the sixteenth century, by his anatomical work, disproved the idea that men had one less rib than women—the missing rib of Adam.

fever had aroused such a storm of contention. In his controversy with Holmes, Meigs had quoted from Simpson, "who was a gentleman," and it was against this same Simpson that he now turned. Reluctance to accept progress, particularly someone else's brand of progress, was not peculiar to the clergy of Simpson's time. It is a general characteristic of human nature and, so far as one can judge, is an instinctive manifestation of a kind of fear and uncertainty of one's own ability to cope with the innovation. Dr. Meigs possessed this instinct to a high degree. Most people, in fact, are conservatives and instinctively hate radicals.

The tone of derision which Simpson had excluded from his papers on religious objections he now let loose in torrents on Meigs and others of the medical profession. Particularly he dwelt upon a statement made by Meigs that the pain of labor was a "natural" or "physiological" pain and should not for that reason be interfered with. A physiological or natural pain was defined as one that was not caused by external violence applied to the body, but was the regular, and therefore presumably normal, accompaniment of bodily function—in this case childbirth. As Meigs expressed it, the pain of childbirth was "a desirable, salutary, and conservative manifestation of life force."

Simpson recognized that the opposition of men in the medical profession differed from that of the clergy only in the line of approach. Both were manifestations of the unfailing resentment aroused by any attempt to change the established order of things. He writes in reply to Dr. Meigs's objection to relieving the "natural" or "physiological" pains of childbirth:

"I have a letter lying before me on the subject of anesthetics in midwifery, by a very highly and very justly esteemed teacher of midwifery in Dublin. 'I do not,' he writes, 'believe that anyone in Dublin has as yet used ether in midwifery; the feeling is very strong against its use in ordinary cases, and merely to avert the ordinary amount of pain which the Almighty has seen fit—and most wisely, we cannot doubt—to allot to natural labour; and in this feeling I heartily and entirely concur.'

"The argument thus used, and so very well expressed by my Irish correspondent, is one which has been often adduced and repeated during the course of the past year. Some minds at first gave immense weight and importance to it. For my own part, I must confess that I never could view it as possessing any great force. Look at it as applied to any other practice which happens to be sufficiently old and established, and then we shall see it in its true import. Supposing, for example, it referred to the *first* introduction of carriages into use; it would then read thus: 'I do not believe that anyone in Dublin has as yet used a carriage in loco-motion; the feeling here is very strong against its use in ordinary progression, and merely to avert the ordinary amount of fatigue which the Almighty has seen fit—and most wisely, we cannot doubt—to allot to natural walking; and in this feeling I heartily and entirely concur.'

"Nay, this frequently-repeated argument against new innovations becomes not only, I think, ridiculous, but really almost irreverent, when we look far backward into the march of civilization, and apply it to any practices that are so very long established as to be very antiquated, and with which, therefore, the human mind has been long intimately familiarized. Someone, but who I cannot pretend to say, no doubt first introduced the practice of wearing hats or bon-nets, or some covering for the head. Supposing this practice, however, stoutly resisted, as doubtlessly it was at first, then the argument of my Dublin friend against this innovation would read somewhat as follows: "I do not believe that anyone in Dublin has as yet used a hat to protect his head; the feeling here is very strong against its use in ordinary weather, and merely to avert the ordinary amount of wetting and cold which the Almighty has seen fit—and most wisely, we cannot doubt—to allot to mankind; and in this feeling I heartily and entirely concur.'

"The truth is, all the tendencies of man, in a civilized state of society, are to intermeddle with and change, and, as he conceives, improve, the action of almost every function of the body. And each such improvement has, at the time of its introduction, been, like the practice of anesthesia, very duly denounced as improper, impious, etc., etc. I might refer to numerous such cases. Let me cite only one example. The human fingers are admirably constructed by our Creator for the function of seizing and lifting objects. The late Sir Charles Bell wrote a whole octavo volume—a Bridgewater Treatise—on the mechanism of the human hand, as beautifully adapted for this and other functions. In the reign of the earlier Stuarts forks were introduced from the Continent to assist our hands in the act or function of seizing and lifting the divided portions of meat, etc., that we wished to eat. But this was a very sad and uncalled-for innovation upon the old and established physiological functions of the human fingers; and, at the time, it was as loudly opposed and decried as the modern employment of anesthetics in aiding the physiological function of human parturition. D'Israeli tells us that the use of forks was so much reprobated in some quarters, that some uncleanly preachers denounced it 'as an insult on Providence not to touch our meat with our fingers.' Nature herself has provided us with fingers of flesh and bone and nerve, and consequently, is it not unnatural and impious in man to attempt, in his human pride and arrogance, to substitute for these, artificial metallic fingers of silver and steel? . . .

"You are well aware that the act of parturition has been often familiarly compared, as the late Professor Hamilton expressed it, 'to the toils of a journey,' and like it divided into stages. 'The sufferings of the mothers,' says he, 'have been in most languages compared to those of travellers.' Now let us for a moment continue this natural simile between the function of parturition and the function of progression. You maintain that 'labour is the culminating point of the female somatic forces.' One of the most illustrious Presidents of your great American Republic—Thomas Jefferson—makes in his memoirs a remark of precisely the same import regarding walking or progression. He describes the act of walking, but not exactly in the same words, as the kind of 'culminating point of the human somatic forces.'

"Few, or none, perhaps, will question the abstract truth of Jefferson's observations on this point. But, because walk-

ing or progression is a 'physiological' function, and the
practice of it is reputed salutary, would this be, with you,
a proper and sufficient reason for never setting aside or
superseding in any way this 'physiological' state, in the
same way as you insist, on the same grounds, that the
physiological pain of labor should not be set aside or superseded? Because progression is a natural condition, would
this be any adequate reason for your medical advisers
adopting your own arguments against anesthesia in midwifery, and insisting upon this, that, the next time you
travelled from your own city of Philadelphia to the cities
of Baltimore or New York, you should walk the distance
on foot instead of travelling it by railway or other con-
veyance? What opinion would you form of the judgment
of any medical adviser to whom you entrusted your own
health if, on going next time to the New York or Baltimore
railway station, he should gravely and solemnly repeat to
you, as his patient, what you tell your midwifery patients,
and, in your own language, advise you to try to accomplish
the intended journey on foot, as (to quote your own words)
'a desirable, salutary, and conservative manifestation of life
force'? And yet this would really be nothing more than
making your *argumentum ad feminam* an *argumentum ad
hominem*. . . .

". . . Suppose you plead with your medical adviser that,
instead of insisting on your going on foot, he should allow
you *for once* to take advantage of artificial assistance, and
proceed on your journey from Philadelphia to Baltimore
or New York by railway, because you were unable to walk
the distance in consequence of being incapacitated by a
rheumatic knee, or a sprained ankle, or an inflamed or
blistered toe, and he replied to you that you should not
care for this, but still proceed and suffer, because the pain
you might thus suffer was (to use again your own language)
still only a 'physiological pain.' Would that argument be
any adequate philosophic consolation under the endurance
of your suffering? or would you not laugh at the logic of
your medical adviser and take your seat in the railway in

spite of his doctrine? And I have a fancy that betimes, in midwifery, patients *will* learn to adopt exactly the same line of practice under the analogous circumstances, and think, and act too, exactly in the same way."

Within two years after his paper describing his first use of chloroform at childbirth, Simpson was able to report that it had been administered to from 40,000 to 50,000 persons in Edinburgh both for childbirth and for surgical operation. Simpson established this advance toward the conquest of death and suffering at birth, and, unlike the unfortunate Semmelweis, lived to see the success of his efforts. He was honored locally, he was knighted, and at his death in 1870 the shops of the city closed while the people went to view the enormous procession of those who attended his funeral. In connection with his title of knighthood it is said that Sir Walter Scott wrote to Simpson and suggested as a coat of arms suited to his work on anesthesia at childbirth, "a wee naked bairn" with underneath the motto, "Does your mother know you're out?"

At the same time that Simpson was fighting for the use of chloroform to alleviate the pains of childbirth, Dr. Channing of Boston was waging a less picturesque but none the less effective struggle to introduce ether for a similar purpose. An objection brought in America against Dr. Channing's work was one that would seem ridiculous today if it were not for the fact that as late as 1921, in the revival of "twilight sleep," the same objection was raised. It can be phrased best in the words of one of Channing's correspondents, who claimed that "the very suffering which a woman undergoes in labour is one of the strongest elements in the love she bears for her offspring." The maternal instinct was engendered by the mother's suffering! In effect it implies that childbirth is in nature something similar to the initiation of candidates into a college club or the hazing of freshmen who from their suffering are supposed to gain a greater appreciation of the exaltation of their new state. The argument that lack of pain would rob the mother of her love for the child was urged, not by expectant mothers, but by women well past the age of child-bearing. Their suppressed desire to have others share the suffering they had undergone was thinly disguised under the sophistry of the loss of maternal instinct. It was the disappointed spinsters, too, who joined the acclaim against anesthesia; the threatened loss of maternal instinct in others gave an excuse for their unconscious malice. Finally, as would be expected, it was men who saw the maternal instinct slipping away with the abolition of pain. Men dislike to see women relieved of any of the burden of suffering and handicaps whose elimination might destroy an illusion of "inferior sex." Nothing was heard on the subject from those women who were about to undergo the pain. They were too busy tending to the wants of the brood they already had, and in making preparations for the new addition, to find leisure for a philosophical discussion of maternal love. They took their chloroform or their ether if they got it, and perhaps wondered what suffering the father must undergo to attain his parental love. Possibly they even covertly wished for a revival of the custom of some native tribes, where the husband was hung up by the feet to dangle head down throughout the hours of his wife's labor.

In the middle of April, 1853, an event occurred which exerted a greater influence on popular acceptance of anesthesia at childbirth, not only in Great Britain, but in America as well, than all the efforts of Simpson. Queen Victoria accepted chloroform for the delivery of her seventh child, Prince Leopold. Nothing could exceed the astonishment with which the announcement was received. The tone of the leading medical journals showed only too plainly what would have been the sentence passed upon Her Majesty's medical attendants had anything untoward occurred. There was not one word of approval for the medical men, for the royal patient, or for humanity. The *Lancet*, May, 1853, said: "In no case could it be justifiable to administer chloroform in a perfectly ordinary labour." Doubtless all concerned felt the "awful responsibility" of the undertaking, but, having been successful, it had the immense influence upon the people exerted by royalty at that time. Again in 1857 the Queen accepted chloroform for her confinement. Formal opposition ceased in Great Britain thereafter, and chloroform was often referred to as *anesthesia à la reine*.

The popularization of anesthesia at childbirth by Queen Victoria was not the first time that royalty had come to the aid of the child-bearing woman. As recorded previously, Louis XIV of France, the "Grand Monarch," had been indirectly instrumental in bringing the physician into the lying-in room and breaking down the age-long hold of the midwives. Incidentally, this was not the only medical contribution of Louis, who seems from all accounts to have been quite a problem for his physicians. He was born with two teeth, much to the worriment of his wet nurses, had smallpox when nine years old, a venereal infection a few years later, and then typhoid fever. This last illness popularized the use of antimony as a remedy; there had been much acrimonious controversy over its use. When twenty-five years old Louis contracted measles from the queen. He was troubled with intestinal parasites, and certain historians, in deference to his station, have endowed him with a tapeworm of proportions to suit his royal magnificence and his royal appetite. His teeth were in bad shape and he was troubled with abscesses about them. At the age of forty-four he developed the gout and in the next year dislocated his elbow in a fall from his horse. Three years later he rendered a great service to the practice of surgery by permitting an operation for fistula of the anus. The operation was successful. The courtiers promptly wished for a similar operation on themselves, even though they did not need it, but in that way to show their sympathy with the king in his delicate affliction. The example of Louis brought about the rehabilitation of French surgery. The king, among his other complaints, was afflicted with malaria, which was carried to him by the mosquitoes which lived in hordes in the ponds at his favorite residence, Marley. He was cured of this complaint by chinchona, quinine, and this fact helped to popularize this remedy. Later he had a serious carbuncle, his gout became worse, and he was troubled with gravel in his urine. He finally developed hardening of the arteries and died of a consequent gangrene of the leg. His greatest contribution to medicine, however, lies in the treatment not of himself, but of his mistress, for whose confinement he called in the physician Boucher instead of a midwife, thereby opening the way for male midwifery.

Simpson's work in introducing anesthesia for labor was a success, but it did not render child-bearing painless. The first optimistic belief that chloroform might safely accomplish this end was soon shattered—occasional deaths of the mother resulted from chloroform in cases where it was administered for too long a time or to a particularly susceptible patient. Simpson apparently did not recognize the fact that anesthetics were potent drugs, as is indeed illustrated by a story told by Lord Playfair at the semicentennial celebration of the use of ether in the Massachusetts General Hospital. Simpson came to Lord Playfair one day and told him he was disgusted with chloroform and would thank him for a satisfactory substitute. Lord Playfair, a few days later, announced to him that he had made the required discovery; the material was di-bromide of ethylene. Simpson smelled the compound, said it was what he wanted, and wished to repair immediately to Lord Playfair's private room and experiment on himself. He was finally dissuaded from the personal experiment by the suggestion that the drug be tried on rabbits. The rabbits were made to inhale the vapors and were then put away to await developments. On the next day Simpson appeared, promptly propped himself up with two chairs, and asked Lord Playfair for the drug, that he might administer it to himself. Lady Simpson, who was present, advised her husband to see how the rabbits had fared under the treatment before he tried it. "When the attendant came in," says Lord Playfair, "we saw him holding by the ears two rabbits—perfectly dead!"

The recognition of the occasionally dangerous qualities of chloroform, particularly in surgical operations, led to a

return to the use of ether. The change was not so greatly
felt in child-bearing, for the parturient woman is apparently—although no one knows why—less than normally
susceptible to the poisonous action of chloroform. Even to
her chloroform cannot safely be given for long periods—
nor can ether. Painless childbirth had not, as Simpson
hoped, been achieved. But if the anesthetics have not robbed
childbirth of all its pain, they have robbed it of its most
intense agony.

The process of birth may last for many hours; eighteen
hours is perhaps an average figure for the first child, and
six hours for the second. The suffering involved varies
greatly in different women. The pains accompany the intermittent contractions of the muscle of the uterus as it attempts
to expel its contents, and arise from this contraction, from
the pressure brought to bear upon joints and tendons, from
the gradual dilatation of the opening of the uterus, and
finally from the stretching of the soft part of the birth canal.
At first these intermittent pains are spaced many minutes
apart, but the time between them decreases as the labor
progresses and their intensity increases. The most severe
pain, the agony of childbirth, comes after the child's head
has passed from the uterus and while it is propelled through
the vagina. The passage is stretched and sometimes torn; the
pain is often extremely severe. It is in these last stages of
the birth that anesthesia by chloroform or by ether has its
greatest benefit. The time involved is not long and these
anesthetics may usually be safely given. When Simpson's
first case, related above, is read carefully, it will seem that
he administered chloroform for only twenty-five minutes,
although labor had already been in progress three and a
half hours. He had robbed the birth of its "agony," and so
great did the difference seem to him that it was by comparison a painless birth.

There are other agonies, too, which ether and chloroform
remove from childbirth. They are the pains that accompany
manipulations of instrumental assistance at the birth. The
version of Ambroise Paré was done in his time without

anesthesia, and so, too, forceps were used in the time of the Chamberlens, without anesthesia. These procedures are in effect surgical operations, but surgical operations were without anesthesia until after the middle of the last century.

The situation today in the use of anesthesia in childbirth has not changed much from what it was in the time of Simpson. The majority of cases have no anesthesia unless instruments or manipulations are necessary. In a somewhat less number of cases chloroform or ether or some other anesthetic is given toward the end of the birth, to rob it of its last and most severe pains. In a few cases an attempt is made to render the whole delivery as nearly painless as is possible. There is no simple, safe, and efficient method as yet of rendering childbirth entirely painless. When the woman in labor is allowed to use an anesthetic it requires more fortitude than most physicians have to deprive her of its use when the labor becomes unduly prolonged; therefore, most physicians wait as long as possible before commencing the anesthetic.

The majority of cases of childbirth are today conducted as they have been conducted since woman first bore children—without any anesthesia. The practical difficulty of giving the anesthetic is one reason for this, and indifference is another reason. Most women unwisely bear their children in their homes instead of in hospitals, and many are delivered without medical assistance of any kind. But even if a physician is present there are difficulties in the giving of an anesthetic. If he is a modern physician his hands are covered by sterilized rubber gloves and he attempts by every effort to prevent their contamination. He cannot properly assist at the birth and at the same time administer the anesthetic. If he is not a modern physician and is today indifferent to the cleanliness of his hands, he is probably equally indifferent to the pain of his patient. The physician, in order properly to conduct his work at childbirth, needs a nurse, and if he is to administer anesthesia he needs also an assistant—the last he rarely finds except in a hospital. Most cases of childbirth conducted in homes are without a nurse or an assistant—both are luxuries to most families and particularly to families which have the most children. The physician may draft to his needs a sister, mother, or a neighbor of his patient instead of the nurse, and call in the unwilling and flustered husband as an anesthetist. There is no situation in life where a husband is so useless and where he shows it as plainly as at the birth of his child. He feels, particularly from the attitude of the sister or mother, and sometimes from the outspoken statements of his wife, a vague responsibility resting on him for the pain his wife is enduring. On every side it is impressed upon him that a husband is out of place and is somehow shirking his duty at a childbirth. The climax comes when he is brusquely told to hold an ether cover over his wife's face, and the physician, to cheer him and to make him feel his responsibility, tells him jovially that he will never have a better chance of disposing of his present wife. The administration of anesthesia at childbirth in the home is, except in rare cases, a difficult procedure. The country practitioner shooing off the persistent advice of the patient's sister or mother, dragging the fainting amateur anesthetist out-of-doors to revive him, and assisting at the birth of the child, makes an heroic picture of the patience of a now passing breed of physician. But such procedures leave much to be desired for the relief of the mother.

Surgical operations, even the most serious, were at one time performed in the home. They are now rarely performed outside of hospitals if the operation is of sufficient severity to require a general anesthetic. When every woman realizes and every physician insists that child-bearing deserves the same consideration as a major surgical operation, when every case of childbirth is cared for in a modern hospital, then and then only will a woman reap the greatest benefits from anesthesia. There, whether she is in a private room or in a ward, she will have some anesthesia. What is even more important to her future health, she will be kept under the anesthesia, after the child has been born, until the physician attending her has had ample time to make a careful examination and to repair injuries which, if left untreated, as they formerly always were, would result in chronic illness.

Although ether and chloroform are still the anesthetics most extensively used in child-bearing, nitrous oxide and the other gaseous anesthetics have replaced them to some extent. Nitrous oxide in particular has the advantage that it can be given for a long time with much less danger to the mother and the child than is the case with chloroform or even ether. Nitrous oxide, which was suggested as an anesthetic by Sir Humphry Davy in 1800 and used in dentistry by Wells in 1844, was recommended for childbirth by Klikowitch of St. Petersburg in 1880. The increasing use of nitrous oxide, either alone or combined with ether, for surgical operations has led to the more general use of this anesthetic in childbirth. While it is unquestionably safer than chloroform and much more rapid in action and less irritating than ether, it has the practical disadvantage of requiring special and cumbersome apparatus for its administration. It is used to some extent in lying-in hospitals and to a much less extent for deliveries in homes, and there only among the comparatively few patients who can afford such service.

The anesthetics which are inhaled have been an inestimable boon to the child-bearing woman; they have been also a step in the search for means to make child-bearing painless. Spinal anesthesia has been one of the methods attempted—and largely given up. About the spinal cord is a layer of fluid, the cerebro-spinal fluid. When cocain, or a drug similar in action, is injected into the spinal fluid the nerve fibers in the spine cease temporarily to conduct nervous impulses, and sensations of pain are blocked. It is possible thus to block the lower part of the spinal cord, and with care the anesthetic action can be prevented from traveling sufficiently high along the spine to interfere with the nerves which send their impulses to the muscles moving the ribs in breathing. A woman treated with spinal anesthesia has, theoretically, no sensation from the lower part of her body, and the anesthesia may be made to last for an hour or so. At present the disadvantages in the use of spinal anesthesia in child-birth are that it is necessary to employ a special technique in which few physicians are trained; it can be carried out properly only in the hospital; and occasionally the after-effects of the anesthesia are unpleasant.

In 1899 the use of morphine combined with scopolamine, a drug closely related to belladonna, was advocated to relieve the pain of surgical operations. The patient was drugged into a semiconscious dreamy state called "twilight sleep," in which pain was felt but not appreciated, and was soon forgotten. In 1902 the method was used in childbirth, and from the first reports it seemed, indeed, as if the painless childbirth so eagerly sought for had at last been attained. The medical profession naturally grasped this opportunity to relieve the pain of the child-bearing woman, and the drugs were soon extensively employed, and soon abandoned in most places. Labor was in many instances prolonged and it was necessary to use forceps in greater numbers of cases. The method was not adapted for use in homes, but only in such hospitals as had an unusually large staff, for it was necessary to watch closely the woman treated. Particularly it was necessary to guard against danger to the child, since the drugs used were harmful to the child. The woman accepting "twilight sleep" as a relief from some of her suffering did so at the price of possible injury or even occasionally the loss of her child. In 1921 there was a revival of interest in "twilight sleep," but at that time it was shown that the increased mortality for the child from the drugs used had not been eliminated.

The latest method attempted for painless childbirth is with the use of magnesium sulphate injections given in conjunction with morphine and with ether dissolved in oil, and absorbed from the rectum. Magnesium sulphate, a purified form of the familiar Epsom salts, when injected into the body with a hypodermic needle, acts as a narcotic. It does not exhibit this action when taken by mouth, for very little is absorbed; its action as a cathartic results, in fact, from this failure of absorption. The mild narcotic action of magnesium sulphate is believed to reinforce that of ether and morphine, to intensify, and particularly to prolong their action. Some measure of success has been attained by the use of these combinations. There is every probability that in the near future a nearly painless childbirth will be effected by this or some other method for those women wise enough to go to hospitals for their delivery, or for those few who are economically able to bring the hospital treatment to their homes. The prospect for painless child-bearing is not promising for the vast majority of women who will not go to the hospitals and who have not the means to procure elaborate medical care in their own homes.

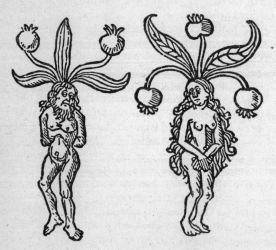

## A PAIR OF MANDRAKES

From an old woodcut. The mandrake was used as an ingredient in soporific potions and love philters. The latter use is suggested here.

## Part Three

# THE PROGRESS OF SURGERY

## CHAPTER VI

## MAKING AN ANATOMY

he earliest known pictures of surgical operations are engraved on the stones over a tomb near Memphis, Egypt. These engravings were made 2,500 years before Christ; their age is more than twice that of the Christian era. The pictures show the operation of circumcision and operations on the legs and arms, and these operations, with the addition of castration, included all the surgical procedures performed by the Egyptians. At this early period all surgery was wound surgery, which included the dressing and treating of wounds, the opening of abscesses, and, as a last resort, the amputation of limbs. All operations were upon the surface of the body or the extremities, for the Egyptians were unacquainted with anatomy beneath the surface. Even if they had possessed such knowledge and had attempted to operate for appendicitis, gall stones, or other disorders in the abdomen, their patients would have died of hemorrhage or infection. The few surgical operations that the Egyptians attempted were undertaken without anesthesia. The attitude of the patients in the pictures on the tomb of Memphis indicates suffering and the hieroglyphics beneath the pictures describe it.

Forty-three centuries after these pictures were made surgery was still wound surgery. In fact, there were no great advances until late in the nineteenth century. Until that time operations were still performed only on the surface of the body, and operations still involved as much suffering, and wounds were as universally infected, as in the early Egyptian period.

The nineteenth century opened with surgery nearly as crude and barbarous and as limited in its scope as it had been in the earliest civilizations, and is now among the most primitive peoples. The nineteenth century closed with modern surgery well developed. Its beginning was not due to any superior manual skill of the surgeons of the nineteenth century, for the Egyptian and European surgeons of the sixteenth, seventeenth, and eighteenth centuries were as skillful manually as are those of today. The development of surgery was prevented by the lack of four attributes more fundamental than manual skill. Modern surgery began when the last of these essentials was discovered. These essentials are (1) a knowledge of anatomy; (2) a method for controlling hemorrhage; (3) anesthetics to deaden pain; and (4) a knowledge of the nature of infection and methods for its prevention.

The first of these essentials, a knowledge of anatomy, was developed in the sixteenth century, and in that same century a method for controlling hemorrhage was introduced. While surgery benefited from these two discoveries, its scope was not extended beyond the surface of the body nor was it freed from pain and infection. There was very little improvement in surgery for three hundred years. Then in the nineteenth century the discoveries of anesthesia and antisepsis rounded out the art of modern surgery, and one of the most beneficent of all the arts rose rapidly to its present development.

The Egyptians had only the most rudimentary knowledge of the structure of the body, a fact which seems peculiar in a people who carried out embalming of the dead. The very fact, however, that they practiced embalming indicated their belief in the sanctity of the body, and under this belief dissection was an offense against the dead. The method of embalming used by the Egyptians varied with the wealth and importance of the deceased. The most expensive process of embalming, costing the equivalent of a thousand dollars, commenced with an incision in the wall of the abdomen. The man who made the incision ran away as soon as the act was completed, to avoid being stoned, a ceremonial gesture to indicate his offense against the dead. The embalmers then took charge of the body; the men of this trade were formed into a guild, or labor union, down to the time of the Roman Empire. They removed the abdominal viscera and preserved them in vases of clay, limestone, or alabaster. They next removed the brain through the nostrils by means of an iron hook. The cavities of the skull and abdomen were filled with spices. The body was next soaked for seventy days in a solution of salt, and afterward coated with gum, wrapped in cloth and placed in a wooden coffin shaped like a man—the sarcophagus—and then deposited in the burial chamber together with the canopic jars containing the viscera. The process of embalming necessitated observation of the abdominal contents, but none of these observations were utilized as anatomical knowledge for surgery.

There was much need for surgery in Egypt, as is shown by archeological surveys, particularly that of 1907 instituted by the Egyptian government in that part of Nubia which was subsequently flooded by the raising of the Assuan dam. In the mummies examined there were found evidences of mastoid disease, appendicitis, fractured bones, fatal sword cuts of the head, and ulcers of the skull due to carrying water jars on the head. The teeth of the mummies of the earliest inhabitants of Egypt were free from decay, probably on account of their diet, for coarse and fibrous foods were found in their intestines. In the mummies of the New Empire, a period of greater luxury, decayed teeth were common and in many instances abscesses had developed and extended into the jaw bone. Evidently there was no dentistry.

Like the Egyptians, the Babylonians had little knowledge of anatomy, although there were surgeons among them. As early as 2250 B.C surgeons' fees were regulated by law; ten shekels was the amount authorized for treating a "gentleman" by opening an abscess of the eye; for a similar operation on a poor man the fee was five shekels, and for a servant two shekels. There were certain conditions written into the law which must have discouraged reckless surgery: If as the result of an operation a gentleman lost his life or his eye, the surgeon had his hand cut off in retaliation. Surgeons often operated under similar penalties in Europe in medieval times.

The ancient Jews likewise had little anatomical knowledge. They gave much attention to hygiene, however, and the Book of Leviticus contains stern mandates against touching unclean objects or committing sexual perversions; it tells of the hygiene of the menstrual period and of measures for the purification of women after childbirth. There are only two surgical operations mentioned in the Old Testament, that of circumcision and the operation on Adam for the formation of Eve. The use of a bandage is noted in the case of Pharaoh's broken arm. There is very little anatomical knowledge in the Bible, but the later Jewish writings as embodied in the Talmud are improved in this respect and give a sketchy kind of anatomy. The bones of the body are variously numbered as 248 and 252, and include the bone of Luz. This bone is the supposedly indestructible nucleus, a sort of seed, from which the body is to be resurrected. The belief in the bone of Luz and the missing rib of Adam persisted until the sixteenth century, when Vesalius showed that both are myths.

A knowledge of human anatomy is the first requirement of surgery, but this was not attained by the Greek physicians. They made valuable contributions to anatomy, but they did not dissect the human body. The Greek religion was even more hostile than the Egyptian toward any interference with the bodies of the dead. The great Greek physician, Galen, who lived in the second century after Christ, derived his knowledge of anatomy from the pig, the ape, the dog, and the ox. He assumed that the structures he found in these animals were identical with the structures in the human body. For thirteen centuries the human breastbone was supposed to be segmented like that of an ape and the liver to be divided into many lobes like that of a hog; the uterus was supposed to be in two long horns as in the dog, and the hip bones to be flared as in the ox. Such was the hold that Galen's work obtained upon the clerics and physicians of the Middle Ages that when Vesalius, in the sixteenth century, showed that Galen's description of the hip bones was wrong, the excuse that was offered for Galen's error was that man had changed his shape through wearing tight trousers.

With the decline of the Roman Empire the Arabs collected the manuscripts of Galen and other Greek physicians and used them in the development of a brief but brilliant period of Arabian culture. Galen had stated that surgery is a form of treatment subordinate to medicine. This conception appealed to the Arabs, for they held the idea, peculiar to Oriental religions, that it is unclean or unholy to touch the human body under certain conditions. The Arabs advanced the study of medicine, but they subordinated the study of anatomy and surgery. In the Western civilization the books of Galen, which were all written in Greek, lay hidden in the monasteries for centuries. When they were finally translated into Latin— then the language of learning—Galen's ideas were accepted by the Church and acquired an authority like that of ortho- dox theology. To question Galen was heresy. Under such con- ditions anatomical knowledge could not be acquired.

During the early part of the Middle Ages there were no trained surgeons in Europe. The only men with any medical education were the Jews; they studied in Arabia. The Church forbade the employment of these men, although the officials of the Church did not hesitate to consult them in case of seri- ous illness. At no time during the Middle Ages or even during the Renaissance did physicians undertake any surgical work. Toward the end of the Middle Ages men began to specialize in surgery, but performed no operations. They confined their work to dressing wounds. Surgical operations were performed only by barbers or by vagrant practitioners who wandered about the country or set up their booths at fairs. The surgery of the time was so crude and barbarous that Gregory of Tours, in the sixth century, advised that the people should emulate the saints and endure their pain with patience rather than to submit to operation.

Even as late as the eleventh century the armies had no sur- geons. The Norwegian king, Magnus the Good, after his battles selected twelve of his soldiers with the softest hands to care for the wounded men. The armies of the ancient Greeks had surgeons; Xenophon in the fourth century before Christ had eight field surgeons for his "Ten thousand." Sick and wounded men were sheltered in villages or cities and on the march were carried in the rear of troops. They were cared for by women from the camp-followers—"from the baggage," as Xenophon says. In Europe in the fifteenth century the nobility took their own physicians to war with them. Standing armies did not then exist, and such surgeons, like Paré, as followed the army retired to their civil practice after each campaign. For the most part the wounded common soldiers were left to the ministrations of their companions in arms or to the camp-followers. These latter were mostly prostitutes and they often equaled in number the regular fighting force.

It is difficult now to comprehend a time when wounded soldiers were killed if the army was forced to march, and prisoners of war were regularly tortured and massacred unless they were of sufficient importance to be ransomed. Yet such was the case in Europe even during the sixteenth century. Possibly something of the spirit of the time can be gathered from a quotation from Paré; he certainly was as humane a man as the century produced. He was at the siege of Metz in 1553, when Emanuel Philbert, general of Emperor Charles V, besieged Therouenne and the château of Hesdin. Paré stood on a rampart and saw "about fourscore or a hundred camp-followers and wenches of the enemy about a spring to draw water." The spring was within range of the French cannon and Paré says: "I prayed Monsieur du Pont, Commissary of Artillery, to fire a cannon-shot at this rabble. He made me a flat refusal, remonstrating with me that all this kind of people were not worth the powder that one would spend on them. Again I begged him to point the cannon, telling him, 'The more dead, the fewer enemies,' the which he did at my request, and by this shot were killed fifteen or sixteen of them and many wounded."

It was during this same battle that one of the first agreements was made between the belligerents to refrain from massacring the prisoners of war. The Spaniards took the city and Paré describes how well the agreement was kept. He says: "Afterward the Spanish soldiers entered by the breach without any resistance, our men thinking they would hold their faith and agreement, that they should have their lives saved. They entered in a great fury to kill all, to plunder, and to sack. They retained some men, hoping to have ransom for them; they tied them . . . with their arquebus cord, which were thrown over a pike that two held on their shoulders, they would pull the cord, with great violence and derision, as if they wished to sound a chime, telling them that they must put themselves to ransom, and to tell of what family they were, and if they saw they would have no profit from them, they killed them cruelly in their hands. . . . But they killed all with their daggers and cut their throats. See then their great cruelty and perfidy; let him trust them that will."

There was some prejudice in Paré's remarks, for the fall of the city brought him into a quandary. When he learned that the common soldiers were to be spared, he disordered his clothes and tore holes in his hose that he might be taken for a person of no consequence and thus avoid paying ransom. He saw, however, that the common soldiers were to be massacred, and he hastened to put himself under the protection of the Compte de Martigues, who had been shot through the chest. Paré went into captivity as his surgeon; the compte died and Paré obtained his freedom by successfully treating a colonel of the enemy who had suffered for six or seven years from an ulcer on his leg. The Spaniards made Paré a flattering offer to join them as a surgeon, but he refused, making, as he said, a "brave answer." In those times it was not uncommon to recruit the captured physicians of the enemy. When the Spanish Armada was defeated a Jewish physician named Roger Lopez was captured and Queen Elizabeth retained him for her personal physician. Subsequently he was convicted of conspiring against the life of the queen and was hanged in Tyburn in June, 1594.

Two centuries after the time of Paré the first true Red Cross agreement ever made was effected between the French and English at the battle of Dettigen in 1743. A physician, Sir John Pringle, was the author of this measure; he proposed it to the Earl of Sair, who in turn suggested it to the French. Pringle says: "But the Earl of Sair, my late illustrious patron . . . proposed to the Duke of Noailles, of whose humanity he was well assured, that the hospitals on both sides should be considered as sanctuaries for the sick and mutually protected. This was readily agreed to by the French general, who took the first opportunity to show a particular regard for his agreement . . . This agreement was strictly observed on both sides all that campaign, and although it has been since neglected, yet we may hope that on future occasions the contending parties will make it a precedent."

Warfare offered the best training available for surgeons in the fifteenth, sixteenth, and seventeenth centuries. But most surgeons did not care for military life and in the English army as late as the seventeenth century it was necessary to impress surgeons into service. The pay of the English army surgeons was good; a first-class surgeon in the fifteenth century received two hundred dollars a year and twelve cents a day for expenses. The wage for a laboring-man at that time was about five dollars a year. The high pay of the army surgeon drew many quacks into the service, as may be judged from a quotation from the writings of the surgeon Thomas Gales, who says: "I remember when I was in the war at Montreuil (1544), in the time of that most famous Prince, Henry VIII, there was a great rabblement there that took upon them to be surgeons. Some were sow-gelders and some horse-gelders, with tinkers and cobblers. This noble sect did such great cures that they got themselves a perpetual name; for, like as Thessalus's sect were called thessalions, so this noble rabblement for their notorious cures were called dogleechers; for in two dressings they did commonly make their cures whole and sound forever, so that they neither felt heat nor cold, nor no manner of pain after. But when the Duke of Norfolk, who was then general, understood how the people did die, and that of small wounds, he sent for me and certain other surgeons, commanding us to make search, how these men came to their death, whether it were by the grievousness

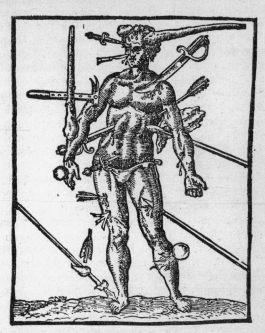

## THE WOUND MAN

A sixteenth-century first-aid chart showing the location and nature of wounds occurring during war. This illustration is from the *Surgery* of Ambroise Paré, but it is in turn a copy of a much earlier picture and therefore no gun-shot wounds are shown. Prior to the use of gunpowder the majority of wounds received in battle were about the head and shoulders, but after the introduction of gunpowder, wounds of the body predominated.

of their wounds, or by the lack of knowledge of the surgeons; and we, according to our commandment, made search through all the camp and found many of the same good fellows which took upon them the names of surgeons, not only the names, but the wages also. We asking of them whether they were surgeons or no, they said they were: we demanding with whom they were brought up, and they with shameless faces would answer either with one cunning man or another which was dead. Then we demanded of them what chirurgery stuff they had to cure men withal, and they would show us a pot or a box which they had in a budget, wherein was such trumpery as they did use to grease horses' heels withal and laid upon scabby horses' back with verval and such like. And others that were cobblers and tinkers, they use shoemakers' wax with the rust of old pans, and they made their withal a noble salve, as they did term it. But in the end this worthy rabblement was committed to the Marshal sea and threatened by the duke's grace to be hanged for their worthy deeds except that they would declare the truth, what they were and of what occupations, and in the end they did confess as I have declared to you before."

The attitude toward men practicing surgery in the Middle Ages and Renaissance was such that the surgeons were continually in jeopardy of life. In 580 Gutram, king of Burgundy, had two surgeons executed upon the tomb of his queen because she died of the plague after they had opened her plague sores. In 1337 a surgeon was thrown into the river Oder because he failed to cure John of Bohemia of blindness, and in 1464 the king of Hungary proclaimed that he would reward the surgeon who cured him of an arrow wound, but would put him to death if he failed. Even as late as the sixteenth century the surgeon might be similarly punished for errors or even unavoidable accidents. Pope John XII burned an unsuccessful surgeon of Florence; after the pope's death his friends flayed the surgeon who failed to keep him alive. The Church mistrusted surgeons and forbade them to bleed a married woman in the absence of her relatives, for fear of adultery. In Prussia up to the time of Frederick the Great it was part of the duty of the army surgeon to shave the officers.

The relations of Dr. Radcliffe and Queen Anne illustrate the physician's attitude of caution for fear of vengeance in case of failure to cure. Dr. Radcliffe was one of the most prominent English physicians in the seventeenth century and had been the physician of William and Mary. His manner was gruff and overbearing, and because of his frankness in telling Queen Anne that her illnesses were only "vapors" he was discharged from her service. When the queen was dying, Radcliffe was sent for "by order of council," but refused to attend her, giving as his excuse "that he had taken physic and could not come." His real reason, however, is expressed in a letter to one of his friends: "I know the nature of attending crowned heads, in their last moments, too well to be fond of waiting upon them without being sent for by a proper authority. *You have heard of pardons being signed for physicians, before a sovereign dies.* . . ." Radcliffe, however, got into trouble for his caution. The people were convinced that the queen would have lived if he had attended her; the queen's death was consequently blamed on Radcliffe and he was in danger of being mobbed. He retired to a country village and died there three months after the queen; it is said that his fear of assassination hastened his death.

The earliest medical school in Europe was founded at Salerno and is first mentioned in the literature of the tenth century. The origin of this school is obscure, but it is certain that the Church was not instrumental in its foundation, for it gave no incentive to medical education. The first instructors at the school were mostly Jews from Arabia. An effort was made to develop surgery. The surgeons, however, were to treat wounds and not to perform operations. The only anatomy that was taught was that of the hog as recorded by Galen. The school was sacked by Henry VI in 1194 and thereafter lost much of its prestige to other schools which had arisen at Naples, Palermo and Montpellier. The school of Salerno was finally abolished by Napoleon on November 29, 1811, after having been in existence for nearly a thousand years.

During the first two centuries of its existence the hospital at Salerno supplied surgical treatment for many wounded crusaders. The following romance is told of this hospital; it pictures the surgery of the twelfth century at the best hospital of the time: "Among the visitors of distinction who honored Salerno with their presence, was Robert, Duke of Normandy [son of William the Conqueror], who, having gone among the first Crusaders to Palestine, and having been wounded there in the arm with an arrow, came to Salerno for medical advice about the year 1100, accompanied by his wife Sybilla, daughter of Count of Conversana, a lady of distinguished beauty and accomplishments, for whose sake Robert had sacrificed his chance of succeeding to the throne of England on the death of his brother, William Rufus, by wearing away his time with her in Italy, when he should have been on his way to England. Robert's wound had, from neglect, degenerated into a fistulous ulcer. Upon a consultation among medical men of Salerno, it was decided that the only means of extracting the poison which prevented the wound from healing was suction, could any person be found bold enough to undertake so disagreeable an office. The high-spirited and generous prince, however, refused to listen to the proposal of a remedy which threatened the operator with danger; but the advice of the physicians coming to the ears of his wife whose affections were wedded with her hand to her husband, she resolved not to yield to him in generosity; and, taking advantage of an opportunity when his senses were locked in opiate slumber, she extracted the poison from his wound with her own mouth, and thus rescued from the grave, at the price of her own existence, a husband without whom she felt the gift of life would have been valueless."

The medical school at Salerno favored its royal visitor with a medical book written especially for his guidance. This book, called *Regimen Sanitatis Salernitanum,* was widely circulated and existed for many hundreds of years in great esteem as a standard textbook. It is the best-known literary survival of medieval medicine. Like most medical literature of the time, it was written in verse. In the sixteenth century it was translated into English by Sir John Harington, a godson of Queen Elizabeth and a tutor of Prince Henry. Sir John was not only an author, but was the inventor of the modern

water-closet, his invention being described in a work entitled
*A New Discourse on a Stale Subject, Called the Metamor-*

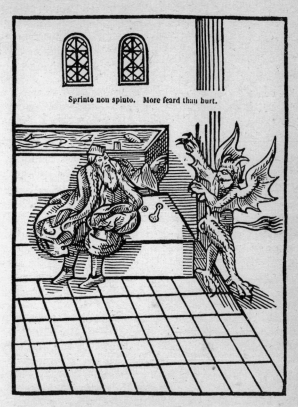

*A godly father, sitting on a draught,*
*To do as need and nature hath us taught,*

### THE FIRST WATER-CLOSET

An illustration from *The Metamorphosis of Ajax,* by Sir John Harington, published in 1596. His invention constituted one of the few
sanitary innovations that came before the nineteenth century. Its general adoption was slow.

*phosis of Ajax*. This title is a pun on the word "jacks," which was then the slang term for a privy. This book, which was the first specimen of Rabelaisian satire in the English language, was printed in London in 1596. The importance of Harington's invention can be judged from the fact that previously the finest palaces had only privies, if indeed they provided any accommodations of this nature.

The title of Harington's translation of the poem of Salerno is: "The Englishman's Doctor or The School of Salerne or Physicall observations for the perfect Preserving of the body of Man in continuall Health." The three verses from the work given below show its style and general character. In changing from the old to the modern typography the words lose some of their quaintness; the original had the tall s, resembling an f, and the transposed u and v. The medical advice presented in these poems may not be as soundly scientific as that in modern popular books of hygiene, but certainly the poems are more readable.

White *Muskadell*, and *Candie wine*, and *Greek*,
  Do make men's wits and bodies grosse and fat;
*Red wine* doth make the voyce oft-time to seeke,
  And hath a binding qualitie to that;
*Canarie, Madera, both are like*
  To make one leane indeed; (but wot you what)
Who say they make one leane, would make one laffe
  They meane, they make one leane upon a staffe
*Wine, Women, Baths,* by Art or Nature warme,
  Us'd or abus'd do men much good or harme.

------

Sixe things, that here in order shall ensue,
  Against all poysons have a secret power,
*Peare, Garlicke, Reddish-root, Nuts, Rape,* and *Rue,*
  But *Garlicke* Chiefe; for they that it devoure,
May drink, & care not who their drinke do brew.
  May walke in aires infected every houre.
Sith *Garlicke* then hath powers to save from death,
  Bear with it though it make unsavory breath;

And scorne not *Garlicke*, like to some that think
  It only makes men wink and drinke and stinke.

---

Some love to drinke new wine not fully fin'd
  But for your health we wish that you drinke none,
For such to dangerous fluxes are inclin'd,
  Besides, the Lees of wine doe breed the stone,
Some to drinke onely water are assign'd,
  But such by our consent shall drinke alone.
For water and small beere we make no question,
  Are enemies to health and good digestion;
And *Horace* in a verse of his rehearses,
  That *Water-drinkers* never make good verses.

The three physicians recommended in the textbook of Salerno are:

Use three physicians still; first Doctor *Quiet*
Next Doctor *Merry-man, and* Doctor *Dyet.*

The physicians of the medical school of Salerno instructed their pupils in the etiquette of dealing with their patients. The precepts they advocated indicate the low social position of the physician of that time. He was to approach the patient with humble mien; to punctuate his remarks at table with frequent inquiries about the patient's condition; to regard the patient's illness as grave in order that a favorable outcome might reflect to his credit as giving good treatment, or, in event of an unfavorable outcome, as giving good prognosis. The physician was not to lessen his professional dignity by staring at the patient's wife, daughter, or servant. The giving of harmless but unnecessary medicine was permissible, since otherwise the patient might not feel that he was getting a return for his money and a recovery without any treatment might reflect upon the necessity of having a physician. It was even suggested that if the patient, after recovery, exhibits ingratitude, it might be wise to sicken him temporarily by some harmless medicine.

The school of Salerno had a quickening influence on

# THE ENGLISHMANS DOCTOR.

## OR,

### *The Schoole of Salerne.*

## OR,

Physicall obseruations for the perfect
*Preseruing of the body of Man in*
continuall health.

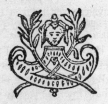

London
Printed for Iohn Helme, and Iohn
Busby Iunior and are to be solde at the little shop
next Cliffords Inne-gate, in Fleet-
streete. 1608.

---

TITLE PAGE OF THE MEDICAL POEM OF SALERNO

As translated by Sir John Harington. The original poem in Latin was dedicated to Robert of Normandy, son of William the Conqueror, who had been treated at Salerno. The book is a manual of diet and household medicine with many shrewd sayings such as "Joy, temperance, and repose slam the door on the doctor's nose."

medicine and surgery that brought a number of priests and monks into the practice of these arts. There followed many abuses; medical fees were sought, to the detriment of regular duties of the priests and often to the detriment of the patients. The Church recognized the fact that a priest or monk might, as the result of his treatment, be the cause of a patient's death. Such an occurrence was at variance with the purpose of holy orders, and the Church instituted edicts aimed at the malpractice of monks. A decree of the Lateran Council of 1139 states that priests and monks "were neglecting the sacred objects of own profession, and holding out the delusive hope of health in exchange for ungodly lucre."

The edicts grew more emphatic, and that of Tours in 1163 went wide of its mark and officially cast surgery into disrepute. The essence of this edict was *Ecclesia abhorret a sanguine*—the Church abhors the shedding of blood. In other words, surgery was not respectable.

Two centuries later another papal bull was misinterpreted to the detriment of anatomical study. Pope Boniface VIII in 1300 decreed that whoever dared to cut up a human body or boil it should fall under the ban of the Church. This edict was intended to prohibit a practice of the crusaders, who, when one of their number died during the pilgrimage to the Holy Land, cut up the body and boiled it in order to obtain the bones, which could be conveniently transported back to relatives in Europe. The papal bull against this practice was misinterpreted as applying to dissection for anatomical study.

Under the influence of the Church the practice of surgery in Europe was relegated to barbers, bath-house keepers, sowgelders, executioners, and any strolling vagabond who cared to try his hand at the art. Surgeons were looked upon as menials. The feeling was so strong against the practice of surgery that the school at Montpellier abolished its instruction in surgery and issued a decree that none of its students should study or practice surgery.

In France from the thirteenth to the seventeenth century there were three classes of men practicing the medical arts. They were the preëminent physicians, the surgeons of the long robe, and the surgeons of the short robes, or barber surgeons. The physicians merely prescribed medicine and gave advice. The surgeons of the long robe dressed wounds with poultices and plasters, but performed no operations. They lived in the towns and could be easily reached for revenge if there was an unfavorable outcome from their work; in consequence they learned discretion and avoided operations. The barber surgeons were looked upon both by the physicians and by the surgeons of the long robe as being merely servants.

Ⓒ Incipit Regimē ſanitatis Salernitanū excellētiſſimū pro cōſerua tione ſanitatis totius humani generis puril:ſſimū:necnó a magiſtro Arnaldo de Villa-noua Cathellano omniū medicoᵹ uiuentiū gēma utiliter:ac ᵱm omniū antiquoᵹ medicoᵹ doctrinā utraciter expo⁄

### THE ℞ IN ANCIENT MEDICAL MANUSCRIPTS

The symbol ℞ used today as the prefix of the physician's prescription is not, as is frequently supposed, an abbreviation of a Latin word meaning recipe or compound, but is an invocation to Jupiter, a prayer for his aid to make the treatment effective. It is one of the superstitious elements that have clung to medicine even though their significance has been lost; it persists now merely as a convention. Sometimes in old medical manuscripts all the R's occurring in the text were crossed as in the few lines shown above taken from the title page of the Latin version of the medical poem of Salerno.

They were originally trained to bleed and shave the monks, and they owed their origin to the decree of 1092 forbidding monks from wearing beards. Occasionally one of the barber surgeons rose to some degree of eminence—Paré was an example—but for the most part they were uneducated and uncouth. Paré, when he became famous, was made a surgeon of the long robe, but even in his case the examination for his admission to this order was dispensed with because he knew no Latin, which was the language used by all educated men in their professional writing. Shortly before the French Revolution the surgeons of the long robe and the barber surgeons united in a common guild, and after the Revolution, in the early part of the nineteenth century, the distinction between surgeons and physicians was broken down and both were required to obtain the degree of doctor of medicine.

In the late Middle Ages and in the Renaissance an occasional dissection, called "making an anatomy," was allowed by ecclesiastical authorities. The subjects for dissection were executed criminals, but the actual dissection was a subordinate part of what was in reality an elaborate social function. The subject for the dissection was selected from among the prisoners, special rites were performed over him, and spiritual indulgences were allowed for the indignities which were to be done to his body. When thus prepared spiritually the prisoner was strangled by the executioner and the body was turned over to the university. Invitations to the dissection were issued to the city officials and other prominent persons. In the presence of the assembled company the papal indulgence permitting the dissection was read and the corpse was then stamped with the seal of the university. Often as a preliminary to the dissection the subject's head was removed in accord with the prejudice against exposing the brain, which, according to the Christian conception, is the seat of the soul. After these formalities an introductory oration was read and the physicians sang in chorus. Then came the dissection, which was a perfunctory affair. The physician in charge did not touch the body. Instead, it was opened by a servant while the physician stood to one side and read aloud from Galen, pointing with a wand to the various structures as they were enumerated in the text. A celebration followed the dissection and there was a concert, banquet, or theatrical performance. The whole affair occupied the greater part of two days and was concluded by ceremoniously burying the slightly mangled corpse.

The first great contribution to anatomy was made by Andreas Vesalius in 1543. Vesalius actually dissected the human body and made accurate observations unblinded by veneration of Galen. Vesalius had undertaken the study of medicine at the age of eighteen, first attending a school at Montpellier and afterward at Paris. Among his instructors in anatomy at Paris was Jacques Du Bois, called Sylvius, who afterward damned his pupil for daring to disagree with Galen, and Guido Guidi, whom Benvenuto Cellini mentions in his memoirs. The instruction in anatomy given in Paris consisted in reading Galen, dissecting a few animals, and observing an occasional very brief demonstration of the easily accessible parts of the human cadaver.

About the time that Vesalius completed his medical studies war was declared between the Emperor Charles V and Francis I of France. It was during this war that Paré obtained his surgical training, serving with the French army. Vesalius left Paris at the outbreak of the war, for he was a Belgian and his father was apothecary to the emperor. He went to Louvain, where he obtained a human skeleton by surreptitiously removing it from the gallows outside of the city. The skeleton was that of a criminal who had been executed and hung in chains for the people to see. The theft of the skeleton was a very daring act, for Vesalius himself would have been executed if he had been detected. His actions, however, were quite in keeping with his impetuous nature and with his intense desire for truth in anatomy.

After a short service in the army of Emperor Charles V, Vesalius, then twenty-three years of age, accepted from the Senate of Venice the appointment of professor of anatomy at Padua. During the next six years he conducted painstaking dissections of a number of human cadavers. In 1543, before he had reached the age of twenty-nine, he was ready to publish his great work on anatomy. The illustrations were drawn, it is generally believed, by Stephan van Calcar, one of Titian's pupils.

As might be expected, the first correct demonstration of the anatomy of the human body was met with a storm of violent protest. Vesalius had dared to cast discredit on Galen! But it was not so much that fact alone as it was the abrupt way in which Vesalius did it. The human mind has an amazing ability of being able to hold simultaneously two distinct and irreconcilable beliefs. For instance, it is possible for a man to believe in the Old Testament Creation and at

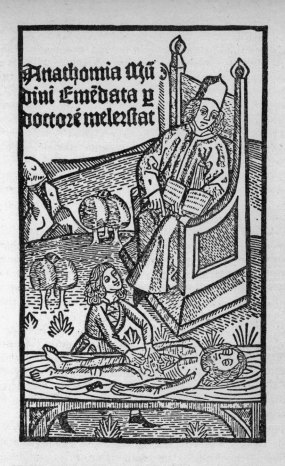

**TITLE PAGE TO THE *ANATOMY* OF MUNDINUS**

Written in 1316 and first published at Padua in 1487. Although this book is in no way comparable to the systematic work of Vesalius in the sixteenth century, it is evidence of an early attempt to revive human dissection. The physician is shown seated in the chair, directing the dissection which is being performed by an assistant. The dissection itself was little more than an examination of the easily accessible organs of the body; more on the order of an autopsy than a dissection.

the same time acknowledge the truth of the evolutionary
rise of man. It was possible for the anatomists to believe and
teach Galen and yet know that the anatomy they saw in
their brief dissections was different from that which Galen
described. The conflict between two opposing views of the
mind comes only when the mind is forced to make a positive
and open choice of one or the other. The conflict results in
indignation against the person who forces the issue. Vesalius
by publishing his book forced the issue; he discarded
Galenic tradition. Intense indignation was aroused among
the physicians; in the words of Sylvius, his former teacher,
Vesalius was "an impious madman who is poisoning the air
of all Europe with his vaporings."

Vesalius was not wholly free from some of the Galenic
superstitions of anatomy, for he upheld the idea that the
nasal secretion came from the brain. It was two centuries
later that its local origin in the mucous membrane of the
nose was discovered, and until that time physicians continued to give drugs to increase the flow of mucus, thereby
"to purge the brains." Nevertheless, the downfall of the
Galenic anatomy was complete in principle. The four abdominal muscles of the ape no longer graced man; the
multi-lobed liver passed away, and so, too, did the segmented
sternum, the double bile duct, and the horned uterus. With
Galenic error went many ancient anatomical superstitions;
the bone Luz, or the resurrection bone, was proved a myth,
and Adam's missing rib was restored.

There was nothing gentle about the blow that Vesalius
dealt Galenic medicine. In his onslaught against the superstitions of his professional brethren he was as intolerant as
they in their errors, but in dealing with the bodily functions
he was less radical. Galen had said that the blood passed
from the right side of the heart directly to the left side
through pores in the wall between the ventricles. The fact
that the blood, instead, flows through the lungs in making
this circuit was fully established later by Harvey in 1624.
Vesalius could not find the pores that Galen had told of,
but in deference to Church opinion he said, merely: "We

are driven to wonder at the handiwork of the Almighty, by means of which the blood sweats from the right into the left ventricle through passages which escape the human vision." To flay his medical brethren was one thing, but it was quite another to knock a little skin off the clergy, for the teleological functions of the organs which formed part of the Galenic conception had been absorbed into medieval theology. Vesalius's discretion was well founded for his contemporary, Servetus, who was less cautious, maintained that the blood passes from one side of the heart to the other through the lungs—as in fact it does. In consequence of this heresy his books were confiscated and he was himself burned at the stake. Nevertheless, the Church was not wholly antagonistic to medical advancement. Three years after the death of Servetus, complaints reached Emperor Charles V that the sin of dissecting the human body was becoming common. He therefore referred the question to the theological faculty of Salamanca for opinion, and received the reply: "The dissection of human cadavers serves a useful purpose, and is therefore permissible to Christians of the Catholic Church."

Vesalius in a fit of temper over the opposition to his work burned all his manuscripts, accepted the post of court physician to Emperor Charles V, married, gave up anatomy, and settled down to be a courtier. His place at Padua was taken by his pupil, Fallopius. In 1563 Vesalius set out on a pilgrimage to Jerusalem, probably to get away from the tiresome surroundings at court. While still in the Holy Land he received an invitation to resume his former position in Padua. This fulfillment of his long-cherished hope fired Vesalius with ardor to undertake again the study of anatomy. On his way home he was shipwrecked on the island of Zante and died there of starvation and exposure.

Vesalius opened the way to the study of human anatomy, but many years passed before anatomy could be taught to medical students by means of dissection, the only method by which physicians and surgeons can fully acquire this knowledge. The religious opposition to dissection was based upon a belief in material resurrection; and it was only as this belief slowly passed away that executed criminals became available for dissection. There were not enough bodies from this source to supply the needs of the anatomist, but

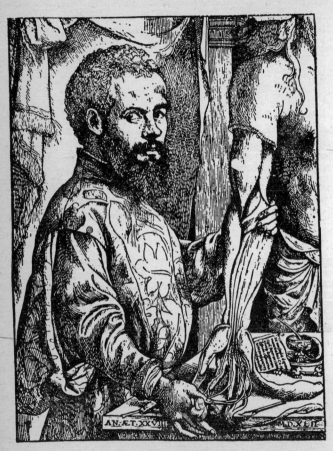

ANDREAS VESALIUS

From a woodcut appearing in the *Fabrica*, his book of anatomy, published in 1543.

there were no other legitimate sources. The common people looked upon dissection as an insult to the body, and paupers were buried at public expense. The scarcity of anatomical material in the seventeenth century may be judged from the fact that Rondelet, a professor of the medical school of Montpellier, for want of other subjects, dissected the body of his own dead child before his classes.

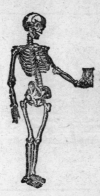

### THE SKELETON FROM PARÉ'S *SURGERY*

Drawn in the same century that Vesalius did his anatomical work. Taken in comparison with the following figure it shows the great advancement which had been made in human anatomy. In medical books of that time the skeletons were presented in picturesque and often grotesque postures.

In time, grave-robbing was resorted to in order to obtain a supply of bodies, and this practice aroused an even stronger public sentiment against dissection. Grave-robbing finally developed into a profession, and men known as "resurrectionists" made a business of supplying medical schools. This practice eventually led to murder as a means of obtaining bodies. To avoid the incentive to crime, laws were enacted in the nineteenth century to provide medical schools with unclaimed bodies. The opposition to dissection has now been largely dispelled under the influence of education and the realization of the real purposes of dissection. It still exists, however, among ignorant and superstitious people.

The development of anatomical teaching in the United States was hindered by this opposition to dissection. In Colonial times it was difficult to obtain bodies, for the country was sparsely settled and executions were infrequent.

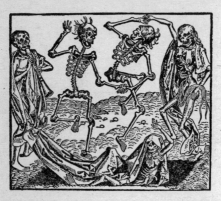

THE SKELETONS OF A MEDIEVAL DEATH DANCE

A woodcut made about 1495 and shown here in comparison with the previous illustration. The inaccurate anatomy, particularly striking in the bones of the pelvis and the joints of the legs, is an example of the lack of anatomical knowledge before the time of Vesalius.

The need for anatomical study is shown by the diary of Judge Samuel Sewell: "Sept. 22, 1676, Spent the day from nine in the morning with Mr. Brakenbury, Mr. Thomson, Butler, Hooper, Cragg, Pemberton, dissecting the middle-most part of the Indian executed the day before. X, who taking the heart in hand, affirmed it to be the stomach." The Mr. before these names does not indicate the laity, for the term doctor was rarely used in the Colonies before 1769. The first public announcement of a course in dissection appeared in the *New York Weekly Postboy* for January 27, 1752:

"Whereas Anatomy is allowed on all Hands, to be the Foundation of PHYSICK and SURGERY, and consequently without SOME knowledge of it, no person can be duly qualified to practice either: this is therefore to inform the Publick, that a COURSE of OSTEOLOGY and MYOLOGY, is intended to be begun some Time in February next, in the City of New Brunswick (for which Notice will be given in this Paper, as soon as the proper number have subscribed toward it). . . . The course is proposed to be finished in the Space of a Month.

"THOMAS WOOD, Surgeon."

In a note below this announcement it is stated that surgical operations will be demonstrated on a "dead body. The use of which will appear to every Person who considers the Necessity of having (at least) SEEN them performed, before he presumes to perform them himself on any living Fellow Creature."

The first successful course of anatomical dissection given in the United States was conducted by Dr. Shippen at Philadelphia. Dr. Shippen has been dealt with in a previous chapter in connection with his school of midwifery, his service as surgeon-general in the army during the Revolution, and his part in founding the medical department of the University of Pennsylvania. Dr. Shippen's instruction in dissection started as a private enterprise in 1762, but three years later it was taken over by the university. Philadelphia at that time was the metropolis of the Colonies; its population in 1790 was 45,250, while that of New York was only 33,113; the population of the entire country was slightly under four million. Philadelphia was then the cultural center of the country. Yet serious disturbances arose when dissection became common, because the people were ignorant of its real purpose. The building in which Shippen performed his dissections was attacked several times and he was forced to conceal himself to avoid personal injury. On one occasion he was attacked on the street by a mob; a gun was fired at him, the bullet passed through his carriage, and he escaped by running up an alley. He repeatedly attempted to allay

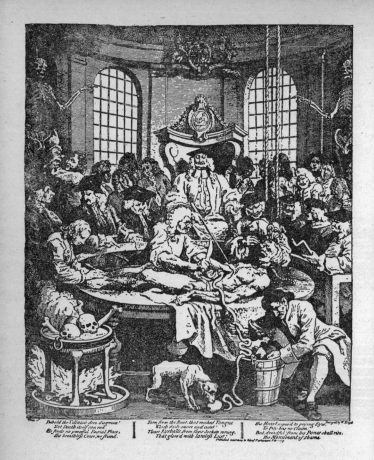

Behold the Villain's dire disgrace!
Not Death itself can end.
He finds no peaceful Burial-Place,
His breathless Corse, no friend.

Torn from the Root, that wicked Tongue
Which dark'ning more and curst
Those Eyeballs from their Sockets wrung,
That glow'd with lawless Lust!

the Heart expos'd to prying Eyes,
To Pity has no Claim,
But dreadful! from his Bones shall rise,
His Monument of Shame.

## AN ANATOMICAL DISSECTION AS REPRESENTED BY HOGARTH

This engraving was the last of a series called "The Stages of Cruelty";
the central figure of the various engravings was shown passing from
one evil deed to another—which finally culminated in an atrocious
murder. He has been convicted and hanged and as a reward of cruelty
his body has been brought to the surgeon's Hall for the dissection
which is shown in progress. In the eighteenth century, the period of

animosity by inserting announcements in the papers assuring the public that reports of violation of private burial-grounds were false and that the bodies were either those of persons who had committed suicide or who had been publicly executed except, he adds, naïvely, "now and then one from the Potters' Field."

The most violent outburst against dissection occurred in New York City in the so-called Doctors' Mob of April 1788. On that day Dr. Richard Bayle, working in the laboratory of the Hospital Society, observed a small boy peering in at one of the windows. In a spirit of medical humor he waved the arm of a cadaver at the boy to frighten him away. The exaggerated tales told by the terrified boy resulted in the collection of a mob which stormed the building and burned the anatomical collection. The physicians of the hospital took refuge in the jail. The jail was attacked and it was necessary to call out the militia in order to quell the disturbance. In the encounter that followed, seven of the rioters were killed and several more were seriously wounded. The following year the Legislature of New York authorized the dissection of the bodies of persons executed for burglary, arson, and murder.

The fact that dissection was formerly looked upon as an insult to the body is indicated in the first "anatomy law" of Massachusetts. Under this law the coroner was authorized to dispose of the bodies of men killed in dueling either by burial, "without a coffin, with a stake driven through

---

this engraving, executed criminals formed the only legitimate source of material for dissection. The Rev. J. Trusler, an annotator of Hogarth's work, has described the scene as follows: "The skeletons on each side of the print are inscribed James Field (an eminent pugilist) and Maclean (a notorious robber). Both of these worthies died by the rope. They are pointing to the physician's crest, which is carved on the upper part of the president's chair—viz., a hand feeling a pulse; taking a guinea would have been more appropriate to the practice. The heads of these two heroes of the halter are turned so as to seem ridiculing the president 'scoffing at his state and grinning at his pomp.' Every countenance of this grisley band is marked with that medical importance which dignifies the profession."

the body . . . or to deliver the body to any surgeon or surgeons to be dissected and anatomized." In 1831, less than a century ago, Massachusetts passed a law making

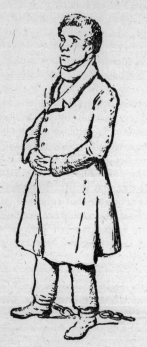

**WILLIAM BURKE IN CHAINS**

Burke enriched the language with the word "burking," which now signifies "to suppress or hush up." Burke and Hare smothered their victims so that there would be no marks of violence on the bodies which they sold under the pretense that they had obtained them by robbing graves.

available for dissection "deceased persons, required to be buried at public expense." Since that time similar laws have been passed in most of the other states. One of the factors which led to the passage of the law in Massachusetts was the notorious murder trial of Burke and Hare, which had occurred three years previously in Edinburgh, Scotland, and which is described herewith.

"Resurrectionists" were particularly active in Scotland in supplying bodies for dissection. Most of these bodies were obtained by grave-robbing or the so-called "body-snatching." Under the Scottish law such acts could not properly be called robberies, for there were no property rights in a dead body. The "resurrectionists" were careful to avoid taking the clothing of the corpse, for that would have been theft. As early as 1752 a murder had been committed in order to obtain a body. Helen Torrence and Jean Valdig, two nurses of the degraded type prevalent in the eighteenth century,

THE SIGNATURE OF WILLIAM BURKE, MURDERER

Taken from the confession he made after his trial. He admitted to some sixteen murders committed for the purpose of obtaining bodies to sell to Dr. Knox of Edinburgh, who conducted a school of anatomical dissection. Burke was executed January 27, 1829.

were employed by a group of medical students to obtain a body. The nurses had been unsuccessful. Finally they enticed a woman and her small boy into their house. One of the nurses supplied the woman with liquor until she was drunk; the other nurse took the boy into an adjoining room and suffocated him with a mattress. They were paid two shillings sixpence for the boy's body and were hanged for their crime.

In 1827 William Hare and William Burke, in partnership, undertook a series of murders to obtain bodies for dissection. Hare and his wife and Burke and his mistress, Helen McDougal, lived together in Edinburgh, where Hare ran a boarding-house for vagrants. One of the tenants of this house, an old man named Donald, died, owing Hare four pounds. The parish authorities sent a coffin for his burial and the body was put into it. Later Hare and Burke ripped off the cover, removed the body, hid it in a bed, and filled the coffin with tanners' bark. They sold the body to Dr. Knox, who conducted a school in anatomy, and received seven pounds ten shillings. This stroke of business started them on their career of murder. Before they were detected they had killed sixteen men and women and disposed of the bodies to the medical school. Their methods are illustrated by the case of Abigail Simpson, a drunken hag who lived on the outskirts of Edinburgh. With the aid of Burke's mistress, McDougal, she was enticed into Hare's house and there was plied with liquor until she was unconscious. She was then carried to a bed, where Burke lay across her to hold her down, and Hare smothered her by holding his hands over her nose and mouth. This method of strangling was later known as "Burking." It was employed in order to avoid any marks on the body which might give rise to a suspicion of violent death. The body was sold for ten pounds.

Burke and Hare confined their murders to people whose disappearance would attract little attention, but suspicion was aroused when they killed Mary Paterson, a girl of wide if unsavory repute, and later James Wilson. He was a good-natured imbecile, generally known as "Daft Jamie," and was a familiar figure on the streets of Edinburgh, where he earned a precarious living by running errands. His disappearance aroused comment, and the disappearance soon afterward of a woman named Dougherty led to a search which resulted in the arrest of Burke, Hare, and McDougal. At the trial Hare turned state's evidence, McDougal was discharged for lack of evidence, and Burke was condemned to death. He was hanged in 1829 before a gathering of twenty or thirty thousand people. After his death the mob turned against Dr. Knox and his school of dissection, and police interference was necessary to save his life. Dr. Knox was technically innocent, but he must have known that the bodies were not legitimately obtained. He defended himself boldly against the charges brought against him, but he was ostracized and finally forced to leave the town. The sensational and disreputable episode of Burke and Hare led to the passage of laws providing a mode of obtaining bodies for medical schools.

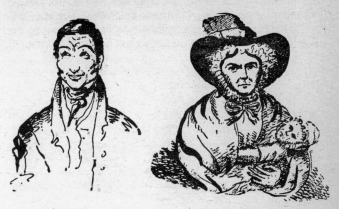

**HARE AND HIS WIFE AND CHILD IN COURT**

Hare and his wife were accomplices of Burke in the "Anatomy Murders" of Scotland. They were arrested with Burke and his mistress, McDougal, but the evidence of guilt was circumstantial. Burke and McDougal refused to give state's evidence, but Hare consented to do so. On this evidence Burke was convicted. Hare was given his freedom, although he was quite as guilty as Burke; in fact, there was considerable agitation in favor of hanging him in spite of the immunity which his evidence gave him. The sketch shown here was made during the trial. The child was kept in court by its mother, although it was suffering from whooping cough.

Little outspoken opposition exists today against dissection, but occasionally an ignorant fanatic creates a momentary sensation by proclaiming that dissections are performed on living people. In reality all bodies used for dissection are first embalmed as thoroughly as those of Egyptian mummies and are quite as dead. This attitude and the type of people who adopt it are illustrated in the words of Dowie, written in 1901. Dowie was the fanatical leader of a religious sect now located at Zion City, a suburb of Chicago; he was opposed to medical treatment and, in fact, to all science; he taught that the world was flat. He writes: "I will tell the story of a dissecting-room where the first touch of the lancet made the supposed corpse rise from her long trance; and as the sight burst upon her of those butchering students with their garments stained with blood, standing around her, all aghast with fear, holding their knives in their hands, she

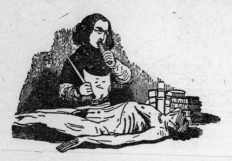

THE ANATOMIST
An etching by Daumier

realized the horrible fact that she had been carried there for dissection, and she instantly died from the shock and the wounds inflicted by their knives. . . . The very best men in the profession will tell you that nineteen-twentieths of the dissections are unnecessary. But they please the devils who are preparing the doctors, and accustom the youths to the atmosphere of profanity as they hear the filthy and unclean remarks which are made as they stand over the dead bodies and handle the sacred secrecies of humanity and laugh with diabolical glee over the consequences of a poor woman's fall or a degraded youth's syphilitic body. I tell you this, that pollution, damnation, and hell are holding high carnival there, and a young man who escapes from that without life-long injury is only one in a large number."

Dowie's charge of dissecting the living body is not the first to be brought against anatomists; Leonardo da Vinci and Michael Angelo were similarly accused in their time, and Pope Leo X in 1519 for this reason denied da Vinci admission to the hospital in Rome, where he wished to study anatomy.

# CHAPTER VII

## THE GREATEST SURGEON

On the foundation laid by Vesalius there was eventually developed the full and exact knowledge of anatomy which was the first requirement of surgery. In telling something of this development in the previous chapter events were carried beyond the time at which the second requirement of surgery was supplied. Paré furnished a means for controlling hemorrhage. It is necessary now to return to the century in which Vesalius and Paré lived.

Vesalius and Paré not only were contemporaries, but they actually met at the deathbed of Henry II of France. The king was wounded during a joust with Comte de Montgomery. The count's lance broke through the king's helmet and was splintered against his orbit. Fragments of the lance penetrated his skull. Paré and Vesalius experimented on the heads of six executed criminals in an effort to determine the course taken by the splinters, but were unsuccessful. After an illness of eleven days the king died. At the autopsy Paré found an abscess on the surface of his brain. He says: ". . . at which place was found a beginning of corruption: which was cause enough of the death of my lord, and not only the harm done to his eye." The king's wound was entirely accidental, but Montgomery fled. Later as a prisoner of war he fell into the hands of Catherine de' Medici, and she had him executed in revenge for her husband's death.

When Paré studied surgery at the Hôtel Dieu at Paris and on the battlefields of France, the cautery was used to stop hemorrhage. Boiling oil, molten pitch, or the red-hot iron were applied to the bleeding surface. The pain from this procedure was agonizing and the wound healed slowly in consequence of the injury from the burn. Paré, instead of cauterizing, tied the ends of the severed blood vessels with cords, as surgeons do today. At the siege of Danvilliers he amputated the leg of an officer and used ligatures to control the hemorrhage. In speaking of the outcome of this case he says: "I dressed his wound, and God healed him. He returned

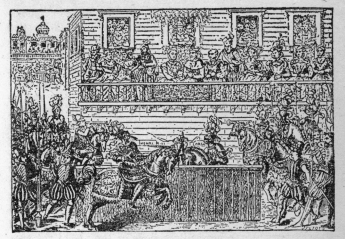

THE FATAL JOUST BETWEEN HENRY II AND
MONTGOMERY

Gabriel de Montgomery, Seigneur de Lorges, captain of the Scotch Guards of the French Court, was persuaded against his will to enter the lists against the king. His lance struck the visor of the king's helmet, splintered, and penetrated the king's eye. The wounded king was attended by Paré; Vesalius was called in consultation. The king died. Montgomery fled to avoid the vengeance of Catherine de' Medici, but years later she obtained him as a prisoner of war and had him tortured and executed.

home gayly with a wooden leg, saying that he had got off cheaply without being miserably burned to staunch the bleeding." The use of the ligature to control hemorrhage did not originate with Paré, but had been used occasionally by Greek physicians before the Christian era; but this procedure had been subsequently discarded. Renaissance surgery was strongly influenced by the methods developed among the Arabs. The Arabs cauterized all wounds. Aside from the immediate suffering, the practice was, at the time, desirable, for the heat sterilized the wound. After Paré's time infection in surgery was more frequent than it had been when the cautery was used. The full benefit of the ligature in controlling hemorrhage was not obtained until after Lister had shown the means of avoiding surgical infection.

Surgery advanced under Paré's guidance, but Paré's surgery was still wound surgery. He did not open the abdomen, and his influence thus prevented for many years any attempts at Cæsarean section. In Paré's time the arm could not be amputated at the shoulder, nor the leg at the hip joint, because infection of these joints was fatal. In writing of the death of the king of Navarre, Antoine de Bourbon, at the battle of Rouen, Paré says: "The King of Navarre was wounded some days before the assault by a bullet-shot in the shoulder. I visited him and aided in dressing him with his surgeon, named Maître Gilbert, one of the chief surgeons of Montpellier, and others. They could not find the ball. I searched for it very exactly. I perceived by conjecture that it had entered by the head of the bone at the top of the arm, and that it had run into the cavity of the bone, which was the cause that they could not find it. . . . Monsieur la Prince de la Roch-sur-Yon, who loved intimately the King of Navarre, drew me aside and asked if the shot was mortal. I told him yes, because all wounds made in the great joints, and especially contused wounds, were mortal, according to all authorities who had written of them. . . ." The king died on the eighteenth day after he had received the wound. The bullet was found as Paré had predicted; it had not entered the chest, but was "just in the middle of the cavity of the bone at the top of the arm." Few surgeons today could make a similar diagnosis without the use of the X-ray.

Paré's success as a surgeon was the result not only of his operative skill, but even more of the care and observation which he devoted to his patients. The treatment he used in the case of the Marquis d'Arnet, to whom Paré was loaned by the king of France, is illustrative of his methods. This treatment forms a contrast with that given to Robert Duke

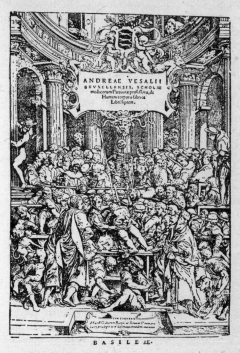

## TITLE PAGE FROM THE *FABRICA* OF ANDREAS VESALIUS

Published in 1543. One of the most celebrated pictures in the history of medicine. Entirely different from his predecessors in anatomy, Vesalius is himself performing the dissection instead of sitting at a distance and pointing out with a rod the organs uncovered by a lay assistant. (See page 151.) The amphitheater, the crowd of men and women, the student reading the book, and the dog and monkey are probably conceptions of the artist. Near the top of the picture is a shield bearing three weasels which form the coat of arms of Vesalius. The illustrations for this anatomy were drawn by von Calcar and are far better than any previously made except those of Leonardo da Vinci.

of Normandy at the hospital of Salerno as recounted in the previous chapter. In each case the treatment was the best afforded in Europe in the twelfth and sixteenth centuries, respectively. Paré's treatment could not have been bettered by any surgeon living before the latter part of the nineteenth century.

Paré traveled from Paris to the farm near Mons where his patient lay, and found him "with great fever, his eyes very much sunken, with a moribund and yellow face, his tongue dry and parched, and all his body very emaciated, his voice low as of a man very near to death; then I found his thigh much swollen, abscessed and ulcerated." This infected wound, which was the cause of the illness, had resulted from an arquebus-shot and had occurred about seven months previous to Paré's arrival. In addition to his wound the marquis had a large bed sore. After examining his patient Paré learned from the five surgeons who had been in attendance upon the marquis that, because of the pain from the wound, they had been unable to move their patient or change his bed linen for two months. Paré then drew aside to consider his line of treatment. He says: "Having seen him I went away to walk in a garden. . . . I discussed in my mind the means it would be necessary for me to use in effecting a cure. They called me to dinner; I entered by the kitchen, where I saw taken out of a great pot, half a sheep, a quarter of veal, three great pieces of beef, two fowls, and a very great piece of bacon, with abundance of good herbs; then I said to myself, that this broth of the pot was succulent and of good nourishment." After dinner Paré held a consultation with the five surgeons and detailed to them his plan for treating the marquis. He says: "This my discourse was well approved by the surgeons. The consultation ended, we went to the patient, and I made three openings in his thigh, from which went forth a great quantity of pus and sanies and at the same time I took from him some little splinters of bone. . . . Two or three hours afterward I had a bed made for him near his own, on which were clean white sheets; then a strong man placed him in it and he was glad to be taken out of his dirty stinking bed.

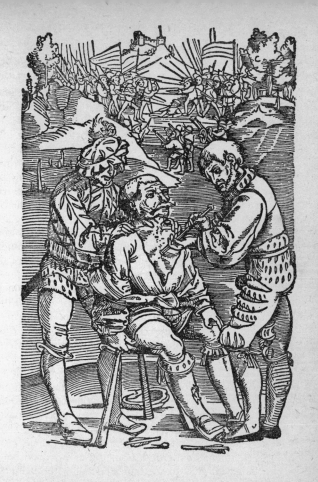

### BARBER SURGEON REMOVING AN ARROW

A woodcut from a surgery published in 1517. Military experience was then the best training available for surgeons. The nobility brought their own surgeons, but the common soldiers were for the most part dependent upon the ministrations of their companions in arms or of the camp-followers, who were usually as numerous as the soldiers.

Soon after he asked to sleep, which he did for nearly four hours; whereat everybody in the house commenced to rejoice, and especially Monsieur le Duc d'Ascot, his brother."

The next day Paré cleaned the wound, put in drains, and applied a plaster. The patient had in that short time improved to such an extent that he discharged three of his surgeons. Paré massaged his patient and supported him on pillows to protect his bed sore. He fed him the broth from the great pot in the kitchen, together with plums stewed in wine, white meat of capons, and wings of partridges. In speaking of the diet, Paré says: "The sauces should be oranges, sorrel, bitter pomegranates; and he should likewise eat good herbs as sorrel, lettuce, purslain, chicory, marigolds, and the like. At night he can take barley-water, with juice of sorrel and water lilies, of each two ounces, with . . . opium (as much as 5 barley grains). Moreover, he should smell flowers of herbbane and water lilies, bruised with vinegar and rose water, with a little camphor wrapped together in a cloth, which should be held for a long time against the nose. . . . Furthermore, one should make artificial rain, by making water run from some high place into a cauldron, that it may make such a noise that the patient can hear it; by these means sleep will be provoked in him. . . ."

After a month of Paré's treatment the marquis was able to sit in a chair. Paré then ordered "viols and violins and some comedian to make him merry." The convalescent marquis was moved "to the gate of the château to see the people pass. The peasants for two or three leagues about, knowing that they could see him, came on fête days to sing and dance, men and women, pellmell for a frolic, rejoicing at his good convalescence, being all glad to see him, and not without much laughing and much drinking. He always caused a hogshead of beer to be given to them, and they drank all merrily to his health." Paré stayed with his patient two months, and before leaving was banqueted by the officials of all the neighboring towns. Paré concludes: "I demanded leave to go from him which he granted me, with great regret (so he said) and gave me a worthy present of great value, and had me conducted again by the maître de hôtel with two pages to my house in Paris."

Paré performed only one slight surgical operation in treating the marquis; the remainder of his work consisted in dressing the wound daily and taking excellent care of the mar-

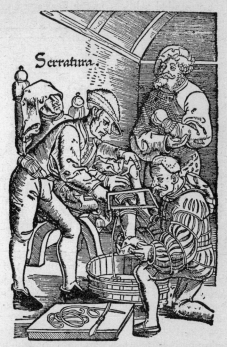

Serratura

A SIXTEENTH-CENTURY AMPUTATION

A woodcut from a surgery published in 1517 and said to be the earliest pictorial representation of this operation. Amputations were frequent then and continued so until Lister introduced the antiseptic principle late in the nineteenth century. After that time many of the infected wounds which formerly led to amputation could be controlled by antiseptics and amputation thus avoided. The patient shown in the woodcut is enduring the pain of his operation without anesthesia, and so did all patients until the middle of the nineteenth century.

quis's health. Aside from the brief operation all of his procedures were those which today are undertaken by a trained nurse. But in Paré's time the trained nurse was unknown. Only once in his writings is feminine aid mentioned, and that was during the siege of Metz by Emanuel Philibert. Paré had charge of the wounded soldiers in the besieged city, and he

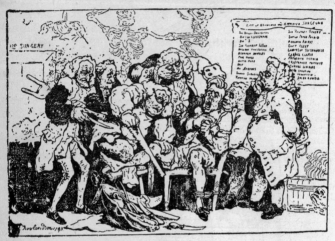

AN AMPUTATION ACCORDING TO ROWLANDSON

Except for the obvious quality of burlesque, the procedure shown in this caricature, made in 1793, does not differ essentially from the surgery shown in the preceding figure, nor, for that matter, from the surgery of the eighteenth century.

called in feminine help to wash bandages for which the supply of cloth was exhausted. He says: "I could not forget the ragged bandages with which they were dressed, which were only rewashed every day and dried at the fire, and therefore were as hard as parchment. I leave you to think how their wounds could do well. There were four big, fat prostitutes to whom was given charge of the washing of the linen, who acquitted themselves of it to the strokes of a stick, and likewise they had no water at their command, and less soap."

The training of women in the art of "helping the patient to live," which is the office of the nurse, began in the nineteenth century. Prior to that time there were nurses in hospitals, but they were untrained. In Roman Catholic institutions the nursing was done by nuns, but in all other hospitals the sick were cared for by the worst type of women conceivable for the service. In 1857 the *London Times* describes the servant nurses in the London hospitals in the following terms: "Lectured by committees, preached at by chaplains, scowled on by treasurers and stewards, scolded by matrons, sworn at by surgeons, bullied by dressers, grumbled at and abused by patients, insulted if old and ill-favored, talked flippantly to if middle-aged and good-humored, tempted and seduced if young and well-looking—they were what any woman might be in the same circumstances." They were, in fact, mostly dowdy-looking females of drunken and dubious habits.

Paré, in treating the marquis, performed his operation and then remained two months to care for him. He helped his patient to get well by gentle ministrations, soothing drinks, clean bed linen, massage, fresh air, and all of those acts which to the patient are mercies. Only the most prominent men of the French nobility could obtain Paré to act as their nurse. Most patients of that time made whatever shift they could, with any help they could find, to supply their wants after the surgeon had operated. Today trained nurses supply to the least important patient in the hospital better care than was available to the king of France in the sixteenth century.

Florence Nightingale made nursing a dignified profession. Under her influence the inefficient and drunken females who worked as servant-nurses in the hospitals were replaced by well-bred and well-trained women with high *esprit de corps* in their profession. The idea of training nurses to attend the sick originated with Theodore Fieldner, pastor of a small German town. In 1833 he turned the garden house of the pastorate into an asylum for discharged female prisoners. With the help of his wife he trained these women to care for the sick. Three years later he founded a school for nursing deaconesses. Florence Nightingale, an English lady living on the Continent, attended this school and received a training in nursing. When the Crimean War broke out in 1854 she went with forty English nurses, trained like herself, to take charge of the barrack hospital at Scutari. Florence Nightingale did not know the part played by bacteria in causing infection, but she did know that cleanliness, fresh air, pure water, and sunlight were necessities in the proper care of the sick. Her attempts to supply these necessities to the wounded men at Scutari were hindered by the bureaucratic army regulations; her work was treated with indifference by war officials in England. But enthusiastic praise came from the officers and men who saw her reforms in operation at the barrack hospital or benefited from her nursing. Under the difficult conditions of war time, she laid the foundation for modern nursing. On her return to England in 1860 a fund of fifty thousand pounds, the "Nightingale fund," was raised by subscription and was used to establish a school at St. Thomas's Hospital for training the "new-style nurses." The nurses trained there were soon in wide demand and other schools were established. Within a few years the slatternly females that had served in the hospitals were replaced by these efficient women who "helped the patient to live." Oliver Wendell Holmes has summed up the importance of nursing in these words: "I confess that I should think my chances of recovery from illness less with Hippocrates for my physician and Mrs. Gamp for my nurse, than if I were in the hands of Hahnemann, with Florence Nightingale or good Rebecca Taylor to care for me." And Holmes had a very low opinion of Hahnemann, who was the founder of homeopathy.

The training of nurses was the first step toward the greatest of the qualities of the modern hospital—its cleanliness. The necessity for cleanliness was demonstrated by Lister a few years after Florence Nightingale had brought cleanliness, light, and comfort into the barrack hospital of Scutari.

Joseph Lister was born at Upton, Essex, in the spring of 1827. His father was a prosperous London wine merchant and a Quaker who devoted his leisure to the study of optics, and was famous for his improvements in the microscope. The son, Joseph Lister, graduated in medicine from the University of London in 1852, and from there went to the Edinburgh hospital to study surgery under Symne. In 1860 he became professor of surgery in the University of Glasgow. Six years later he published his paper, "On the Antiseptic Principle in the Practices of Surgery."

Lister thus supplied the last essential to modern surgery—a means of preventing infection. He gave to surgery the dignity of a science, and every surgical operation today is a monument to Lister. In the little more than half a century that has passed since he introduced antisepsis the number of lives his work has saved are numbered in the millions. Antisepsis, like all innovations, was met with opposition at first. Surgeons failed to grasp the essential of the idea of antisepsis and thought that Lister was trying merely to introduce a new type of surgical dressing. Lister continued his work, and one by one the leading surgeons accepted his ideas of antisepsis. The full recognition of the value of his work came during his lifetime; when he retired in 1896 his fame was international and he was the first medical man to be raised to the English peerage. His body lies in Westminster Abbey and the stone there marks the resting-place of the greatest surgeon the world has known.

Lister's problem was much the same as that which confronted the unfortunate Semmelweis when he sought to prevent puerperal fever. Early in his hospital experience Lister became deeply impressed with the high mortality from the diseases which followed surgery. In those days no surgeon could feel sure of the results of his work; it did not matter how much care he took in planning and performing his operation, nor how good the patient's condition was at the completion of the operation. The patient might do well for a day or two, but then, even in the most favorable cases, pus appeared in the wound. The presence of pus was considered a sign of healing, and it was called "laudable pus." This belief had persisted from the Galenic and Arabic teachings. The appearance of pus might indeed in those times have been called favorable, for many patients lived too short a time after the operation for pus to form. They died of blood-poisoning, which was the same as the puerperal fever which Semmelweis had sought to prevent in the wards of the hospital at Vienna. The appearance of pus or the occurrence of blood-poisoning depended upon the type of infection; all wounds were infected, but some with organisms called staphylococci, which produce pus, and others with the more virulent streptococci, which do not produce pus but cause blood-poisoning. Occasionally the streptococci spread in the skin surrounding the surgical wound, causing erysipelas. This disease would then spread from patient to patient in the hospital until all were infected and many died. Death from infection occurred as readily from the small wound of a minor operation as from the large wound of such an operation as amputation. Before antiseptic surgery the amputation of a leg or an arm was a frequent operation, for nearly all compounded fractures necessitated amputation. In Lister's own statistics of amputation between the years 1864 and 1866, 45 per cent of the patients died. A compound fracture in 1866 was nearly as dangerous as the bubonic plague.

In hospitals today all wounds which are not infected before the time of operation heal by "first intention." At the close of the operation the wound is sewed shut and the flesh quickly grows together. Infected wounds heal by "second intention"; the wound is open, the healing starts at the bottom, and tissue slowly builds up to fill the gap. Healing by second intention requires a much longer time than does healing by first intention, but before antisepsis and asepsis the slower method was the method to be preferred, for if the surface healed together, pus formed in the deeper part of the wound and a second operation was then necessary to drain it.

Semmelweis developed his methods for the prevention of infection by a laborious process of elimination; Lister made a practical application of Pasteur's work on the fermentation of wine. Pasteur, whose work is discussed more fully in a subsequent chapter, had then recently demonstrated that all forms of fermentation were due to the presence and growth of minute organisms, and that putrefaction is essentially the same process. He found that if care were taken to exclude these organisms from the liquids in which these changes occurred, no fermentation took place. If the organisms were present in the liquid, their activities could be stopped by heat. Lister observed that when an occasional wound healed without pus formation, there was no putrefaction. He conceived the idea that pus arose from infection. He saw a possible practical application of Pasteur's work and set out to determine whether by preventing the development of organisms in wounds he could prevent infection. He realized that Pasteur's heat treatment could not be used for living tissue, and instead he tried chemical antisepsis. After experimenting with several substances he selected carbolic acid. His attention was drawn to it by the fact that it had been employed a short time before for the purpose of deodorizing sewage at the town of Carlisle.

Lister's first experiment was on a compound fracture. Such a fracture is one in which the ends of the broken bone have been forced through the flesh and skin, forming a wound in which the bone is exposed. They are therefore nearly always infected. Such a fracture even today is more serious than a simple fracture in which the bone does not protrude and hence is not infected. In Lister's time a compound fracture nearly always necessitated an amputation, for unless this was done the infection of the shattered bone and injured tissues usually resulted in death. Lister had observed the fact that a simple fracture was not accompanied by the formation of pus, and that a compounded fracture was. Both were wounds, but one was exposed to the air and the other was not. He felt that Pasteur's work offered an explanation for the pus formation in open wounds, for Pasteur had found that the germs which caused wine to ferment came from the air. Lister thus felt justified in trying to disinfect a compounded fracture, for results could not be made worse even if his efforts failed. His first attempt at antisepsis was made in March, 1865. The result was a failure and, as Lister said later: "It proved unsuccessful, in consequence, as I believe, of improper manage-

ment. . . ." In August of the same year he again applied
the antiseptic method to a compound fracture, painting the
wound with pure carbolic acid and dressing it with cloths
dipped in the dilute acid. This case justified his persistence,
for the wound healed without infection.

In his paper reporting the results of two years' experience
with the antiseptic method of treating wounds Lister says:
"There is, however, one point more that I cannot but advert
to, *viz.*, the influence of this mode of treatment upon the
general healthiness of an hospital. Previous to its introduction the two large wards in which most of my cases of accident and operation are treated were among the unhealthiest
in the whole surgical division of the Glasgow Royal Infir-
mary, in consequence, apparently, of these wards being unfavorably placed with reference to the supply of fresh air;
and I have felt ashamed, when recording the results of my
practice, to have so often to allude to hospital gangrene or
pyæmia [blood-poisoning]. It was interesting, though melancholy, to observe that whenever all or nearly all the beds
contained cases with open sores, these grievous complications
were pretty sure to show themselves; so that I came to
welcome simple fractures, though in themselves of little
interest either for myself or for the students, because their
presence diminished the proportion of open sores among the
patients. But since the antiseptic treatment has been brought
into full operation, and wounds and abscesses no longer poison the atmosphere with putrid exhalations, my wards,
though in other respects under precisely the same circumstances as before, have completely changed their character;
so that during the last nine months not a single instance of
pyæmia, hospital gangrene, or erysipelas has occurred in
them."

Lister thought that the infection was carried into wounds
by the air, as is evident from this extract. This assumption
was natural both from the ideas prevailing in regard to
"miasmas" and the harmful effects of night air and also from
Pasteur's work. Lister did not recognize at first that the real
source of infection was on the surgeon's hands and instru-

ments. He went to great lengths in his attempts to abolish the germs in the air, and for this purpose he injected a spray of carbolic acid into the air of the entire operating-room. The carbolic acid was unpleasant and often dangerous to inhale. It was the basis of the objections made by many surgeons to the adoption of Lister's work; they mistakenly thought that he had introduced a medicine, carbolic acid, and failed to grasp the fundamental principle of his work. Lister continued to develop the antiseptic method, and finally gave up the carbolic spray and the elaborate dressings used to exclude air from the wound. The antiseptic method gradually merged into the aseptic.

The aseptic methods of modern surgery are a combination of antisepsis and asepsis. All instruments and dressings are treated antiseptically; they are rendered sterile of germ life by heating. Likewise the surgeon's hands are treated with chemical antiseptics, as is also the patient's skin in the field of the operation. The rest of the operation is aseptic—that is, infection is prevented from getting into the wound by using instruments and dressings that have been sterilized. Air-borne bacteria do not cause infection in wounds unless the bacteria are present in large numbers, as in the spray of saliva; the surgeon covers his nose and mouth with a gauze mask to protect his patient against danger from this source. Lister taught surgeons to wash their hands and instruments before they operated, instead of only afterward. And when they had learned to do this the control of surgical infection was won and modern surgery became possible. Surgery ceased to be only wound surgery and the cavities of the bodies could be operated upon as well as the surface. Surgery of the chest, abdomen, brain, and joints became possible. Before the time of Lister appendicitis was as common as today, but it could not be operated on; the patient died instead. There had been Cæsarean sections on living women before the time of Lister, but they were almost always fatal for the women. Even Paré in all of his varied surgical experience never once opened the abdomen. Today Cæsarean section is one of the common life-saving procedures in surgery.

The triumphs which have come to modern surgery can be appreciated from an extract from a textbook of surgery published in 1876, scarcely fifty years ago; at the time abdominal operations were still rare. The extract in question deals with the consequences at that time of tubal pregnancy. It sometimes happens that the embryo develops in the tube leading to the uterus. As it grows it ruptures the wall of this tube. Serious hemorrhage follows and usually an abdominal operation is the only means by which life can be saved. The text of 1876 says: "The gravest accident that can happen to the victim of misplaced pregnancy is rupture of the gravid cyst. This is attended with the most alarming symptoms and frequently terminates in death within a short time. The almost universal opinion of the profession is that this accident is uniformly fatal, and, if not so, that we have no reliable means of combating its dangers. True, some have raised their voices and used their pens to advocate surgical interference, but as yet no one has been bold enough to hazard an operation under the circumstances. Operative interference is condemned by the highest authorities upon the subject, and he who would subject a woman under these circumstances to the dangers of gastrotomy would have to possess the courage of McDowell and his immediate followers."

The words in this text of 1876 might as well have been written three or even ten centuries ago, for they express no advance in treatment from these periods. The author deplored these deaths, but he was helpless in the face of the inadequacies of surgery. He says: ". . . A few women have recovered, though the number is very small—so small that when one is called to a case of this kind it is his duty to look upon his unhappy patient as inevitably doomed to die, unless he can by some active measure wrest her from the grave already yawning before her. The history of human injury and disease presents no condition parallel to this one. However fatal the disorder, science and art have found some means of prolonging life or soothing the stormy passage to the grave . . . ; but here is an accident which may happen to any wife in the most useful period of her existence, which good authorities have said is never cured, and for which, even in this age when science and art boast of such high attainments, no remedy, either medical or surgical, has been tried with a single success. From the middle of the eleventh century, when Albucasis described the first known case of extrauterine pregnancy, men have doubtlessly watched the life ebb rapidly from the pale victim of this accident as the torrent of blood is poured into the abdominal cavity but have never raised a hand to help her."

This statement was made in 1876; only seven years later Dr. Lawson Tait, in Birmingham, England, performed an operation for tubal pregnancy. Within a few years thereafter forty more such operations were performed. Only one of these women died; thirty-nine were saved. Previously all forty would have died without the operation. Today tubal pregnancy possesses none of the terrors that it did in 1876; nor, in fact, do any of the major surgical operations.

*Part Four*

# THE PASSING OF PLAGUE AND PESTILENCE

## CHAPTER VIII

## THE BLACK DEATH

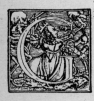 ibbon, the historian, writing in the last part of the eighteenth century, makes this statement: "If a man were called upon to fix the period in the history of the world, during which the conditions of the human race were most happy and prosperous, he would without hesitation name that which has elapsed from the death of Domitian to the accession of Commodus." The period thus defined is from 96 to 180 A.D. Let us consider certain aspects of life during this period and see if today we would agree with Gibbon. In the year 68 A.D. an epidemic of bubonic plague occurred in Rome. Eleven years later there was a second epidemic. In 125 A.D. and again in 164 A.D. the disease raged, and after the latter date continued without interruption for sixteen years. This "most happy and prosperous" period commenced with a plague which at its height killed ten thousand persons in a day at Rome. Tacitus says of it: "Houses were filled with dead bodies and the streets with funerals." The same period closed with sixteen years of plague of such severity that it threatened to exterminate the Roman army. A writer of the time says: "A great pestilence raged throughout Italy at that time but with most violence in the city. . . . The Emperor, by advice of physicians, retired to Laurentium."

In this same period malaria spread through Italy. A nation

can recover from the mortality and demoralization caused by plague, but it is enervated by malaria. The attacks of plague are intermittent and in the pauses reconstruction of society can occur. Malaria is continuous. Its victims do not die at once, but by their deterioration they slowly sap the strength of the society of which they are a part. Malaria is most prevalent in rural districts. The farmers infected with the disease neglect their land. The country population flows into the city to swell its slums. After three centuries of malaria, Rome was pillaged by the barbarian tribes from the forests of Germany. Malaria and plague were as much its conquerors as were these Goths and Vandals.

In this "happy and prosperous" period, the golden age of civilization, leprosy was common. Diphtheria took its toll of the young. Tuberculosis carried off entire families. Anthrax killed men and animals. Typhoid fever and dysentery were continuous scourges. There was no dentistry worthy the name, except extraction, and its methods were brutal. Surgery had no operation for appendicitis; if the appendix ruptured, death always resulted. Cancers were not removed. Such surgery as existed was brutally rough, and for its pains there was no relief by anesthesia. Infant desertion was a common practice and there were no asylums for orphans.

Viewed in the light of modern conditions, Gibbon's statement seems as paradoxical as the remark of Herodotus on ancient Egypt, which, he said, was the healthiest country and filled with physicians. Nevertheless, Gibbon, at the time he wrote, 1776-1780, at the same time as the American Revolution, was justified in his statement. A hundred years before, England had emerged from three centuries of the plague; fifty years before, Marseilles had been devastated by it. Diphtheria, typhoid fever, typhus, and consumption were prevalent, and rickets was on the increase. Syphilis, cholera, and smallpox had been added to the list of pestilences. Jenner had not yet demonstrated the effectiveness of vaccination. There were still no operations for appendicitis, nor for cancers except when they occurred on the surface of the body. Antisepsis and asepsis did not come into use for nearly a century after Gibbon's time. If the surgeon of his time had a greater skill in "cutting for the stone" or in

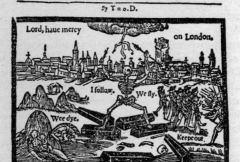

A Rod for Run-awayes.

# Gods Tokens,

Of his feareful Iudgements, sundry wayes pronounced vpon this City, and on seuerall persons, both flying from it, and staying in it.

*Expressed in many dreadfull Examples of sudden Death, falne vpon both young and old, within this City, and the Suburbes, in the Fields, and open Streets, to the terrour of all those who liue, and to the warning of those who are to dye, to be ready when God Almighty shall bee pleased to call them.*

By Tho. D.

Printed at London for Iohn Trundle, and are to be sold at his Shop in Smithfield. 1625.

## "A ROD FOR RUN-AWAYES"

The title page of one of Thomas Dekker's plague pamphlets, 1625. The plague was almost continually present in London until late in the seventeenth century, but in some years, the so-called plague years, the disease broke out in a violent epidemic; 1625 was one of these plague years. In his pamphlet, "A Rod for Run-awayes," Dekker describes the conditions in London during the epidemic. The illustration on the title page shows the wrath of God descending as lightning from the clouds, and in the center death stands represented as a skeleton. On the left are men and women dead in the fields and over them is the inscription, "Wee dye"; on the right is a group of people fleeing from the plague and in response to their words, "We fly," death answers with, "I follow." The people of the suburban districts realized the truth of death's "I follow" and attempted to prevent the infected Londoners from contaminating their towns, as is shown by the armed men marked with the inscription, "Keepe out."

amputating limbs than surgeons in Roman times, the advantage was offset by the likelihood of infection in the hospital. There was still no anesthesia. Childbed fever was epidemic and Semmelweis had not yet shown the method of prevention. The convulsions of childbirth were prevented no better in the time of Gibbon than in the time of the Roman Empire. Infanticide was forbidden and severely punished, but for the host of women who bore illegitimate children in a licentious age death was often preferable to the treatment they received in charitable institutions.

Gibbon could not see the advances of civilization which would result in the control of the pestilences. He looked at his own time and he looked back to the past. From the elevation which civilization had attained he looked back across the morass of the Middle Ages to the mountain that was Rome in its golden age. He was far enough above the Middle Ages to see across the mist of ignorance and disease that hung over them. Beyond them the days of Rome, plague-ridden as they were, seemed clean and clear in the sunlight of knowledge and civilization. He looked back to the Middle Ages when the lepers crept about the streets, when the "sweating sickness" raged, and men were contorted by the "dancing mania." He saw the times when diphtheria was called "garotillo," or the strangler, by the Italians, and the years which were named from its ravages. He saw men consumed with the dry rot of consumption and he saw men burned with the disease of "holy fire" seeking the shrines of St. Anthony to leave their withered limbs upon the monastery walls. When Gibbon wrote he could say that the Roman epoch he had chosen from among the centuries was truly "the period in history during which the conditions of the human race were most happy and prosperous."

Now that the pestilences are largely held in check, it is difficult for us to picture to ourselves their ravages in former days. We can form only a slight conception of what they were; the only experience on which we can base such a conception is the destruction wrought by that pestilence which still comes with each generation. That pestilence is the influenza. At intervals it starts in the Far East; from there it travels slowly but inevitably around the world as a pan-

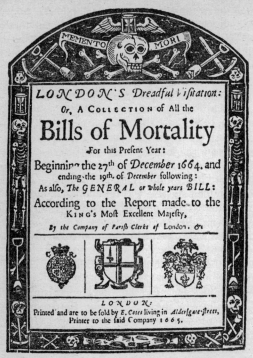

TITLE PAGE OF THE LONDON BILLS OF MORTALITY FOR 1665

The year of the great plague. The people of the city followed with anxiety the rise and fall in the number of deaths from the plague, hoping always to see the sharp decline which they knew from past experience indicated that the epidemic was nearing its end. When the decline came the refugees, mostly from the nobility and wealthy merchants, returned to the city, and then for a time the mortality rose again as the disease attacked these new arrivals. The plague of 1665 started in June; its peak came in September and its decline in October. The secondary rise occurred in November and cases of the disease were reported as late as March of the following year.

demic. It affects about 400 in every 1,000 of the population, but out of those 400 only two die. As a pestilence it is mild in comparison with the "great mortality," the bubonic plague, which may affect 100 per cent of the population and kills from 20 to 80 out of every 100 of those affected. Influenza is relatively a mild pestilence which comes and passes on in the course of six weeks; but 400 in every 1,000 among a population of 150,000,000 people is 60,000,000 sick; and of these sick, 240,000 die. Among the dead are many child-bearing women, for with the pregnant woman that plague, like all others, is deadly. The pandemics of influenza in 1836, 1847, 1889, and 1918 give only a faint idea of what the world has suffered through the ages from the greater pestilences and plagues.

From the earliest recorded times epidemic diseases have ravaged civilization. These epidemics, rising to the proportion of pestilences, have ranked with war and famine in keeping down the population. They have been efficient allies of the high infant mortality of past civilizations. In times of peace and when free from pestilence the population grew, owing to the prodigious rate of reproduction. In times of pestilence the population decreased at such a rate that the extermination of whole nations was sometimes threatened. The periods of increase of population barely compensated for the periodic ravages of the pestilences. For centuries the population could not increase, for any increase predisposed to pestilences. Now at last the pestilences are largely held in check; it is only now, therefore, that we can realize the social and cultural retardation which resulted from them. The people could not expand and develop; they could only struggle to hold their numbers against the pestilences. The average life of the individual was short. Three centuries ago the usual span of life was only twenty years. A short average life results in a rapidly changing population, and this condition is detrimental to general advancement. Every individual spends many years of his life in infancy and childhood, during which period he is dependent upon others before he reaches an age at which he becomes productive. Variation in length of life does not affect the length of the dependent period. It affects only the period of productivity. Thus a dependent period of fifteen years leaves for an average life of twenty years only five years of productivity. For an average life of sixty years, approximately that in civilized countries today, the dependent period, remaining the same, leaves a productive period of forty-five years. Thus a threefold increase in the average length of life results in a ninefold increase in productivity. This prolongation of the productive period is an economic and social asset of enormous value to the advancement of civilization.

The benefit derived from the control of the pestilences has been even greater for women than for men. The burden of holding the population against extermination by war, infant mortality, and pestilence falls upon the women. The number of births necessary to balance the number of deaths varies in exact proportion with the average length of life. To effect this balance three centuries ago women were forced to bear three times as many children as they would be to maintain a stationary population today. Large families were once a necessity for the preservation of the human race. Many of the laws and religious precepts in effect today express this necessity of the past; this is particularly true in respect to voluntary efforts to limit the number of offspring.

A reduction in the number of children borne by each woman results in a decrease in the mortality from childbirth. This decrease does not, however, appear in the statistics for the number of mothers who die for each thousand children born, which is the usual way of estimating the mortality from childbirth. Such statistics do not show the actual mortality of the mothers. That depends upon the number of women bearing the children, which in turn resolves itself into the number of children each woman bears. If 5 women die for every 1,000 children born, the mortality for the mothers is 5, 10, or 15 deaths per 1,000 women, depending upon whether each woman has one, two, or three children. Thus, for mothers, the number of children born is quite as important a factor in the hazards of childbirth as is the number of deaths per thousand children. Pestilences, aside from their direct bearing in shortening of life, have an indirect bearing on the hazards of childbirth by increasing the number of children that women must bear. The control of pestilences is thus an important factor in decreasing mortality of mothers at birth.

Diseases were once regarded as an affliction from the Deity, a punishment for sin. Even today in law certain forms of disaster are termed "acts of God," such as those due to the uncontrollable forces of nature in hurricanes and the eruption of volcanoes. In particular the diseases that rose to the proportion of pestilences were considered to be an outpouring of the wrath of a vengeful Deity. They were thought to occur as a punishment for the sins of men, and the Church taught that they were to be accepted with resignation. Job attributed his suffering to the arrows of the Almighty. Boccaccio, in describing a plague at Florence in 1348, has expressed the prevailing belief as to the cause of such pestilences. He says: "Such was the cruelty of Heaven and perhaps of men . . . that upwards of 100,000 souls perished in the city." Martin Luther said: "Pestilences, fever, and other severe diseases are naught else than the devil's work." In 1495 Emperor Maximilian issued an edict in which he stated that the "new French disease," syphilis, was an affliction from God for the sins of men. Two centuries later in New England, Cotton Mather saw in the same disease a punishment "which the just Judgment of God has reserved for our late Ages. . . ." In a previous chapter the clergy of Scotland were quoted as maintaining that "smallpox was an affliction from God."

Under the belief in the divine origin of pestilences the preventives were prayers, incantations, charms, and the sacrifice of animals and even of human beings with which to propitiate the angry God. With the advance of civilization the credulity as to the divine origin of most diseases was gradually replaced by the belief that disease arises from cosmic disturbances. Even down to modern times, such occurrences as eclipses, comets, earthquakes, and tidal waves

| | | | |
|---|---|---|---|
| Abortive | 4 | Impostume | 8 |
| Aged | 45 | Infants | 22 |
| Bleeding | 1 | Kingsevil | 4 |
| Broken legge | 1 | Lethargy | 1 |
| Broke her scull by a fall in the street at St. Mary VVoolchurch | 1 | Livergrown | 1 |
| Childbed | 28 | Meagrome | 1 |
| Chrisomes | 9 | Palsie | 1 |
| Consumption | 126 | Plague | 4237 |
| Convulsion | 89 | Purples | 2 |
| Cough | 1 | Quinsie | 5 |
| Dropsie | 53 | Rickets | 23 |
| Feaver | 348 | Rising of the Lights | 18 |
| Flox and Small-pox | 11 | Rupture | 1 |
| Flux | 1 | Scurvy | 3 |
| Frighted | 2 | Shingles | 1 |
| Gowt | 1 | Spotted Feaver | 166 |
| Grief | 3 | Stilborn | 2 |
| Griping in the Guts | 79 | Stone | 2 |
| Head-mould-shot | 1 | Stopping of the stomach | 17 |
| Jaundies | 7 | Strangury | 3 |
| | | Suddenly | 2 |
| | | Surfeit | 74 |
| | | Teeth | 118 |
| | | Thrush | 6 |
| | | Tissick | 9 |
| | | Ulcer | 1 |
| | | Vomiting | 10 |
| | | Winde | 4 |
| | | Wormes | 20 |

Christened { Males — 90, Females — 81, In all — 171 }
Buried { Males — 2777, Females — 2791, In all — 5568 } Plague — 4237

Increased in the Burials this Week — 249

Parishes clear of the Plague — 27  Parishes Infected — 103

*The Assize of Bread set forth by Order of the Lord Maior and Court of Aldermen,*
*A penny Wheaten Loaf to contain Nine Ounces and a half, and three*
*half-penny White Loaves the like weight.*

## THE DISEASES AND CASUALTIES DURING THE PLAGUE YEAR

A bill of mortality for the week August 15 to 22, 1665. During this week 171 children were christened, but 5,568 persons died, and 4,237 of these deaths were attributed to the plague. The causes of death as recorded were ascertained by old women employed by the parish authorities to inspect the body at each death. As may well be imagined, the diagnoses were often mere guesses; except in time of plague the only reliable statistics were for accidental deaths and executions. The latter, however, do not figure in this bill of mortality because courts and executions were suspended for the duration of the epidemic; when it was over most of the prisoners, both those condemned and those awaiting trial, had died of the plague.

were regarded as warnings of impending pestilences. We have only in recent years learned that the mists from marshes and the night air are not the cause of disease. As cosmic disturbances are beyond human control, religion was still supposed to offer the only relief from the pestilences. When theological practices failed to ward off the pestilences, men naturally sought to avoid or to escape from them. Their efforts to this end were unorganized. They fled before the pestilence or hid from it as one would flee or hide from a storm. They avoided the sick, as the tangible evidence of the locality in which the rain of the pestilence fell or as centers from which the blighting atmosphere of the pestilence blew.

Belief in the supernatural origin of disease inevitably placed all of the prevention of disease in religion. Medicine was not preventive, it was only a healing art. The part it played was merely accessory to theology. It attempted to relieve the suffering or to save the lives of those from whom the priests or clergymen had been unable to ward off the pestilence. Frequently the practices of religious functions and medical functions were combined. This combination of medicine and theology has existed from the earliest times; from the Egyptian priest to the medicine-man of the American Indian the association has been maintained in one form or another. Mr. Ward, the Vicar of Stratford-on-Avon, writing in the fifteenth century, says: ". . . In King Richard the Second's time physicians and divines were not distinct professions, for one Tydeman, Bishop of Landaph and Worcester, was physician to King Richard the Second." Thomas Thacher, the first minister of the Old South Church of Boston, wrote the earliest medical treatises printed in this country. The bigoted Cotton Mather was not a physician, nevertheless he practiced medicine along with theology in Massachusetts. Being a clergyman, he naturally derived disease from sin. He says: "Sickness is in Fact the whip of God for the sins of man." In his writings on the care of infants he encourages the distracted mother of the ailing child with these reflections: "Think; oh the grevious Effects of Sin!

This wretched Infant has not arrived unto years of sense enough, to sin after the similitude of the transgression committed by Adam. Nevertheless the Transgression of Adam

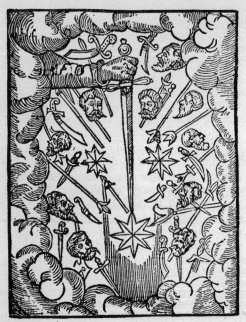

"THE FIGURE OF A FEARFUL COMET"

From Paré's *Surgery*. Comets, particularly when accompanied by a cloud of swords, daggers, coffins, and men's heads, were considered to be omens of impending plague. Pepys, in his *Diary*, mentions the comet of December, 1664, at which King Charles II and his queen looked from the windows of Whitehall and of which there was "mighty talk." The comet appeared again in the February following and once more in March. After these preliminaries the plague broke out in June.

. . . has involved this Infant in the guilt of it. And the poison of the old serpent, which infected Adam when he fell into Transgression by hearkening to the Tempter, has corrupted all mankind, and is a seed unto such disease as this

Infant is now laboring under. Lord, what are we, and what are our children but a Generation of Vipers?" The medicine with which he followed this comforting eulogy was a stiff dose of the tincture of "sowbugs," millipedes. He says: "Poor Sowbug! . . . Take . . . half a pound, put 'em alive into a quart or two of wine." The dose of this concoction was two ounces twice a day.

Two generations ago children wore about their necks bags filled with asafetida. This practice was a sort of compromise between superstition and medicine; they were worn as an amulet, but were filled with drugs. In accord with the prevailing tradition, the drugs were the most unpleasant that could be found, thus the more effectively to discourage the approach of the disease or at least the approach of those who had the disease.

So long as medicine was subordinate to religion, it could not advance. Medicine is most effective in prevention and is least effective in the cure of epidemic diseases. Even today the best medical treatment would not be able to stop any of the pestilences once they got started in a modern American city by merely caring for the sick. The control of the pestilences became possible only when medicine rose from its subordinate position and replaced theology as a means of preventing disease. The prayer for the sick gave place to pills and elixirs, and these in time have given place to quarantine and other measures of prevention. The striking difference between treatment and prevention and the subordinate value of the form is seen in the contrast between the two branches of medical science—surgery and medicine. Surgery actually treats disease and often cures it; it repairs damage, but only after injury. Surgery struggles hand to hand with the enemy, disease. But this struggle occurs only after the enemy has attacked; for surgery is not preventive. Its benefits are for the individual only. Medicine, by contrast, can do little to repair damage from disease. Except in a few diseases, medicine cannot cure. It can only support the strength and lessen pain for the sufferer and at best it keeps him alive until nature heals him. Medicine confers its greatest benefits in the prevention of disease; the benefits are for both the individual and the community.

Modern urban civilization is founded on preventive medicine. The great pestilences no longer rage in the more civilized countries, but the fact that they are excluded does not mean that they have died out. Unremitting vigilance and continual activity are necessary if the country is to be

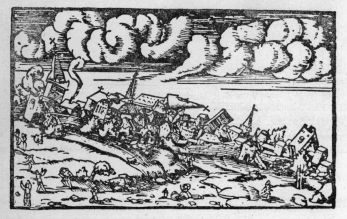

AN EARTHQUAKE

that came before the outbreak of the plague. Disasters of various kinds were formerly supposed to be portents of the plague. Before the plague of Justinian in 543 A. D., the harvest failed and there was an earthquake at Antioch which is said to have killed 25,000 people.

kept free from them. If the preventive measures were relaxed the pestilences would quickly return and even the most civilized countries would be ravaged now as they were in the Middle Ages. The rate at which the pestilences would spread, their extent, and the demoralization which would follow them would be greater today than they were in the Middle Ages. The railroad and other means of rapid communication would expedite the spread of disease. The crowding of people in cities would allow the spread to be extensive.

Urban communities are dependent upon sustained commerce and transportation for even food and water; the means of commerce and transportation would fail under the pestilence. Hunger, thirst, fire, and darkness would add to the panic and death from the disease itself. Exclusion of the pestilences is one of the supreme benefits conferred upon mankind by the advancement and application of knowledge.

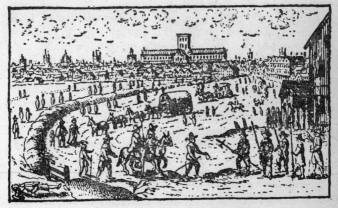

BURYING THE PLAGUE VICTIMS

Posters were published in 1665 and 1666 to illustrate events of the plague in London. The scene here represented shows the trenches which were dug in the fields to bury the dead. The bodies, a few in coffins, but most in coarse shrouds or naked, were brought from the city in heavily loaded horse-drawn carts.

The progress of medicine has supplied knowledge which can be used for the prevention of disease. But medicine alone cannot apply the knowledge; that can only be done by civilization. Before civilization can apply the knowledge to prevent pestilence it must advance beyond the belief that disease is of supernatural origin. Pestilences have occurred in those times when theology was at its greatest heights of faith. Human life was held of little value then. The essential features of the advance of civilization are the acquisition of knowledge and the application of this knowledge. When knowledge is thus utilized for the advancement of civilization, more knowledge becomes available. It is no mere coincidence that Hippocrates, who gave medical knowledge the form it held for twenty centuries, lived in the same age as Pericles, Socrates, Plato, and Phidias. Galen, who has left his imprint on medicine to this day, was both a contemporary and a friend of Marcus Aurelius. Vesalius and Paré, the founder of anatomy and the reformer of surgery, lived in the same period that Martin Luther lived in. Harvey, who described the circulation of the blood, lived in that brilliant period, the age of Shakespeare and Queen Elizabeth; Bacon was both his teacher and his patient. Pasteur, Lister, Simpson, and Semmelweis made their contributions to medical knowledge in the period of the steam engine, the steamboat, and the railway, the telegraph and the telephone, electric lights and the automobile.

Knowledge is the basis for the advancement of civilization, but civilization exists only to the extent that the knowledge is applied. The Greeks and Romans left a store of knowledge to the world, but the medieval Europeans did not utilize it. Electricity affords illumination, but this fact of itself lights no houses in countries which are satisfied with oil-lamps and candles. As knowledge alone, the demonstration by Semmelweis of the cause and transmission of childbed fever has only academic value, but when applied in the practice of obstetrics it saves thousands of lives.

The extent of the application of knowledge is the outstanding feature of any stage of civilization. Thus at any time different countries may show wide divergences in their applications of knowledge. In the case of childbed fever the extent of application appears in the hazards of childbirth and is measured by the deaths of mothers. Similarly, the prevalence of a pestilence such as smallpox shows that knowledge as to its prevention is not applied. Thus the prevalence of smallpox affords a measure of cultural retardation. About one-fifth of all the smallpox in the world occurs in the

United States; India is the only country that has more small-pox than we do.

The pestilences are held in check only to such extent as civilization has progressed and has put into effect the knowl-edge supplied by medicine. Their prevalence is a symptom of at least a latent belief in the supernatural origin of disease. Outside of the protection which civilization now affords against the pestilences still lie these ancient enemies. Once

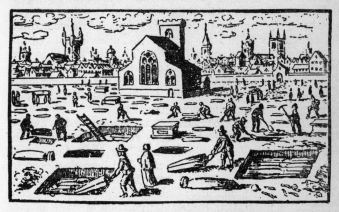

### THE CROWDED CHURCHYARD

From a plague poster. During the plague many bodies were buried together in large graves and when the plague subsided the level of the yard was sometimes raised a foot or more above its original height.

they stalked openly through the land. Generation after gen-eration they took their ghastly toll of human life and suffer-ing, in spite of prayers, charms, holy relics, and all the futile efforts of theology to propitiate the angry deities. The test of the supreme control over pestilence comes in time of war; for at such times civilization declines, the preventive measures are relaxed, and pestilences rise again. In the memory of men now living the prevention of disease has progressed enor-mously. Formerly typhoid fever often reached the dimensions of a pestilence. It was known as such even in the time of Hippocrates. It has always flourished in encampments during war. In each year of the Civil War of the United States 1,000 out of every 100,000 died of typhoid, and this was not thought extraordinary. In the Spanish War (1898) the prevalence of typhoid was considered a disgrace, although only 100 men in every 100,000 died of it. In World War I, 5 died of typhoid in every 100,000. This decrease in the prevalence of typhoid was due to preventive medicine and not to theology. The care of drinking-water took the place of incantations. The sanitary disposal of excrement became a ritual. Prophylactic inoculation against the disease replaced the wearing of charms and holy relics. The part played by flies in the spread of disease was suggested by Paré in the sixteenth century. In the twentieth century the screening out of flies was found more effective in preventing the spread of typhoid than all the prayers of the pious.

Leprosy was the first pestilence to be controlled in Europe. It was a disease which was easily controllable even by the methods available in medieval times. The method of control, avoidance of contact with the sick, had been developed by the ancient Jews and is set forth in the Bible. Leprosy is transmitted with difficulty; usually it requires intimate contact of long duration. Systematic isolation of those afflicted eventually brings an end to the pestilence. When the medieval Europeans set out to eradicate leprosy they did so with characteristic brutality. In 1313 Philip the Fair ordered that all the lepers in France should be burned. But this radical measure was not fully carried out and instead the monasteries of Saint Lazarus were set aside for the lepers. These institutions were named lazarettos. Into them were crowded "Christ's poor," as the lepers were called, to be cared for by priests who were themselves lepers. In western Europe alone there were 19,000 of these lazarettos. The lepers were the living dead; as they were torn from their friends and families to be entombed in the lazarettos, the burial ritual was read over them; they were dead for all civil affairs and buried so far as their wives and children were concerned. When they crept

out from their filthy quarters they dressed in a manner to
show their illness. They wore masks to hide their deform-

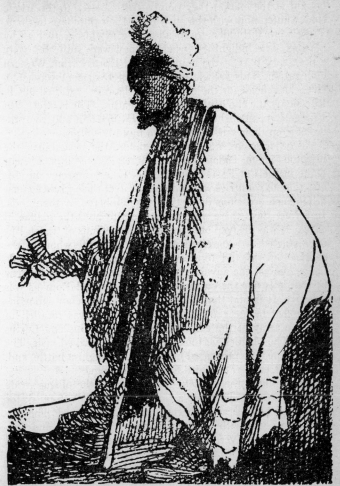

THE LEPER, AFTER REMBRANDT

ities. In their hands they carried a bell or rattle to mark their coming and to warn the healthy from their path. If they bought at the market they pointed with a stick to the article they wanted and with the stick drew their purchase to them. They were forbidden to speak above a whisper to healthy persons. The indignities to which they were subjected were a necessary part of the eradication of leprosy from Western civilization. This calculated cruelty of treatment was effectively beneficial for the country, for leprosy had died out in Europe by the end of the sixteenth century. The lazarettos of France were abolished by Louis XIV in 1656 and the proceeds from their sale were used to build hospitals.

All other scourges seem feeble before the great killer, the bubonic plague. Today it still exists sequestered in its ancient home in the Far East. From there it takes an excursion now and then to countries which do not protect themselves against it. On such occasions its victims are numbered by thousands. In former days there were no barriers to hold the plague in check. It was delayed only by the slow methods of travel. But once started, it progressed inevitably over the whole of the civilized world and its dead were then numbered by millions. Against the advance of the plague neither the hygiene of the Jews nor the culture of the Greeks and Romans was effective. It is said that Galen, the great physician, ignominiously fled before the plague in Rome. He was recalled to join the army of the emperors Marcus Aurelius and Lucius Verus. The plague overtook the army. Verus died of it. The army turned about, routed before it had fought a battle, and, retreating, carried the dead Emperor to Rome.

All through "the Golden Age" of Rome the plague made periodic attacks. Then for a time the epidemics stopped, for Rome fell before the barbarians and travel ceased. The empire rose again with Constantinople as its capital, and Justinian, the lawgiver, was on the throne. Peace and travel prevailed. Then began a series of those calamities in which the superstitious saw omens of the impending plague and warnings of the divine wrath that was to culminate in the plague. Christian superstition was then in all the vigor of its youth. An earthquake destroyed in a few moments the greater part of the city of Antioch, and 25,000 people were buried in the ruins. A comet appeared. The sun was darkened for a whole year. A famine occurred in Italy and multitudes were starved. After these preliminaries the plague broke out in lower Egypt. In 542 it spread slowly up the Nile and crept

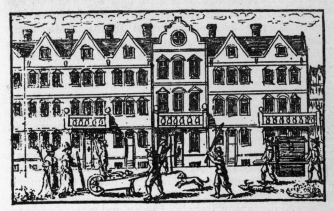

### LONDON DURING THE PLAGUE

A scene from a plague poster. A street in London is shown; the doors of the houses are marked with red crosses to indicate that there is plague among the inmates, and armed guards stand in the street to prevent anyone from coming out. To the left are two searchers, each carrying the staff which indicates her position; their duty is to enter the houses and certify to the cause of death. In the middle is a dog-killer slaughtering every dog he meets; near him is a raker carrying away a wheelbarrow full of dogs. Dogs were believed to carry the plague and thousands of them were killed, but no attention was paid to the rats which were responsible for the epidemic. Before every sixth house a fire is burning in the street to help purify the air.

from there into Asia Minor. At first it followed the coast line where the traffic was most active. Gradually it worked into the interior. It reached Constantinople. There at its height it killed 5,000 to 10,000 persons daily.

In its relentless advance the plague extended over Greece

and into Italy; it entered Gaul and reached to the Rhine. This spread of the plague took fifteen years. Then it slowly receded and on its return struck again at Constantinople. It had lost none of its virulence from its travels. The piled-up dead of Constantinople were disposed of by unroofing the towers of the walls, cramming the space thus exposed with corpses, and replacing the roof. Gibbon writes of this less "happy and prosperous" period: "In time the plague's first malignancy was abated and dispersed; the disease alternately languished and revived, but it was not until the end of a calamitous period of fifty-two years that mankind recovered their health, and the air resumed its pure and salubrious quality." It is evident from this passage that in Gibbon's time the conception of a divine origin of disease was being replaced by that of a cosmic origin and it was thought that diseases arose from miasmas and fetid air. He continues: "No facts have been preserved to sustain an account, or even a conjecture, of the number that perished in this extraordinary mortality. I only find that during three months, four and at length ten thousand persons died each day at Constantinople, that many cities of the East were left vacant, and that in several districts of Italy the harvest and vintage withered on the ground. The triple scourge of war, pestilence, and famine, affected the subjects of Justinian, and his reign is disgraced by a visible decrease of the human species, which has never been replaced in some of the fairest countries of the globe."

As if replete from its harvest of the sixth century, the plague, except for minor outbreaks, lay dormant for eight hundred years. Mohammed made his hegira; Haroun al-Raschid held the caliphate of the *Arabian Nights* untroubled by the plague. Charlemagne built the empire of the west. Jerusalem fell to the Mohammedans and the crusades started and continued for two centuries. Still there were no great outbreaks of the plague. In the thirteenth century Roger Bacon, the scientist, Thomas Aquinas, the theologian, and Dante, the poet, left their immortal work. All this time there were no outbreaks of the plague. In the fourteenth century the city of Lubeck appointed a city physician; this first non-theological health officer of Europe earned his fee of four dollars a year without interference from the plague. In 1330 gunpowder was used for the first time in the west; in 1336 the Hundred Years' War started, and in 1345 the first apothecary's shop was opened in London. That same year the bubonic plague was epidemic in Africa and Asia. Two years later it spread to Constantinople and then to Greece and Italy, and so gradually but inevitably from there throughout Europe. It was during this great epidemic that the plague was named "the Black Death," because of the dark areas formed by minute hemorrhages which appeared in the skin of those affected. With each generation the epidemics recurred. As they swept over Europe panic went before them, and demoralization followed in their train. The ravages of the Black Death during the next three centuries equaled those in the last century of the western Roman Empire and in Constantinople in the time of Justinian. But the records are better for the more recent period and the actions of men in the face of the plague can be seen at closer range.

The customs that held men together in commerce, law, and order fell apart before the approach of the plague and left raw human nature to follow its own dictates. Some men gave way to the wildest panic; others to the deepest despair. Some rose to heights of heroism in their self-sacrifice, others indulged in unbridled revelry. This last, wild festivity in the face of death, always appears when life is in great uncertainty. The Bible tells us that Jerusalem, when threatened by the attack of Sennacherib, gave itself over to revelry: "and in that day did the Lord God of Hosts call to weeping and to mourning, and to baldness, and to girding with sackcloth: but behold joy and gladness, slaying oxen, and killing sheep, eating flesh and drinking wine: let us eat and drink, for tomorrow we die." The tales in Boccaccio's *Decameron* are of a merry group of young people who were in seclusion in the hope of avoiding the plague which was epidemic in Florence in 1348, but the introduction to that account reads: "Such was the cruelty of Heaven and perhaps of men, that between March and July following, it is supposed and made pretty certain, that upwards of a hundred thousand souls perished in the city only, whereas, before that calamity, it was not supposed to contain so many inhabitants. What magnificent dwellings, what noble palaces were then depopulated to the last person, what families extinct, what rich and vast possessions left, and no known heir to inherit, what numbers of both sexes in the prime and vigor of youth—who in the morning Galen, Hippocrates, or Æsculapius himself would have declared in perfect health—after dining heartily with their friends here have supped with their departed friends in the other world." From another writer of that time we have: "Shrift there was none; churches and chapels were open but neither priest nor penitent entered—all went to the charnel house. The sexton and the physician were cast into the same deep and wide grave; the testator and his heirs and executors were hurled together from the same cart into the same hole together."

During times of the plague comfort was provided to the dying people by absolutions granted by the popes. In the year 1348 Clement VI granted absolution from all sins of all Christians who should die on a journey to Rome, where, in spite of the plague, a Holy Year was being celebrated. Not only was absolution given, but the souls of those who died were to be carried straight to heaven without first passing through purgatory. By Easter 1,200,000 people from all parts of Europe had gathered at Rome. Some of these pilgrims brought the plague with them; it spread rapidly through the crowded people. Scarcely 10 per cent lived to return to their homes. But the offerings that the pilgrims made to the Church amounted to an enormous sum. The pope did not contract the plague. He was at Avignon, which he had just purchased from Queen Jane of Naples, and when the plague reached that city he isolated himself in one room for the duration of the epidemic. This excellent advice was given him by the famous physician Guy de Chauliac, who himself died of the plague. The mortality at Avignon reached such heights that Clement consecrated the river Rhone so that corpses could be sunk in it instead of being buried. Among the victims of this epidemic at Avignon was Petrarch's Laura.

A frantic wave of piety sometimes overwhelmed the people as the plague approached. They often gave all of their pos-

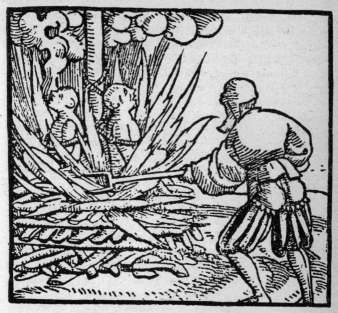

**BURNING PLAGUE-SPREADERS**

From an old woodcut. During epidemics of the plague anyone accused of spreading the disease was dealt with summarily. The absurdity of the evidence upon which such accusations were based made little difference; even a suspicion was sufficient to excite the frightened people to a frenzy of revenge.

sessions to the Church. The Church in turn sometimes took advantage of the rising piety to enforce moral regulations. Thus as the plague neared Tournai the Council issued an edict that all concubines were to be expelled and that both the manufacture and use of dice were to be discontinued. The dice factories were adapted to the tendencies of the time and for a while manufactured rosary beads.

During the fourteenth century, in Europe alone, twenty-five million persons perished, and in all, about one-fourth of the entire population was swept off by recurrent epidemics of the plague before it subsided for a generation because of a lack of susceptible victims. During epidemics of the plague the medieval cities were in an indescribably horrible condition. The dead and dying blocked the streets. They were carted away in some cases by liberated convicts, to be thrown into pits or vaults or even into the sea, from which the bodies were washed back to pile up on the shores. Among the dying multitudes there were scenes of courage, devotion, and self-sacrifice, reminiscent of the early Christians who had won the admiration of the Romans by the heroism they displayed during the plague at Rome. There were scenes, too, of the most despicable brutality as the people sought to find an escape in their panic by the torture and execution of the Jews. At that time, in the Christian countries, the Jews were excluded from nearly all professions except that of money-lending, for they were not allowed to join the trade guilds; most of the banking was under their control. They took interest for loans, a practice which then was forbidden under Biblical authority to Christians. The resentment aroused by this practice, together with religious hate and prejudice of race, made the Jews ready victims of the most absurd suspicions, and these suspicions were furthered by the nobility who owed the Jews money. They were accused of causing the plague by poisoning the wells. In some places they were systematically murdered or driven to their death by persecution. In Mayence 12,000 threw themselves into fires kindled to burn them.

The Jews were not the only persons accused of spreading the plague, and anyone suspected on even the most absurd evidence was tortured and put to death. An instance of this kind occurred during the plague in Milan. On the morning of June 1, 1630, Guglielmo Piazza, commissioner of health of Milan, was observed walking down the street writing from an ink-horn at his belt and wiping his ink-stained fingers against walls of houses. Ignorant women of the neighborhood accused him of smearing the houses with virus of the plague.

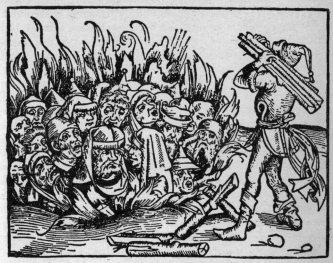

BURNING THE JEWS

From an old woodcut. In the Middle Ages the Jews were oppressed by both ecclesiastical and civil regulations. They were denied admission to trade guilds and it was forbidden to employ them as physicians, although the nobility and clergy did so because of the superior knowledge of the Jews. Many Jews turned to money-lending, for taking interest was then forbidden to Christians on Biblical authority. When epidemics of the plague occurred, the Jews were usually accused of spreading the disease by poisoning the wells or by black magic. The people burned them in retaliation for their supposed infamy and the nobility, who owed money to the Jews, made no effort to prevent their deaths.

They took their complaint to the City Council and Piazza was arrested and tortured. This torture was a survival of feudal times and was carried out in a ceremonial procedure prescribed by law. Many of the village officials to whom the legal aspects of torture were intrusted could not read and to supply them with the necessary information the *Constitutio Criminalis* of Maria Theresa in 1768 had seventeen copper-plate engravings to illustrate the various modes of torture. As a preamble to torture the victim was shaved and

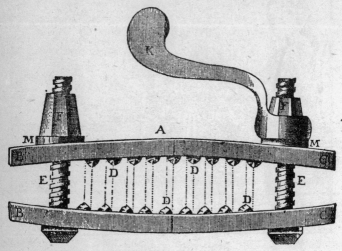

THE THUMBSCREW OF MARIA THERESA

This figure and the three following are taken from the legal code prepared for Maria Theresa of Austria in 1768. In order that her judges, some of whom were illiterate, might carry out the approved methods of torture, the procedures were represented pictorially. In using the thumbscrew, the tips of the victim's thumbs were inserted into the space marked D; the nuts F and F were then adjusted to hold the pointed studs across the base of the thumb nail; and finally the executioner turned the lever K.

purged. If he survived the atrocities inflicted upon his body three times, God was supposed to intervene for him in a miracle showing the victim's innocence. The Commissioner Piazza withstood two applications of the torture, but yielded to the "third degree." To save himself from further torture he said that he had spread the plague, and on being threatened with torture unless he divulged the name of his accomplices he accused a barber named Mora. The latter likewise yielded to torture and gave the desired confession of guilt.

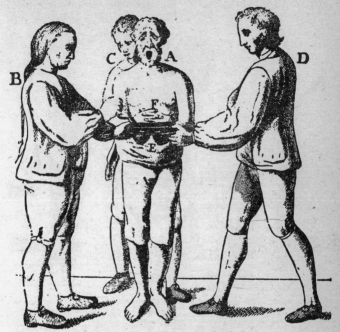

APPLYING THE THUMBSCREW

*Constitutio criminalis Theresiana.* The executioner is here shown tightening the lever of the thumbscrew. The victim is marked A, a quite unnecessary thoroughness of designation. If the thumbscrew failed to elicit a suitable confession from A, he was exposed to a second degree of torture.

He incriminated Don Juan de Padilla, son of the commandant of the fortress, whom the barber had treated for syphilis. The victims of this Renaissance justice were then sentenced to death; they were torn with red-hot pincers, had their right hands cut off, their bones broken, were stretched on the wheel, and after six hours of suffering were burned. Their ashes were thrown into the river and their possessions sold; the house which had been touched with ink was razed and on its site was erected a "column of infamy," to com-

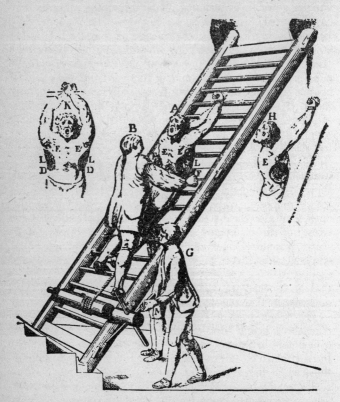

**TORTURE WITH THE RACK AND CANDLE**

*Constitutio criminalis Theresiana.* The victim, A, of eighteenth-century justice is here stretched on the rack, which is being tightened by the executioner's assistant, G. An added refinement consists in the application of the candle flame to the area marked, L. The area **L** is further carefully located by the inserted figure in front and side view.

memorate the part these men were supposed to have played in the spread of the plague. These events happened less than three hundred years ago.

Those artists who were witnesses of the Black Death have handed down to us some of its horror in the pictures they have painted. Among these is the "Peste de Marseille," by François Gerard. It shows the tragedy of a family; the father on the ground writhes in agony while the mother, seated on a chest by his side, clasps to her body her eldest boy, wrapped in a blanket, too weak to stand; a younger child leans against his mother, watching in terror his dying father. To one side the dead are lying heaped under an awning while convicts are dragging corpses away to burial. In the background stands Bishop Belsunce, religious hero of that plague, who fed the poor, visited the dying, and with full ritual of the church exorcised the plague. "La Peste dans la Ville de Marseille en 1720," painted by J. F. de Tory, the younger, shows the convicts cleaning the esplanade of La Tourette of the decomposing corpses which they are throwing into the open vaults of the bastions. The famous picture by Baron Gros, now in the Louvre, entitled "Les Pestiferes de Jaffa," shows Napoleon touching the pest sores, or buboes, of his stricken soldiers. The part played by Napoleon is somewhat exaggerated in this picture, it would seem, for it is denied that he touched the sick and stated that he ordered them poisoned so that the disease would not spread.

The plague which had existed in London from 1349 reached its height in the great epidemic of 1665. The story of it is told in Defoe's *Journal of the Plague Year*. Although purporting to be an exact account, it is in reality strongly influenced in its pictorial qualities by the epidemic at Marseilles, which occurred some years after that of London. A less exaggerated account of the London epidemic is found in *Pepys' Diary;* he was an eyewitness of it and an adult, while Defoe at the time was only six years old. Pepys, true to his character, was more concerned over the great fire of London in 1666 and the loss of property than he was over the plague and the loss of life. This fire of London did for

England what men had been unable to do. The fire destroyed the infected rats which were the carriers of the disease, and brought an end to the plague in that country.

The relation of rats and mice to the plague was observed

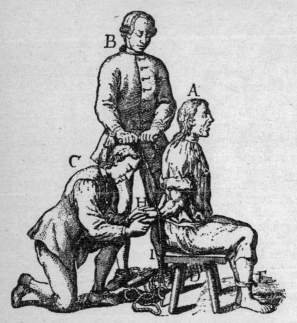

TYING A VICTIM FOR THE STRAPPADO

*Constitutio criminalis Theresiana.* The victim, A, is shown here preparatory to being exposed to the strappado. The rope attached to his arms was run through a pulley in the ceiling, and the executioner, by pulling on the end of the rope, held A suspended from the floor with his arms twisted in their sockets. If mere suspension failed to produce the desired effects, the executioner pulled on the rope and then released it suddenly, thus jerking the victim's arms. If obdurate under this treatment, the victim was weighted down with iron blocks and the procedure repeated. If he survived the application of the three varieties of torture, he was judged innocent and allowed to die of his injuries rather than being executed.

at a very early period, for it was noted that when these animals died in large numbers the plague soon followed, but the causal relation between the two events was not recognized. Only in modern times was it discovered that plague is a bacterial disease of rats which is commonly transmitted to

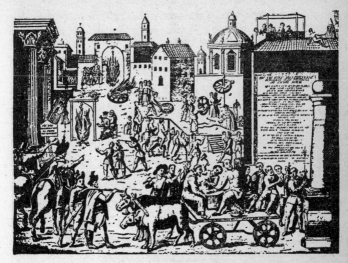

TORTURE AND EXECUTION OF THE PLAGUE-SPREADERS

Milan, 1630; from an engraving of the time. The artist has crowded the events of many days and places all into one picture. On the right is the shop of the barber, Mora, and by it the "column of infamy" already erected. Mora and Piazza, together with the executioners and priests, are shown in a cart in the foreground. The pincers with which the flesh of the victims is to be torn are heating in the charcoal brazier; Mora is having his hand cut off. In the center, but farther back in the picture, the victims are shown having their limbs broken (D) and bent to conform to the wheel (E) upon which they are also shown exposed—the exposure lasted six hours. To the left at M, G, and N are shown the fires in which the bodies were finally consumed, and on the same side, in front of the pillars, is the stream into which their ashes were cast. The column of infamy, which was erected to commemorate the supposed spreading of the plague by these men, was wrecked by a storm in 1788, and in 1803 a house was erected on the site.

man by fleas. The fleas leave the dying rats, and infest men, whom their bite inoculates with the disease. With this knowledge medicine was able to devise the measures that now protect Western countries from the plague. The essential feature of these measures consists in keeping out infected rats.

Even before the rat was recognized as an agent in dissemination of plague, efforts were made to check the

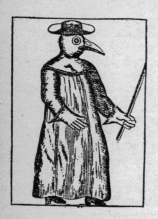
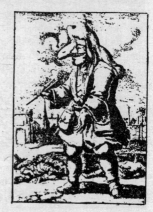

THE PLAGUE DOCTOR

The costume used by physicians during the plague in Marseilles in 1720. The snout was filled with spices presumed to purify the inhaled air. On the right is a German caricature of this dress.

spread of the disease by quarantining travelers at the boundaries of the countries. While this measure impeded the spread of the plague, it was not entirely effective, since no attention was paid to the rats which landed from the infected ships. After the epidemic of 1348 the Venetian Republic established the first official quarantine against suspected persons or ships. The period of detention was forty days and this choice of time had a Biblical significance; Christ and Moses had both remained isolated in the desert for that number of days. The word quarantine is derived from the Italian words *quaranta giorni* meaning forty days. This protection by quarantine was practiced in most countries by the eighteenth century. Jean Jacques Rousseau tells in his *Confessions* of his quarantine at the port of Geneva in the year 1743. Napoleon infringed the quarantine regulations of France on his return from Egypt in 1798; in consequence Abbé Sieyès made a motion in the National Assembly that Napoleon should be shot for his crime.

The effective quarantine developed after it was discovered that the rat was a factor in the transmission of the plague has kept most Western countries free from the disease. The plague caused sixty thousand deaths in Manchuria in 1910-11; it broke out again in 1918, and there were twenty thousand deaths. But there has been no plague in the United States since 1900, when the disease was introduced into San Francisco. The ravages of even the most serious epidemics are quickly forgotten during times of security, and it happens over and over that local authorities attempt, for political or commercial reasons, to deny that the disease has gained a foothold in their community. This occurred in 1900 in San Francisco. The officers of the Federal Health Service insisted, against the denials of the local authorities, that the plague had entered the city. The claim was substantiated by an investigating commission. More than a million rats were caught and destroyed in the city of San Francisco alone, but the disagreement of the local and federal authorities had caused a delay which allowed the disease to spread to the ground squirrels in the neighboring country, and it was necessary to destroy twenty million of these animals. Although a nucleus of the plague still remains with the squirrels, these measures were effective in checking the epidemic; the sacrifice of human life to the plague was limited to less than two hundred deaths. If there had not been this concentrated drive for its eradication the plague would have spread and it is possible that the entire United States might have been devastated by the disease as Europe was in the fourteenth century.

To attempt to stop the plague by treating the sick would today be nearly as futile as were the efforts in medieval times. The physicians of those days protected themselves against the disease by means of suits of leather with leather gauntlets and masks with glass coverings for the eyes and a long snout filled with fumigants for the nose. They carried a wand to feel the pulse so that they might not be forced to touch the sick. They attributed the disease to miasma or corrupt vapors which entered the skin through the open

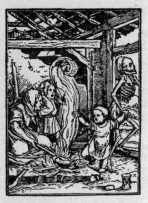

DEATH AND THE CHILD
A woodcut by Hans Holbein.

pores, and forbade bathing for fear that the pores would open wider. They lit fires on which were burned aromatic substances to purify the air; and for the same purpose sprinkled perfumed water in the rooms and on their clothing. Eau de Cologne is a survival of one of these plague waters or essences. The physicians told the healthy to "flee in haste and take much physic," if indeed these two activities could be combined. The best preventive of the plague in those days was administered as "three adverbial pills, quick, far, and late." That is, go quick, go far, and return late. This advice was followed thoroughly by the nobility, and in times of plague they deserted the cities. During the epidemic in London in 1665 George Monck, Duke of Albemarle, remained in the city as the sole representative of the government of King Charles II.

# CHAPTER IX

# PESTILENCE AND PERSONAL LIBERTY

pidemics of pestilence still rage unchecked in countries less civilized than our own, but such epidemics do not arouse concern for our own safety. It is taken for granted by most people that we are immune or that from some law of geographic distribution these diseases cannot extend to our country. In reality we are no more immune than were the people of the Middle Ages. There are few diseases against which geographic barriers are effective. It is only modern preventive measures that keep these diseases out. Asiatic cholera is a disease which is endemic in India, but which does not occur in America now. Nevertheless, in 1832 this disease spread from its Asiatic focus and extended over the greater part of Europe and America. It entered through Quebec and spread from there along the lines of traffic up to the Great Lakes, reaching as far west as the military posts of the upper Mississippi. In the same year it entered New York and by 1840 there were nearly 4,500 deaths from cholera in New York City. In the next two decades some 9,000 persons died in that city from the disease. In 1883 a pandemic started. The disease again reached New York, but by this time the protective measures were in operation. There were only nine deaths in the city. Since then there have been no deaths from cholera in New York, although great epidemics have occurred in other parts of the world. The health examination and quarantine of immigrants are an effective barrier to this disease.

Yellow fever prevented the French from building a canal across the Isthmus of Panama. So great was the mortality from the disease during their work there, that it is said there is a Frenchman buried under every tie of the Panama Railway. Yellow fever was the disease which made Panama the "White man's grave" until General Gorgas introduced the measures which overcame it. No one in this country worries

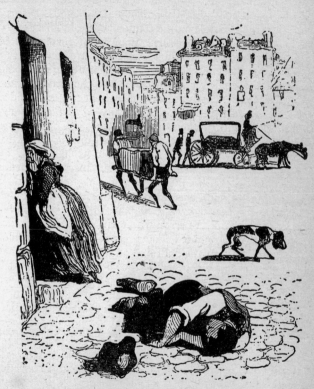

"SOUVENIRS OF THE CHOLERA"

An etching by Daumier. Although cholera has long been known in the Far East, it did not spread to the Western Hemisphere until the nineteenth century; possibly the invention of the steamboat and the consequent greater speed of ocean travel account for this extension of the disease. In the years 1853 and 1854 Asiatic cholera killed 150,000 people in France and in the same decade about 4,000 people in New York City.

now about the possibility of yellow fever occurring here. Yet this disease, during an epidemic in 1793, killed 10 per cent of the population of Philadelphia. The following account describes the conditions: "The consternation of the people of Philadelphia at that period was beyond all bounds. Dismay and affright were visible on the countenances of almost every person. Of those who remained, many shut themselves in their houses and were afraid to walk the streets. . . . The corpses of the most respectable citizens, even those who did not die of the epidemic, were carried to the grave on the shafts of a chaise, the horse driven by a negro, unattended by friends or relatives and without any sort of ceremony. People hastily shifted their course at the sight of a hearse coming toward them. Many never walked on the footpaths, but went into the middle of the street to avoid passing by houses wherein people had died. Acquaintances and friends avoided one another in the street and only signified their regard by a cold nod. The old custom of shaking hands fell into such disuse that many shrank back with affright at even the offer of the hand. A person with crêpe or any appearance of mourning was shunned like a viper, and many prided themselves highly on the skill and address with which they got to the windward of every person they met. Indeed, it is not probable that London, at the last stage of the plague, exhibited stronger marks of terror than were to be seen in Philadelphia from the 24th or 25th of April until pretty late in September. While affairs were in this deplorable state and the people at the lowest ebb of despair, we cannot be astonished at the frightful scenes that were enacted, which seemed to indicate a total dissolution of the bonds of society in the nearest and dearest connections. Who, without horror, can reflect on a husband deserting his wife, united to him perhaps for twenty years, in the last agony; a wife unfeelingly abandoning her husband on his deathbed; parents forsaking their only child without remorse; children ungratefully flying from their parents and resigning them to chance, without an inquiry after their health or safety . . . ?"

While the population of Philadelphia fled in terror before

the disease or shrank from the approach of their fellow-citizens in fear of direct infection, they paid no attention to the mosquitoes which were actually carrying the contagion.

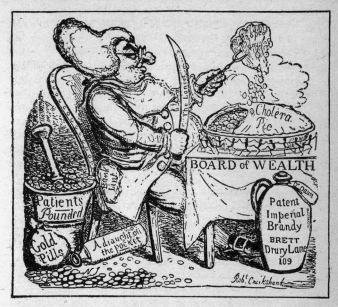

"CHOLERA PIE"

A caricature by Cruikshank indicating a popular belief of the past that physicians became wealthy as a result of epidemic pestilences. Rowlandson drew a similar cartoon showing physicians paying homage to influenza. In the Middle Ages the physicians were sometimes accused of spreading pestilential disease, since they were the only people who profited. The mortality among physicians during these epidemics was, however, extremely high.

The coming of freezing weather—"pretty late in September"—put an end to the epidemic by stopping the activity of the mosquitoes.

It was not until 1881 that the part played by the mosquito in the transmission of yellow fever was suspected, and not until 1900 that it was proved. The prevention of yellow fever then became possible. It was effected by eradicating the stegomia mosquito, which is the carrier of yellow fever.

The treatment of those afflicted with yellow fever is not much more successful under the best medical care today than it was in 1793 when Benjamin Rush stayed in Philadelphia and tried his remedies against the disease. Without the knowledge of the manner in which the disease is transmitted the cities of today would be as defenseless against yellow fever as they were formerly. Ships would still go round Cape Horn instead of taking the shorter route through the Panama Canal. Even if, after immense loss of life, the canal had been built, the continuance of yellow fever in the Canal Zone would lead New York and San Francisco to enforce an absolute quarantine against all ships which had passed through it.

The control acquired over plague and pestilence is an achievement for civilization no less valuable than the control of mechanical power through steam and electricity, upon which all modern industry rests. Just as man has controlled and turned these forces to his aid, so also has he found a beneficial use for one of the pestilences, St. Anthony's fire. Formerly this disease was a cruel affliction that left thousands of maimed victims throughout Europe; today it has been prevented, and not only has it ceased as a pestilence, but its active agent has been turned to the service of the child-bearing woman.

From the ninth to the fourteenth century, and to a less extent until the nineteenth century, there existed in epidemics, particularly in the eastern provinces of France, a plague whose consequences were more horrible than those of leprosy. This plague was called "holy fire," "hell's fire," or "St. Anthony's fire." The last name was given in the eleventh century when the Order of Saint Anthony was founded to take care of the sufferers.

For the medieval Catholics each disease had its patron saint, just as for the ancient Romans each disease had its god. These saints were thought to have the power of both inflicting and curing the disease. In Sir Walter Scott's "Marmion," the impatient Blount addresses Squire Eustace, who is listening to a long tirade from the Abbess:

> "Saint Anton fire thee! Wilt thou stand
> All day, with bonnet in thy hand
> To hear the lady preach?"

St. Valentine, in addition to his kindly interest in lovers in the springtime, had especial care of epileptics. Thomas Neogorgus writes in "The Popish Kingdom" (1570):

"St. Valentine, besides, to such as does his power despise
 The falling sickness sends, and helps the man that to him cries."

The association of a saint with a disease was usually determined by the manner in which the saint died. St. Agattin was tortured cruelly before she was put to death. Her breasts were cut off. Hence, disease of the female breast fell to her charge and she was the patron saint of nursing-women. St. Apollonia had her jaw broken and her teeth dashed out. Prayers were directed to her for her intercession in toothache. She was represented in paintings as holding a tooth or a pair of pincers in her hand. Occasionally the disease was named for its patron saint, as in the cases of St. Vitus' dance and St. Anthony's fire. The use of the saint's name extended sometimes to fields other than that of medicine; the carriage called a fiacre was named after St. Fiacre, the patron saint of diseases of the rectum.

The disease, St. Anthony's fire, existed in several forms. In one form the abdominal viscera were affected and, although the victims suffered much pain, death was fortunately speedy. In its common form the disease affected the extremities; an icy chill developed in the arms and legs and this was succeeded by a torturing burning sensation. As though consumed by internal fire, the limbs became black, and then shriveled and fell from the body. Some of those afflicted with the disease died, but many recovered, maimed and distorted even by the loss of all their limbs, so that there was left only the trunk and head. The disease struck hardest at the pregnant woman; abortion followed even mild attacks.

Until the end of the sixteenth century the only recourse for the sufferers was in pilgrimage to the shrines of St. Anthony. They were cared for there by the holy men who wore as their distinguishing mark a letter T in blue on the left shoulder of their robes. The T probably represented the crutch of those who sought their care. The portals of the hospitals of St. Anthony were painted red or flame-colored. An old woodcut of St. Anthony shows him with a hog, which was his inseparable companion, peering from behind his robe, while before him stands a maimed sufferer braced on his crutch, holding up an arm from which burst flames to typify the sensations and destructions of his disease. As late as the eighteenth century the hospital of the Order of St. Anthony in Vienna had a collection of withered and blackened limbs, relics of the afflicted who had received succor there.

In 1597 the medical faculty at Marburg investigated all the likely causes of the disease. They came to the conclusion that it was due to eating bread made from rye blighted with a fungous growth called ergot. This fungus affected the rye particularly in seasons that were wet and cold. It appeared in the heads of grain as greatly enlarged black kernels. In France the physician to the Duke of Sully in 1630 independently reached the same conclusion and proved the poisonous nature of ergot by animal experimentation. The epidemics of ergotism continued for a century and a half more before recognition of their cause became general. Medicine had won knowledge which could be used to control the scourge of St. Anthony's fire; but in times of famine, dire need has occasionally prevailed over knowledge, and epidemics have occurred among the peasants of Russia down to 1888.

The fact that poisoning by blighted or spurred rye caused abortion in pregnant women was known for many centuries by those "wise women" who were midwives. At a very early date they gave from five to nine of the grains, but by reason

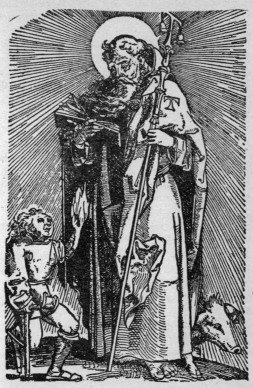

ST. ANTHONY AND A VICTIM OF HIS DISEASE

The monastic order of St. Anthony was devoted to the care of sufferers from ergotism. The sufferer is shown here using a crutch to support a withered leg while his raised hand has burst into flames, symbolic of the sensations of the disease. On the left shoulder of St. Anthony's robe is the T representing his order and probably also designating the crutch of those afflicted with St. Anthony's disease. The hog which was the inseparable companion of this saint is shown here peering from behind the robe.

of superstition never an even number, to hasten the birth of children. In the eighteenth century the fact that small doses of ergot caused the uterus to contract forcibly without poisoning the women to whom it was administered became known to some of the physicians of Europe. They used it to a limited extent in their obstetrical practice. The most valuable use of ergot was, however, developed in America. The drug was first used here by Dr. Stevens of Massachusetts, but Dr. Hosack of New York was the first to use it to stop hemorrhage from the uterus. After the child is born, the area on the wall of the uterus from which the placenta is detached is left raw and bleeding. The hemorrhage from this area is normally stopped by contraction of the uterus. If this contraction is feeble, profuse and even dangerous hemorrhage continues. The powerful contraction which results from the administration of ergot assists materially in stopping the hemorrhage.

The control of the pestilence of Saint Anthony's fire by measures designed to prevent the use of blighted rye met with no active opposition. Most people are familiar with poisoning; the relation between eating poisonous material and the pain and suffering which follow is learned in early childhood both by experience and from the warnings of others. The cause and effect are obvious in poisoning; no supernatural element need be called in to account for them. The mere spreading of the information that blighted rye was a poison was sufficient to prevent pestilence. When the people had obtained this knowledge they ceased to eat blighted rye, avoiding it as people avoid eating toadstools. Likewise the control of pestilential diseases transmitted to man from parasitic insects meets with no great opposition. The relation between fleas and bubonic plague, between anopheles mosquitoes and malaria, between stegomia mosquitoes and yellow fever, and between body lice and typhus fever is not so obvious as is the cause of poisoning. But parasitic insects are of themselves annoying. For this reason, if for no other, the population as a whole raises no objection if the more enlightened of its members bring forward laws embodying measures for the eradication of these insects. Such measures do not affect the ideas of personal liberty of those who pass the laws. They are general, civic matters. When such laws are in effect most people are unaware of the activities which are carried out under them. Similarly, the public readily agrees to the quarantine of immigrants who carry cholera. The quarantine affects only the freedom of the immigrants; it does not disturb the citizens. On the other hand, the control of pestilence meets not only with lack of coöperation, but even active opposition, when the measures designed to prevent disease involve the participation of each individual. The prevention of smallpox by vaccination is an example of this personal participation in the struggle to prevent pestilence. Many persons are neglectful of vaccination and some resent the enforcement of the laws requiring that they submit to vaccination. For this reason such laws have even been repealed in some communities.

Smallpox has been present in India from remote times, and its marks are found on Egyptian mummies entombed three thousand years ago. The slowness of transportation in ancient times kept the disease from spreading widely. A traveler infected with smallpox in Egypt either died or had passed the stage where he could transmit the disease by the time he had made the journey to Europe. Smallpox did not reach Greece and Rome during the period of classical civilization. It came into Europe about the tenth century. Five more centuries passed before it was widely distributed there. The first great epidemic of the disease in London occurred in 1628. Smallpox, once established in Europe, showed itself to be no respecter of persons. Charles IX of France had his nose so badly scarred by it that he appeared to have two noses; Louis XIV had the disease and Louis XV died of it. Queen Mary II of England died of smallpox in 1694. In the century following her death 60,000,000 persons in Europe died of smallpox. The historian Macaulay, commenting on the death of the queen, gives this description of its ravages: "That disease, over which science has since achieved a succession of glorious and beneficent victories, was the most terrible of all the ministers of death. The havoc of the plague had been far more rapid; but plague has visited our shores only once or twice within living memory; and smallpox was always present, filling the churchyard with corpses, tormenting with constant fear all whom it had not yet stricken, leaving on those whose lives were spared the hideous traces of its power, turning the babe into a changeling at which the mother shuddered, making the eyes and cheeks of the betrothed maiden objects of horror to the lover. Towards the end of the year 1694 this pestilence was more than usually severe. At length the infection spread to the palace and reached the young and blooming Queen. She received the intimation of her danger with true greatness of soul. She gave orders that every lady of her bedchamber, every maid of honor, nay every menial servant, who had not had the smallpox should instantly leave Kensington House."

The Queen was thirty-three at the time of her death. Her husband, William III, survived her by eight years. He was sickly and was continually worried about his health. He sometimes wrote to foreign physicians under an assumed name in order thus to obtain an unprejudiced opinion of his illness. The opinions were always unfavorable. He suffered with malaria and probably had tuberculosis, for he was for a long time tormented with a racking cough and at autopsy the left lung was found diseased. He also suffered with boils, and to treat them he dusted his skin with a mixture of flour and dried and powdered eyes of crabs. His death was hastened by a fall from his horse, from which he suffered a fracture of the right collarbone.

The Colonists of New England were brought in contact with smallpox from two sources. In the early part of the sixteenth century the Spaniards introduced the disease into Mexico. Within a short period thereafter three and a half million people there died of the disease. It spread to the American Indians, and one-half of them are said to have died of it in a short time. The Indian tribes along the New England coast were greatly weakened by an epidemic of the disease which occurred a short time before the Pilgrims of the *Mayflower* landed. In the words of Cotton Mather, who saw good for his people in evil to others: "The Indians in these Parts had newly, even about a Year or Two Before, been visited with such a prodigious Pestilence, as carried away not one-tenth but Nine Parts of Ten (Yea 'tis Nineteen of Twenty) among them; so that the woods were almost clear of these pernicious creatures to make Room for a better Growth." The disease of the Indians spread to the Colonists. During the next century six epidemics occurred in Boston. The last of these started from a case brought into Boston in 1721 on the English ship, *The Sea Horse,* sailing from the Barbados. More than one-half of the population of Boston, then about 11,000, took the disease. It was during this epidemic that the practice of inoculation was used in America for the first time.

Prior to the introduction of vaccination, inoculation was the only preventive for smallpox. This practice had been used for centuries among the people of the Far East. It consists of infecting a minute wound with pus taken from a smallpox sore. A mild case of smallpox develops in the person thus inoculated. Although the disease acquired in this manner is rarely fatal, it nevertheless confers as much immunity as does the disease when acquired from contact with a case of smallpox and transmitted in the usual mode by way of the saliva and nasal secretions. Inoculation was introduced into England by Lady Mary Montagu, wife of the British ambassador at the Turkish court. In 1717 she wrote to a friend: "I am going to tell you a thing that I imagine will make you wish yourself here. The smallpox, so fatal and general amongst us, is here entirely harmless by the invention of ingrafting, which is the term they give it. There is a set of old women who make it their business to perform the operation every autumn in the month of September, when the great heat has abated. People send to one another to know if any of their families has a mind to have smallpox. They make parties for this purpose, and when they meet (commonly 15 or 16 together) the old woman comes with a nutshell full of matter of the best sort of smallpox, and asks what vein you pleased to have opened. She immediately rips open that which you offer to her with a large needle (which gives you no more pain than a common scratch), and puts into the vein as much venom as can lie upon the end of a needle, and after binds up the little wound with a hollow bit of shell; and in this manner opens four or five veins. The children or young patients play together all the rest of the day and are in perfect health until the eighth day, then fever seizes them and they keep their beds two days, very seldom three. They have rarely about twenty or thirty [pocks] on their faces, which never mark, and in eight days' time they are as well as before their illness. Everywhere thousands undergo this operation and the French ambassador says pleasantly that they take the smallpox here by way of diversion, as they take the waters in other countries. There is no example of anyone that has died in it, and you may well believe I am satisfied of the safety of the experiment, since I intend to try it upon my dear little son. I am patriotic enough to take pains to bring this useful invention into fashion in England."

The prevention of smallpox, however, was not received in England with the same patriotic spirit which led Lady Montagu to try to introduce it. Both the practice and its sponsor were denounced violently. Lord Wharncliffe, in his edition of the letters and works of Lady Montagu, says: "What an arduous, what a fearful, and, we may add, what a thankless enterprise it was, nobody is now in the least aware. Those who have heard her applauded for it ever since they were born, may naturally conclude, that when once the experiment had been made, and had proved successful, she would have nothing to do but to sit down triumphant and receive the thanks and blessing of her countrymen. But it was far otherwise. Lady Mary protested, that in the four or five years immediately succeeding her arrival at home, she seldom passed a day without repenting of her patriotic undertaking; and she vowed that she never would have attempted it if she had foreseen the vexation, the persecution, and even the obloquy it brought upon her. The clamors raised against the practice, and of course against her, were beyond belief. The faculty all rose in arms to a man, fore-telling failure and the most disastrous consequences; the clergy descanted from their pulpits on the impiety of thus seeking to take events out of the hands of Providence; the common people were taught to hoot at her as an unnatural mother who had risked the life of her own child."

In Massachusetts, Cotton Mather played the rôle of Lady Mary Montagu and, like her, aroused great antagonism from his attempt to introduce inoculation. The story of his efforts can be told no better than in the words of Oliver Wendell Holmes: "In 1721, this disease [smallpox], after a respite of 19 years, again appeared as an epidemic. In that year it was that Cotton Mather, browsing, as was his wont, on all the printed fodder that came within reach of his ever-grinding mandibles, came upon an account of inoculation as practiced in Turkey, contained in the *Philosophical Transactions*. He spoke of it to several physicians, who paid little heed to his story, for they knew his medical whims and had probably been bored, as we say nowadays, many of them, with listening to his 'Angel of Bethesda.' . . .

"The Reverend Mather—I use a mode of expression he often employed when speaking of his honored brethren—the Reverend Mather was right this time, and the irreverent doctors who laughed at him were wrong."

One physician, Dr. Boylston, followed Mather's suggestion. Holmes continues: "On the 27th day of June, 1721, Zabdiel Boylston, of Boston, inoculated his only son for smallpox—the first person ever submitted to the operation in the New World. The story of the fierce resistance to the introduction of the practice; of how Boylston was mobbed and Mather had a hand grenade thrown in at his window; of how William Douglas, the Scotchman, 'always positive, and sometimes accurate' as was neatly said of him, at once deprecated the practice and tried to get the credit of sug-gesting it; and how Lawrence Dalhonde, the Frenchman, testified to its destructive consequences; of how Edmund Massey, lecturer of St. Alban's, preached against sinfully endeavoring to alter the course of nature by presumptuous interposition, which he would leave to the atheist and the scoffer, the heathen and the unbeliever, which in the face of his sermons, afterwards reprinted in Boston, many of our New England clergy stood up boldly in the defense of the practice. . . . Set this good hint of Cotton Mather against that letter of his to John Richards, recommending the search after witch-marks and the application of the water ordeal, which means throw your grandmother into the water, if she has a mole on her arm;—if she swims, she is a witch and must be hanged; if she sinks, the Lord have mercy on her soul!'"

The practice of inoculation was gradually extended and did much good in the prevention of smallpox. It has, however, one great disadvantage. The individual inoculated has true smallpox, and although the attack is very mild, nevertheless other persons may acquire the disease from him just as they would from an ordinary case of smallpox. The small-pox acquired from an inoculated person is as severe and fatal a disease as when acquired from an active case of smallpox. The inoculated person, in protecting himself, might at the same time become the center from which an epidemic of smallpox started. The very mildness of inoculated smallpox made it dangerous. People had always avoided houses where there was a case of smallpox. It was natural to flee from a pestilence which killed off a third or a fourth of those it attacked. But the inoculated smallpox was so mild that they lost the horror of the disease and no longer avoided the spread of the infection. Inoculation was successful in preventing an outbreak of the disease only when everyone in the community was inoculated; otherwise the inoculation of a single person might start an epidemic of smallpox in which many persons would lose their lives. For this reason the practice of inoculation was forbidden by law after the introduction of vaccination.

Two centuries ago when inoculation was practiced the quarantine of those with smallpox was not carried out effectively, as it is today in most countries. People were left largely to their own resources in avoiding those who had disease. The inadequacy of the quarantine against smallpox at as late a date as 1864 is made evident from a few examples

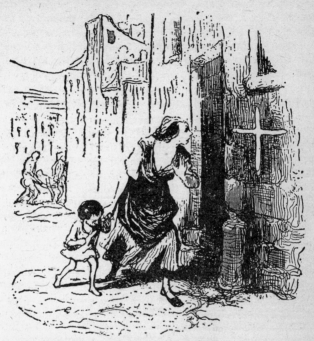

THE QUARANTINE

An etching by Daumier. In the time of Queen Elizabeth houses infected with plague were marked with a green cross, and during later epidemics with a red cross and the words, "Lord Have Mercy on Us." The word quarantine is from the Italian meaning forty days, which, for Biblical reasons, was the duration of isolation.

given by Sir James Simpson during an effort on his part to introduce compulsory isolation. At the time he wrote vaccination as a preventive of smallpox had replaced the practice of inoculation. Commenting on the prevalence of smallpox in

Great Britain and the indifference of the public toward the deaths which could be prevented, he says: "Such figures as these (9,425 deaths in the year 1864) scarcely convey to the mind an adequate idea of the deplorable loss of life still resulting among us from the ravages of this one malady; the more so as the mortality of the disease is distributed through the whole scattered population of the island. But if in any one year some overwhelming catastrophe destroyed all the living population of the counties of Nairn or Kinross; or swept away every living inhabitant of the cathedral cities of Litchfield, Ripon, or Wells; or slaughtered four or five regiments of soldiers; or smothered as many as five or six times the number of members of the House of Commons— such an event would assuredly appall and terrify the public and its guardians; and the strongest measures would, no doubt, be called for, with the view of preventing the recurrence of the catastrophe, provided its prevention were at all possible. Is the similar amount of human slaughter to which our population is constantly subject by smallpox—not once, but continuously, not one year, but each year—preventable? I believe that it is so; and I believe further that the hygienic measures required for effecting this prevention would be found neither specially difficult nor expensive to the country, while they would save annually hundreds, if not thousands, of our population from death, by a disease which, even when it spares life, too often leaves permanent lesions and a broken and damaged constitution.

"The Legislature has no scruples in interfering in some other diseases to as great or indeed to a greater extent. It enforces, for instance, the isolation of any individual affected with insanity, be he rich or poor, who is a homicidal lunatic, endangering the lives of others. If, by a law which no one thinks harsh or severe, lunatics are prevented from destroying the lives of their fellow-men, why should it be thought harsh or severe that people affected with smallpox should be prevented from dealing out destruction and death to all the susceptible with whom they happened to come in contact? Homicidal lunatics do not destroy in Great Britain some eight or ten, on an average, of their fellow-men. Smallpox patients yearly destroy, on the contrary, hundreds instead of units of their fellow-men in the islands.

"The great object of preventing the diffusion of smallpox in any city, or village, or hamlet, by the stamping-out measure which I have ventured to suggest in this communication would consist, of course, chiefly, when practicable, in isolation of the very first cases. Some time ago a professional friend, to whom I was explaining these views, objected to them, that in the case of the town of Leith, which was the habitat of smallpox in 1861 and 1862, the disease was at one time too diffuse to apply them. Dr. Patterson of Leith, however, has kindly informed me that at the time of the visitation of the malady he made an official inquiry into its origin, and found it to be this: A beggar woman, or tramp from Newcastle, brought in the course of her wanderings, to Leith, a child lately affected with smallpox, and with the crusts of the eruption upon it. In Leith she became an inmate of a lodging-house in a 'bank' or block of buildings full of lodgings for the poorest of the poor. Many of the lodgers in these other houses, with their children, visited the room where the woman and the sick child resided. By the time Dr. Patterson was requested by the magistrates to inspect the tenement, several persons were already dead of smallpox caught from this imported case. The disease soon spread to Leith; and, as I am informed by the registrar of the town, 99 human beings were destroyed by it, and much suffering and sickness produced among the many hundreds in the town who caught the disorder and recovered. But if that first case or cases had been obliged to be reported on at once, and had been forthwith isolated in the hospital or elsewhere, all this unnecessary amount of human mortality and disease would have been avoided; nor could the isolation and maintenance of the first case, or of the first ten or twenty cases, have cost as much money as the purchase of the coffins for the 99 who died. The blowing up of the powder magazine in the fort of Leith would not likely produce nearly so much danger and destruction of life among the inhabitants of Leith as the advent of the beggar woman and her infected child. Yet how carefully do we guard against the one danger, and how carelessly do we treat the other!"

The reporting of all cases of infectious disease, required by law, and the isolation of such cases, are so much a matter of course today in civilized countries that it is difficult to understand the indifference and even opposition to these matters that existed only a few years ago. Such circumstances as the following, given by Simpson, would be inconceivable today: "Several instances have been communicated to me of beggars, in the streets of Edinburgh and elsewhere, importuning for charity by lifting up their children with smallpox encrustations still upon them, almost against the very faces of those from whom they ask alms, and infecting with the malady those whom they subjected to this outrage. Not long ago, a woman with her face and hands encrusted with smallpox was seen selling sweetmeats to the children of a school in Glasgow. . . ."

Today every physician is required by law, under heavy penalty, to report to the health authorities all cases of acutely contagious disease that come under his observation. As soon as the report is made the health authorities isolate the person affected with the disease. This isolation takes place without the participation of each individual citizen. It is directed against the personal liberty of only those who have the disease, and against them there is, along with pity, always a feeling akin to animosity. Isolation of those sick with smallpox cannot alone hold the disease in check, for many cases are not detected until the disease is well advanced and there has been opportunity for its spread. Vaccination is a necessary part of the prevention. But vaccination involves active participation by everyone. The laws for compulsory vaccination and the enforcement of these laws are a better indication of the intelligence of a community and its civilization than is the thoroughness of the quarantine which is enforced by civic officials as part of their duty.

The practice of vaccination was introduced in 1798 by Edward Jenner of Gloucestershire, England. In the countryside where he lived there had long been a tradition that dairymaids who had contracted cowpox from the cows that they milked did not take smallpox. Cowpox produces sores both on the udder of a cow and on the human skin which resemble the sores of smallpox, but the disease is very mild. It is not contagious. Early in his medical studies Jenner conceived the idea of applying on a large scale this method of preventing smallpox. Later when he studied under John Hunter in London he told him of his idea. Hunter gave him advice that was characteristic of that great surgeon and investigator. He said: "Don't think, try; be patient, be accurate." Jenner returned to his home. For eighteen years he patiently collected his observations on the protection against smallpox given by cowpox. In 1796 he was ready to try his idea. He performed his first vaccination upon a country boy, James Phipps, using matter from the arms of a milkmaid, Sarah Nelmes, who had acquired the cowpox from the animals she milked. Two months later he inoculated the boy with pus from a case of smallpox. The boy did not contract the disease.

Jenner's enthusiasm led him to prepare a report based on this one experiment. He submitted this report for publication in the *Transactions* of the Royal Society. It was rejected. In the next two years Jenner collected twenty-three cases of successful vaccination and in 1798 he published his book, *Inquiry into the Cause and Effects of Variolæ Vaccinæ*. This book established the thesis that vaccination with cowpox protects from smallpox.

The reception accorded to Jenner's work was the same as that usually accorded to great humane innovations. A few people received it with great acclaim, a somewhat greater number opposed it violently, and the vast majority were indifferent. Napoleon at once had all of his troops vaccinated if they had not already had smallpox. In America the President, John Adams, presided over the American Academy of Arts and Sciences, at a meeting during which the announcement of Jenner's work was made. In 1800 Dr. Waterhouse of Cambridge, Massachusetts, performed the first vaccination in this country on his five-year-old son. In the next year

Thomas Jefferson had the members of his family vaccinated. The practice spread thereafter. In 1812 a tribe of American Indians sent Jenner a belt and a string of wampum, as they

AN

# *INQUIRY*

INTO

## THE CAUSES AND EFFECTS

OF

## THE VARIOLÆ VACCINÆ,

A DISEASE

DISCOVERED IN SOME OF THE WESTERN COUNTIES OF ENGLAND,

PARTICULARLY

## *GLOUCESTERSHIRE,*

AND KNOWN BY THE NAME OF

# THE COW POX.

BY EDWARD JENNER, M.D. F.R.S. &c.

——— — QUID NOBIS CERTIUS IPSIS
SENSIBUS ESSE POTEST, QUO VERA AC FALSA NOTEMUS.

LUCRETIUS.

London:

PRINTED, FOR THE AUTHOR,

BY SAMPSON LOW, Nº. 7, BERWICK STREET, SOHO:

AND SOLD BY LAW, AVE-MARIA LANE; AND MURRAY AND HIGHLEY, FLEET STREET

1798.

TITLE PAGE OF JENNER'S PAPER ON VACCINATION

The application of the facts presented in this paper has probably saved more lives than the total of all lives lost in war.

said: "In token of our acceptance of your precious gift, and we beseech the great spirit to take care of you in this world, and in the land of spirits."

The gratitude to Jenner shown by the American Indians was not shared by everyone. The practice of vaccination was opposed, particularly in England. This opposition at once resorted to the usual formula. "Smallpox is a visitation from God and originates in man, but cowpox is produced by presumptuous, impious men. The former Heaven ordained, the latter is perhaps a daring and profane violation of our holy order." The society of anti-vaccinationists was founded in the year that Jenner published his work and still continues actively. Its recruits come from that large class of persons who mistake fanatical opposition for intelligent criticism. Many of its members continue to confuse vaccination and inoculation. They still believe that vaccine virus is transmitted from person to person as it was in Jenner's early experiment. In reality vaccine virus is obtained from calves and is a vastly purer product than the cleanest milk.

Indifference and forgetfulness have been the greatest obstacles to vaccination. Unfortunately, experience is not a hereditary quality. Each generation has to have the necessity of vaccination impressed upon it by an epidemic, and often several epidemics, at the cost of many lives. In 1896, on the hundredth anniversary of the discovery of vaccination, there was a severe epidemic of smallpox in Gloucestershire, where Jenner lived and where he did his work. Ignorance and low valuation of human life are revealed by the prevalence of smallpox in America. In two states the laws requiring vaccination have been repealed in the face of a rising mortality from this preventable disease.

Simpson, writing in 1847, says of vaccination: "During the long European wars connected with and following the French Revolution, it has been calculated that five or six millions of human lives were lost. In Europe, vaccination has already preserved from death a greater number of human beings than were sacrificed during the course of these wars. The lancet of Jenner has saved far more human lives than the sword of Napoleon destroyed. On these devastating European wars England lavished millions of money and freely bestowed honors, peerages, and heavy annual pensions upon the soldiers who were most successful in fighting her battles and destroying their fellow-men. She grudgingly rewarded Jenner with 30,000 pounds for saving 30,000 of her subjects annually."

What a contrast: Napoleon and Jenner! Napoleon so well known that even the idiosyncrasies of his posture and dress are common knowledge. Jenner unknown even by name to most people. Few indeed would recognize a portrait of this English country gentleman, blond and blue-eyed, a bird-fancier, a musician on the flute and violin, a minor poet of some distinction, and one of the supreme benefactors of all humanity. Perhaps if personal worth were weighed in the scales of human welfare, Napoleon's greatest claim to distinction would come from the fact that he was an ardent supporter of Jenner.

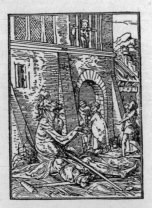

THE CRIPPLED BEGGAR
From a woodcut of Hans Holbein.

# CHAPTER X

## PESTILENCE AND MORALISTS

ost civilizations are willing to accept protection from pestilence when the measures involved require only the eradication of insects, quarantine, the draining of swamps, and similar general measures. Whenever the control of pestilence requires the personal participation of those who are to be protected, as in smallpox, opposition develops in all but the most enlightened civilization. But when concepts of morals are involved in the prevention, fanaticism is aroused even in the highest civilization. There are two pestilences which thus unfortunately involve moral conceptions. They are the plagues of syphilis and gonorrhea. Against them medicine has developed methods of control. They could be eradicated. But as yet civilization has not advanced entirely beyond the ancient belief that disease is imposed by God in vengeance for sin. It still rejects protection. Until the protection is accepted these plagues will continue to exact death and suffering on a scale which probably exceeds that of any one of the medieval plagues.

Those who today still look on syphilis and gonorrhea as punishments for sin have not progressed beyond the ideas of medieval Europe. There was an excuse for the Emperor Maximilian when he issued his edict in 1495 declaring syphilis to be an affliction from God for the sins of men. The civilization of his time had not progressed beyond such beliefs. Cotton Mather declared syphilis was a punishment "which the Just Judgment of God has reserved for our late Ages. . . ." His ignorance was as great as his religious bigotry which led him to drown helpless old women for witchcraft. Ignorance and bigotry are the twin allies of the plagues of syphilis and gonorrhea.

The reason that syphilis and gonorrhea are not viewed as pestilences, which they really are, lies in the fact that they are involved in one of the greatest problems of civilization—the relation of the sexes. The very name "venereal diseases" —diseases of Venus—imputes to them a divine origin and brands them with the stigma which purists have always given to sex. The venereal diseases are involved in that great sex problem about which the ideals and ethics of Christian civilization center. Its ethics, its art, and its literature are instinct with prurient caution in regard to sex. Thus sex is kept a problem. A true perspective on sexual matters is lost because the facts are obscured with secrecy and distorted in the imagination.

The word moral has been corrupted from its proper meaning. It was originally the knowledge of right and wrong. It has come now to signify only right and wrong in the conventions applied to sex. If one were to say correctly that a man who robbed him was immoral most persons hearing the remark would deduce a sexual crime. False conception of morals gives to the word a significance of sex. Moralists who use the word in this sense carry their thoughts of sex only as far as the act which concerns both the male and the female. Their interest centers there. This conception may be an end in itself for these moralists, but it is not the end for woman. She, not the moralists, bears the children. It is certainly not moral in any sense of the word that women and children infected with syphilis or gonorrhea shall pay in the coin of suffering for some man's lack of morality. Our conventional morality sees in the venereal diseases a punishment for sin even to the third generation.

These false moralists use the fear of syphilis and gonorrhea as a bar against illicit sex relations. The very presence of the plagues shows the failure of this bar. The diseases are no more controlled under the moral standards of today than they were two centuries ago, when a moralist expressed the standard prevailing then by saying that the prostitute was the "angel that spread her protecting wings over the virtue of pure women." The moralists and the ignorant are themselves the panderers, the pimps, of the venereal plagues. There is neither sense nor justice in founding morals on disease. Here is no question of right or wrong. All disease is immoral; but no one

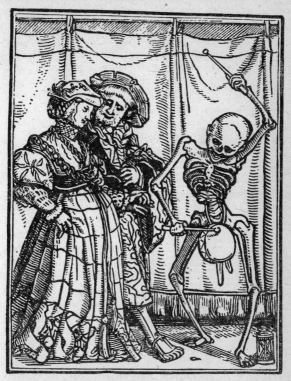

**DEATH AND THE NEWLY MARRIED LADY**
From a woodcut of Hans Holbein.

disease is more so than another. The morality of the body is health.

A continuous epidemic of syphilis has lasted now for at least five centuries. Its origin is a question over which historians argue. Some maintain that syphilis occurred in Europe at an early date and was known to ancient civilizations. According to this view the great epidemic which started in the fifteenth century was simply a recrudescence and general dissemination of an old disease. Others maintain that syphilis was a new disease brought into Europe from the island of Haiti by the sailors of Columbus, and spread throughout the civilized world by the travelers, soldiers, and explorers. The preponderance of evidence points to America as the source of the disease; but the evidence is not absolute.

Syphilis often attacks the bones and leaves definite marks by which it can be recognized after death. Skeletons of ancient peoples in China, Egypt, and Europe have been examined with this point in view. While the marks of many other diseases, such as deforming rheumatism, are found in the skeletons, these marks have also been found in the skeletons of cave bears. Thus far no prehistoric or even pre-Columbian skeleton found in Eurasia shows evidence of syphilis. There are marks on them which have been mistaken for those of syphilis, but these marks are now definitely proved to have occurred post mortem through the action of insects and fungus growths. Furthermore, the physicians of medieval times, whatever may be said of their methods of treatment, were keen observers of illness and it is improbable that they would have failed to detect a disease which at times presents such striking symptoms as does syphilis. If syphilis existed it would not have been overlooked by such keen observers in respect to sexual matters as were Boccaccio and Chaucer; Rabelais mentions it frequently in the sixteenth century. Many of the early references to venereal disease, as in the Bible or other ancient writings, have been believed by some observers to indicate syphilis, but they were more probably gonorrhea. The diseases were often confused. There is no question about the antiquity of gonorrhea in Europe and Asia.

One of the earliest records of tropical medicine was made by Gonzalo Fernandez de Oviedo. He was raised among the pages in the palace of King Ferdinand and Queen Isabella, and was at Barcelona in 1493 when Columbus returned from the island of Haiti. He was intimately acquainted with most of the men who had made the voyage and many of them he knew were ill of a disease which they had contracted in America. Twenty years after Columbus's voyage Ferdinand sent Oviedo to America as superintendent over the gold and silver mines. After a residence of twelve years Oviedo wrote a natural history of the Spanish possessions and dedicated it to Emperor Charles V. He describes a disease known as bubas, or yaws, which, he says, is a very ancient disease in those localities. Oviedo identifies bubas with syphilis, for he says bubas is "no other than the pocks [syphilis] which rageth and hath power over all Europe, especially among the Frenchmen. . . . I can assure your Imperial majesty that this disease which is new in Europe, is well known in the Antille islands lately discovered, and so very common there, that almost everyone of the Spaniards who lay with the Indian women contracted it from them. Thus it was imported from thence into Spain, by those who returned with Columbus after his first or second voyage."

Dr. Roderic Diaz is believed to have witnessed the landing of syphilis in Europe. He wrote a book on the subject dedicated to John III, king of Portugal, which is headed: *Treatise Entitled, Fruit of All Saints Against the Disease of the Island of Española . . . to the Common and General Good of those Suffering from the Disease in Question; Commonly Called Bubas.* . . . Diaz had treated syphilis in several of the sailors of Columbus; among these was the pilot, Pinzon, of Palos.

Gabriel Fallopius, the anatomist, after wandering all over Europe "in order to discover the hidden Secrets of Nature," a practice very common with the medieval physicians as it had been also with those of Greece, wrote in regard to the origin of syphilis: ". . . Amongst the Genoese was Christopher Columbus, a Man of remarkable Genius, who is called Colonus by Peter Martyr, a careful Writer concerning the Indies. . . . For this Columbus, Ferdinand and Isabella ordered a Frigate to be fitted out, and three Pinnaces . . . with which he arrived at the West Indies. . . . There was found there, 'tis true, most precious Gold, and great Plenty of it was brought from thence, together with Aboundance of Pearls; but there was also a thorn joined to the Rose, and Aloes mixed with the Honey. For Columbus brought back his Vessels laden with the French Disease. There the Disease is mild, like the Itch amongst us, but transplanted hither it is become so fierce and unmerciful, as to infect and corrupt the Head, Eyes, Nose, Palate, Skin, Flesh, Bones, Ligaments, and at last the whole Bowels."

The belief that syphilis was the same disease as yaws of the West Indies was until recently generally accepted. In an American book of popular medicine of the year 1730, *Every Man his own Doctor or the Poor Planters Physician*, it is stated: ". . . And because the symptoms are much the same, it is very probable that one was a graft of the other. The pious Spaniards catched it from their negro mistresses in the West Indies and had the honor of propagating it from there to all the rest of the world."

Unfortunately, the relation between bubas or yaws and syphilis is not as clear as would appear from these early statements. Recent investigations have shown that although the organism causing yaws resembles the organism of syphilis, there are nevertheless slight differences. Possibly the natives had both yaws and syphilis, or possibly the organism of yaws caused syphilis in Europeans and by the general process of evolution became the organism of modern syphilis—or possibly syphilis did not come from the natives, after all.

If syphilis was brought into Europe by the sailors of Columbus, certainly conditions were ideal for its reception. In 1493 Charles VIII of France "who from the largeness of his head was called Great Head, and also sur-named hump-backed," claimed the kingdom of Naples as his by hereditary right on the death of Charles, Count of Main. His claim was disputed by the Neapolitans, and Charles VIII gathered an army of mercenaries to take the kingdom by force. In August of 1494 he led his army into Italy and entered Naples in the following February. Toward the end of May he left the kingdom in charge of Gilbert, Count de Montpensier, with an army of 6,000 men. A few days later king Ferdinand broke a treaty he had made some years before with Charles VIII and sent an army into Naples. In this army there were a number of men who had been to the West Indies the previous year and who were still infected with the disease they had contracted there. In recounting the subsequent transfer of the disease to the French, John Astruc, "Physician to his present Majesty the King of France," Louis XIV, says: "And therefore it is by no means strange that many of the Neapolitans should be infected with the same Distemper, as they served under the same Colours, and had to do with the same women who followed the Camp. And for the same reason the Contagion would not but soon be communicated by one or both of them to the French, for as the success of the War continued doubtful the same towns were taken and recovered by both Parties, 'tis plain, that the French also must have had Communication with the same Women who had lain with the Spaniards and Neapolitans, and thus the seeds of the Venereal Disease must have naturally passed from one to the other."

In 1496 Count Gilbert who had been left by Charles VIII died; his army fell into factions, and was expelled from Naples. Those that remained of the 6,000 mercenaries ultimately scattered to their own countries. Their various routes were marked by the spread of syphilis. It appeared in France, Germany, Switzerland, Holland, and Greece in 1496, in Scotland in 1497, and in Hungary and Russia in 1499. The spread of syphilis to the remaining parts of the known world was effected by the great voyagers of the fifteenth and sixteenth centuries. Vasco da Gama carried it on his ships to India in 1498, Europeans brought it to China in 1505, and by 1569 it had been smuggled into Japan. The Jews and Mohammedans, who were driven out of Spain by Ferdinand and Isabella after the conquest of Granada, carried the disease to Africa. There is no similar record of such a sudden establishment of any other disease throughout the world. Since the fifteenth century, this gift of the down-trodden natives of Española has been the constant companion of civilized man.

He has spread it wherever he has gone. It has been truly said that civilization and syphilization have advanced together.

Attempts were made to arrest the disease as it spread to new countries, but all of these attempts failed. The venereal transmission of the disease was not recognized at first, and it was thought to be spread by contagion. Under this idea, Cardinal Wolsey was accused of giving syphilis to King Henry VIII by whispering in his ear. Henry VIII unquestionably had the disease, but there were other and more likely sources than the cardinal's words. In 1497, by act of the parliament of Paris, all persons infected with the new disease were prohibited, "under pain of death, from conversing with the rest of the world." The diseased persons who lived in the city were isolated in the suburbs of St.-Germain. Those who were not residents were ordered to leave the city within twenty-four hours and four Paris sous were given to each one to assist the return to "the Countries and Places where they were born, or where they had their Abode when they caught the Distemper or else where they please, under Pain of Death." Evidently the Parisians did not care who was exposed to the disease so long as they were spared. The decree continues: "No person shall presume to take the said four Sous, unless he be a Stranger or quit the city upon condition never to return to it. . . ." The quarters in St.-Germain became congested and a number of persons failed to obey the edict. Summary orders were given that anyone infected would be "thrown into the River, in Case they are ever hereafter found. . . ." After it was discovered that the disease was not transmitted by contagion the law requiring isolation was no longer enforced. The Scotch seemed to have recognized the venereal character of the disease at an early date, for in 1497 the town council of Aberdeen ordered that: "For protection from the disease which has come out of France and strange parts, all light women desist from their vice and sin of venery and work for their support, on pain, else, of being branded with a hot iron on their cheek and banished from the town."

The Europeans, faced with a new disease, were hard pressed for a name. Each country blamed some other and named the disease accordingly. The Spaniards called it the disease of Española; the Italians called it the French disease; the French called it the Italian disease; the English credited it to the French; the Russians named it the Polish disease; for the Turks it was the French disease; and for the Indians and Japanese the Portuguese disease. France for some reason bore most of the onus until Fracastoro, a physician, poet, physicist, geologist, astronomer, and pathologist wrote his poem "Syphilis sive Morbus Gallicus," published in Venice in 1530. He immortalized himself with this, the most celebrated of medical poems, and invented the name syphilis. The poem was a summary of the knowledge of the disease and its treatment. The fabled hero of this poem, "Syphilos," a swineherder, was represented as the first man to have the disease. By general agreement he has even since borne the blame and relieved the various countries of their nominal responsibility.

Syphilis appeared late among the American Colonists, as would be expected. The stern morality of the early settlers repressed sexual irregularity; the frequent combination of the duties of physician, pastor, and school-teacher in one man opposed the confession of venereal disease. The first known outbreak of syphilis in the Colonies occurred in Boston in 1646, twenty-six years after the landing of the *Mayflower*. The event is recorded in the diary of John Winthrop. It was preceded by an unusual phenomenon of nature, as is frequently supposed to be the case with such outbreaks. In this case a calf was born with three mouths, three noses, and six eyes. As Winthrop says: "What these prodigies portended the Lord only knows, and in his due time will manifest." The next year syphilis came! Of it we have from Winthrop's diary: "There fell out also a loathesome disease at Boston, which raised a scandal upon the town and country, though without just cause." According to Winthrop's story a local seaman went on a voyage; on his return his wife was infected with syphilis. She bore a child and at the same time developed a sore on her breast. "Whereupon," says Winthrop, "divers neighbors resorted to her; some of them drew her breast and others let her children suck them (no such disease being suspected by any), by occasion whereof about sixteen persons, men, women and children, were infected. . . . And it was observed that although many did eat and drink and lodge in

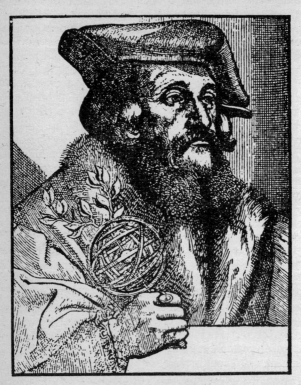

GIROLAMO FRACASTORO

who in 1530 wrote a medical poem entitled "Syphilis sive Morbus Gallicus," from which syphilis derived its name.

bed with those who were infected and had sores, and etc., yet none took it of them, but by copulation or sucking. It was very doubtful how the disease came at first. The magistrates examined the husband and wife, but could find no dishonesty in either, nor probable occasion how they should take it by any other. . . . So it was concluded by some that the woman was infected by the mixtures of so many spirits of men and women as drew her breast (for it so began)."

The commentator of this diary, James Savage, in 1826, remarks: "Whether the results, as stated in the text be the truth or not it is of less consequence than to observe how the

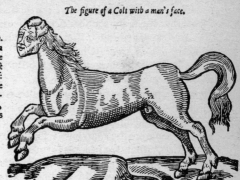

*The figure of a Colt with a man's face.*

At *Verona Anno Dom.* 1 2 5 4. a mare foaled a colt with the perfect face of a man, but all the rest of the bodie like an horf: a little after that, the war between the *Florentines* and *Pifans* began, by which all *Italie* was in a combuftion.

"FIGURE OF A COLT WITH A MAN'S FACE"

From Paré's *Surgery*. Like the unusual calf recorded by Governor Winthrop, the colt shown by Paré was supposed to be a portent of disaster, in this case a war in Italy. The drawing was made for Paré three centuries after the event.

ignorance of our fathers on this topick gives confirmation to the general opinion of their blameless manners." The sophistication of the commentator suggests that the country had fewer with "blameless manners" by 1826.

The age in which syphilis made its appearance in Europe was one of extreme laxity in matters of sexual behavior. The new disease at first involved nothing derogatory to a gentleman's reputation, and this general attitude toward syphilis lasted even into the seventeenth century. It was said at one time that a man who had not had the disease at least once was to be regarded "as boorish and no gentleman." The ethics of the matter have changed since the seventeenth century, but the unfortunate prevalence of syphilis has not. In the early days of syphilis in Europe men had no moral compunction about admitting their infection. The mother of Francis I of France said that her son was punished where he sinned. According to the story, Francis was infected by the wife of a Parisian tradesman. Francis solicited her favors, but was repulsed. After consulting with the court lawyers he decided to exercise his royal prerogative and notified the lady to that effect. With her husband's assistance she acquired a syphilitic infection and revenged herself on the king by its subsequent transmission. He is said to have died of the disease. Benvenuto Cellini, with characteristic frankness, says that he caught the "French evil" when he was a young man. The physician to whom he went for treatment assured him that he did not have the disease, but Benvenuto preferred his own diagnosis. He cured himself with a dose of *lignum-vitæ* and a day of shooting on the marshes, a feat quite as remarkable as many others that Cellini performed.

When the venereal transmission of syphilis was recognized generally the disease was quite naturally attributed to many people through malice. Accusation of sexual irregularity seems to be a favorite means of conveying opprobrium, particularly in religious strife. The Puritans had hardly settled in the American Colonies before they began accusing each other of sexual offenses. Pope Alexander VI was said to have acquired syphilis; his posterity were the Borgia family. To judge from the lives of many kings, and even queens, in the age in which syphilis first became prevalent, it would be remarkable if they were not infected. The commentators of the life of Louis XIV state that he acquired venereal infection in his early youth. In his case no indication of the later manifestations of the disease appeared. Henry III of France is said to have acquired syphilis at Venice on his return from Poland after the death of his brother Charles IX. He was supposed to have been cured by a decoction of burdock root. Vesalius, the anatomist and the physician to Emperor Charles

V, strongly implied that his royal patient had the disease. It appears also that the Duke of Mayenne, head of the French League, was infected. History has been profoundly influenced in some cases by the effects of syphilis upon rulers. Ivan the Terrible of Russia suffered from cerebral syphilis, which drove him to deeds of horrible cruelty. The reign of several of the Tudors of England was marked by the almost unmistakable effects of syphilis. Henry VIII had a series of stillborn children, strongly suggestive of the syphilis with which he was said to be infected. His son, Edward VI, died at an early age of what appeared to be a combination of congenital syphilis and tuberculosis. His daughter Mary—Bloody Mary—shows in her pictures the facial expression quite typical of the congenital disease. Henry himself had an abscess in his thigh, probably syphilis of the bone, which troubled him for many years. His marked sensuality developing in middle life and his blood-thirsty habits of divorce are strongly suggestive of cerebral syphilis. What a difference in the Tudor reign modern methods of treating syphilis might have made! Even Henry VIII, after enduring the heroic treatment for syphilis current a hundred years ago, might have been thus converted into a misogynist as Arthur Schopenhauer was said to have been.

Several characters famous in history and known to have disease of the genital region have been accused of syphilis in an effort to prove the antiquity of the disease. Herod, king of the Jews, is said to have had a malignant disease of the genitals which resulted in his death. John of Gaunt, Earl of Richmond, fourth son of Edward III, is said to have been similarly affected. A manuscript supposedly written by Thomas Gascoigne, chancellor of Oxford in the fifteenth century, states: "I, Thomas Gascoigne, an unworthy Doctor of Divinity, who wrote and collected these Observations, have known several Men who died of Putrefaction of the Genitals and of the whole Body; which Corruption and Putrefaction; as they said, was owing to carnal Copulation. For that great English Duke, viz. John of Gaunt died (1408) of a Putrefaction of this Kind, occasioned by Coition. For he was much

addicted to Venery, as was well known all over England, and
when he was upon his Death-bed, he shewed that Mortifica-
tion to King Richard II. This was communicated to me by
an honest Batchelor of Divinity, who was the only person
in the Secret." Such cases as these in no way invalidate the
belief that syphilis was unknown in Europe before the last
part of the fifteenth century. They were undoubtedly instances of cancer or tuberculosis of the genital organs and
were fatal because there was no surgery at the time by which
they could be treated.

The appearance of syphilis in Europe gave rise to a series
of speculations as to the cause of the disease. As the part
played by bacteria and other organisms in infectious diseases
was not established until the middle of the nineteenth century
these early speculations were somewhat far fetched. They
serve here, however, to illustrate the general conceptions of
disease current in the sixteenth century. Both a divine and
a cosmic origin were given to syphilis. St. Job, because of his
skin affliction, became the patron saint of those with syphilis.
The conjunction of Saturn and Mars and the rainy weather
in Italy were both blamed for the disease. The astrologers,
having observed that syphilis invaded those parts of the
body which they believe to be under the influence of Venus,
called the disease *lues venerea,* or venereal infection. The disease was also attributed to the radical innovation of wearing
linen shirts which were coming in at that time to replace
woolen and leather garments. The physician to Pope
Clement attributed the disease to poisoning. This theory was
advocated to account for most of the epidemics of pestilence
and for the death of many royal persons. This physician says
he was told of a town called Comma, "where there is Plenty
of generous wine, called Greek, that was quitted privately by
the Spaniards in the night-time while the French were be-
sieging it; but first they tainted the Wine, with Blood drawn
from the Patients in the Hospital of St. Lazarus. The French
afterwards entered it, and drinking plentifully of the Wine,
began to be seized with most violent symptoms. . . ." The
idea that syphilis was a venereal form of leprosy was fre-

quently brought forward. In the words of the famous Paracelsus whose teachings are much followed by modern mysticists: ". . . The French disease derives its Origin from the Coition of a leprous Frenchman with an impudent whore, who had venereal Bubas, and after that infected everyone that lay with her; and thus from the Leprosy and venereal Bubas, the French Disease arising, infected the whole world with its contagion, in the same manner as from the Coition of a Horse and Ass the race of Mules is produced."

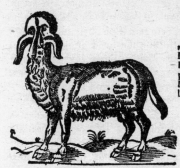

*Celius Rhodoginus* write's that at *Sibaris*, a heard∫-man called *Chraibis* fell in love with a Goat, and accompanied with her, and of this detestable and brutish copulation an infant was born, which in legs resembled the dam, but the face was like the father's.

### A MONSTROSITY ACCORDING TO PARÉ

The older medical literature contains many examples of the supposed result of bestiology. The belief that man can form hybrids with beasts still persists as a legend and the face which "was like the father's" was conceived in the imagination of the artist.

Bestiology and the eating of lizards were blamed for the disease and even Francis Bacon brought forward a dietary origin. He says: "The French from whom the Neapolitan Disease derives its Denomination say, that there were at the Siege of Naples, certain dishonest Merchants who sold human Flesh, new killed in Mauritania, pickled and put up in Vessels, instead of Tunny; and that to this abominable and heavy Food, the Origin of the Venereal Diseases ought to be ascribed. Nor does this Opinion seem to be without just Foundation. For Cannibals in the West devour human Flesh;

and this disease is very frequent in the West Indies when they were first discovered." On this theory of Francis Bacon a writer of the seventeenth century remarks: "Whence we see the Truth of Tully's Observation that nothing can be so absurd but some of the Philosophers have said it."

John Astruc, physician to Louis XIV, reviews the absurd theories which had been advanced for the cause of syphilis. Some are so completely at variance with the ideas of his time that he dismisses them offhand. For instance, he says: "There are some, however, whom I forbear now to spend Time in imputing, such as Augustus Hauptman and Christian Langius, who think that the Venereal Poison is nothing else but a numerous School of little nimble, brisk invisible living things, of a very prolific Nature, which when once admitted, increase, and multiply in Aboundance; which lead frequent Colonies to different Parts of the Body; and inflame, erode, and exulcerate the Parts they fix on; . . . in short, which without any Regard had to the particular Quality of any Humour, occasion all the Symptoms that occur in the Venereal Disease. But as these are mere visionary Imaginations, unsupported by any Authority, they do not require any Argument to invalidate them . . . if it was once admitted, that the Venereal Disease could be produc'd by invisible living things swimming in the Blood, one might with equal Reason alledge the same Thing, not only of the Plague, as Athanasius Kircher, the Jesuit, formerely, and John Saguens, a Minim, lately have done, but also in the small-pox, Hydrophobia, Itch, Tetters, and other contagious Diseases, and indeed of all Distempers whatsoever; and thus the whole Theory of Medicine would fall to the Ground, as nothing could be said to prove the Venereal Disease depending upon little living things which might not be urged to prove that all other Diseases were derived from the like little living things though of a different Species, than which nothing can be more absurd."

What a tragic thing it is when a man lives too early for his ideas! Two and a half centuries later Pasteur demonstrated that contagious diseases were caused by little living things, bacteria. In 1905 Schaudinn and Hofmann found the organism of syphilis "swimming in the Blood." It is known today that the symptoms of syphilis are due to these organisms, which are of "a very prolifick Nature, which once admitted increase and multiply in Aboundance; which lead frequent Colonies to different Parts of the Body; and inflame, erode, and exulcerate the Parts. . . ." The humoral theories of disease and the veneration of their sponsor, Galen, blinded men to many of the facts of disease for fifteen centuries.

The search for the organism of syphilis started when bacteria were discovered by Pasteur to be a cause of disease—a little more than half a century ago. The organisms causing the infectious diseases were discovered in rapid succession, but that of syphilis stayed hidden. The twentieth century started with the organism still undiscovered. Among others, the famous Russian biologist, Metchnikoff, tried his skill in discovering the organism. He failed to find it, but he made a great step forward in the search; for in 1903 he demonstrated that syphilis could be transmitted to the higher apes. This discovery furnished a means for studying the disease experimentally. The higher apes are the only animals which, when inoculated, develop syphilis resembling the disease in man. Even animals as closely related to the apes as are monkeys have only a slight local infection when they are inoculated. The fact that calves cannot acquire syphilis is of more than passing interest, for the opponents of vaccination have on occasion talked of "bovine syphilis," an entirely imaginary disease, which they claim is transmitted by vaccination. Besides his work on animal inoculation Metchnikoff showed that the organism of syphilis is large enough to be seen with a microscope. He did not see the organism, but he found that when he passed the material used to inoculate animals through a porcelain filter the filtered material no longer caused the disease. The organism of syphilis was stopped by the filter, and particles large enough to be thus stopped can be seen under the microscope.

The organism of syphilis could not be made visible under the microscope by means of staining. Most bacteria absorb dyes readily and the color thus imparted to them allows them to be differentiated from the material containing them. The organism of syphilis does not absorb dyes, but remains colorless and transparent and hence invisible under the microscope as it is ordinarily used. Two German investigators, Schaudinn and Hofmann, working at the University of Berlin in 1905, sought for the elusive organism by another method of using the microscope. They used what is known as dark stage illumination. In the ordinary use of the microscope a brilliant source of illumination is arranged, so that its beams shine through the object to be examined. The observer looks through the object just as one looks through a camera film held up to a window. Examined in this way, transparent and colorless objects are invisible; the organism of syphilis is both colorless and transparent. Schaudinn and Hofmann placed a black background under this microscope to cut off all light coming through the material they were examining. They moved their source of illumination to one side and brought its beams horizontally across the field. With the light thus shining in a direction at a right angle to that in which they were looking they could see only such light as was reflected from objects which the rays struck. The principle involved in dark stage illumination is the same as that by which dust particles ordinarily unobserved in the air of a room become visible in a beam of sunlight. Under this method of examination the organism of syphilis could be seen. It was a spirochete, that is, an organism spirally shaped. It was, in fact, like a very tiny but very perfect corkscrew, usually with fourteen turns. In material in which the spirochetes were still living they could be seen to move about, whirling, lashing, and bending. The organism was named *spirochæta pallida*, the colorless spirochete.

The spirochæta pallida is a frail organism. It has a relatively short life outside of the body; under ordinary conditions it dies in less than six hours. Moreover soap and water serve to destroy spirochetes that may be deposited on such articles as drinking-glasses. If the spirochete had the resistance of the tubercle bacillus, syphilis would be a vastly more

prevalent disease than it is. It is possible to transmit the
organism by articles in common use, if they are passed almost
immediately from the syphilitic to another person. The spirochete is transmissible from the syphilitic only during those
stages of the disease when there are sores on the skin or
mucous membranes, but as such sores, particularly on the
mouth and lips, may be so small as to escape detection, there
is little satisfaction to be gained from this fact. The stage
of the disease during which the sores appear lasts from a few
weeks to two or three years, depending on whether the disease is properly or improperly treated. After this stage,
the disease, although it may persist, can no longer be transmitted in the usual manner.

The spirochetes when successfully transferred to a new
host—infection—cannot force their way through the un-
broken skin or mucous membrane. They can enter only
through a break in the surface; but again there is little satisfaction to be gained from this fact, for the break need only
be of microscopic size. Although theoretically the invasion
may occur at any point on the body, it rarely does so outside
of the genital organs and lips. About 5 to 10 per cent of all
cases start from the lips and such cases are usually caused
by kissing. The mouth of every syphilitic person which contains a sore from the disease—the sore may occur in his
mouth no matter in what fashion he acquired the disease—
is a virulent source of contagion. The kissing of such a person
is a very dangerous pastime. How dangerous it may be is
shown by an instance of the infection of seven young girls by
one man at a party where a kissing game was played. While
it is true that syphilis may be acquired "innocently," as the
"moralists" say, it is likewise true that 90 to 95 per cent of
the cases are acquired through sexual contact, which group
includes women who are guilty of marrying syphilitic men.

When infection occurs, events follow a characteristic order.
The spirochetes at first show none of the aggressive characteristics which mark their later activity. These they develop
about a month after infection has occurred. During this in-
cubation period there is no indication of the impending dis-

ease. In fact, the invading spirochetes are so slow in gaining a foothold that during the first twelve hours they can be eradicated and the disease prevented. This fortunate opportunity for preventing syphilis makes possible an effective prophylaxis. It is an opporunity afforded by very few diseases.

Syphilis is a mild disease, but, paradoxical as it may seem, the mild diseases are often the most persistent. In an acute disease, such, for instance, as pneumonia, there is an intense reaction of the body to the organisms causing the disease. It is this reaction by the human body which appears to the patient and his physician as the disease. The man is acutely ill; his fever rises high. All the forces of his body are marshalled to contend with the invading organism. The battle is sharp but brief. Either the germs win and the man dies; or the man wins and the germs die. In acute diseases the defense, once successfully developed by the body, often persists after the disease is over. This persisting defense prevents a second attack of the disease; the man is immune. This immunity occurs particularly in such diseases as measles and smallpox.

Mild diseases do not elicit an acute reaction on the part of the body. Consequently, they persist, and in persisting they become chronic diseases. If the reaction between invading organisms and the human body in acute disease may be compared to a war, the chronic diseases may be likened to an immigration. After the immigrants have become established they multiply and overrun their new home. In time they own it. If they are stopped by curing the disease, they cause no immunity, and a second immigration may occur whenever the opportunity is offered.

Syphilis is initially a mild disease and then becomes chronic. There are no acute stages in its progress. Its duration is marked by years rather than by days. In its course it shows the various stages of its invasion. First there is a local disturbance at the point where the spirochetes enter the body; this period is called the primary stage. Next there is a general but mild disturbance of the body. The spirochetes are spreading to all parts of their new home. This period is called the secondary stage of the disease. Finally, the spirochetes, after having involved all parts of the body, may concentrate in various localities and cause serious damage in these parts. This last period of the syphilitic invasion is known as the tertiary stage of the disease.

The first symptom of syphilitic infection is a chancre, a round ulcerated area which appears at the point of infection. The margin of this ulcer is swollen and feels hard under the touch. It is painless, is associated with no feeling of illness, and gives no indication in itself of the serious nature of the infection. It is an indolent ulcer; it gets neither better nor worse, but persists for three or four weeks before it shows any tendency to heal. The chancre of syphilis is sometimes called a Hunterian chancre, after the famous English physician of the eighteenth century. John Hunter, indeed, needs some posthumous recognition for the heroic but misleading experiment to which he subjected himself. He maintained that gonorrhea and syphilis were caused by the same virus and were simply different manifestations of the same disease. According to his idea, infection by this virus produced syphilis if the skin was infected and gonorrhea if a mucous membrane was infected. To prove his point he deliberately inoculated his skin with pus taken from a case of gonorrhea. He developed syphilis! What he had overlooked was the possibility of the two infections occurring at the same time in the subject from which he had obtained his material for inoculation. His erroneous idea, supported by his heroic demonstration and the prestige which he had in medicine of his time, caused the two diseases to be confused for many years. In his later life John Hunter suffered from the constitutional effect of the disease.

Hunter's erroneous idea of the identity of gonorrhea and syphilis was overthrown by Philippe Record in 1838. Record was born in Baltimore, Maryland, but studied and practiced in Paris. As a result of his professional experiences he was pessimistic in regard to the morality of the human race and he was outspoken in his pessimism. Oliver Wendell

Holmes said he was "the Voltaire of pelvic literature—a skeptic as to the morality of the race in general, who would have submitted Diana to a treatment with his mineral specifics and ordered a course of blue pills [mercury] for the vestal virgins."

During the primary stage of syphilis the spirochetes are mostly in the area about the chancre and for the first week the disease cannot be detected by testing the blood with the Wassermann reaction. Nevertheless, an examination of the material from the chancre under a microscope with dark stage illumination shows the spirochetes in great numbers. Under proper treatment applied early in its primary stage the disease can be stopped so quickly that no manifestation other than the chancre develops. The treatment of syphilis becomes more difficult and the results of the treatment less certain as the disease advances through the secondary and into the tertiary stage.

From their focus in the chancre the spirochetes spread into the blood and are carried throughout the body. The general manifestations of the disease develop and give rise to the secondary stage of the disease about two months after the original infection and at about the time the chancre is healing. An eruption appears on the skin and the mucous membrane of the mouth becomes raw in places. The intensity of the skin eruption varies between the widest limits. There may be only a few pink spots on the skin of the trunk or there may be an eruption of such severity that it resembles smallpox. There is rarely any disablement and usually the skin eruption is not of a character to cause alarm in the sufferer. Even without treatment the secondary stage of the disease passes away in time; it may last a few months or it may persist for a year or two. Treatment, even of a kind which does not eradicate the disease, frequently brings an end to the secondary stage.

If syphilis produced no effects except its primary and secondary stages it could almost be ignored, for there is little inconvenience or physical suffering. The serious nature of the disease appears years later. Insanity, paralysis, and disease of the heart and blood vessels and other conditions of the so-called tertiary stages develop. It has also severe effects on children who acquire it from their mothers during pregnancy. The lack of suffering during the early stages of syphilis is one of the most dangerous features of the disease. Severe pain and illness force men to seek relief or at least to keep to their beds where they are out of contact with other people. The evidences of some diseases are clearly marked and can be readily recognized and the sick thus avoided. None of these events occur in the early stages of syphilis, and it is only during these stages that it can be transmitted. Even if a man recognizes the disease, he may hide it from fear of the odium which is attached to the venereal diseases. The spirochetes can be completely eliminated from the body by proper treatment during the early stages of the disease, but in the late stages, even if the spirochetes are eliminated, the damage to the body cannot be repaired.

In the late stages of syphilis the spirochetes are not distributed throughout the body; colonies of them persist in various tissues. These persisting foci of infection destroy the tissue and as it heals scars replace it. The walls of the arteries are the commonest locality for this action of the spirochetes. Hardening of the arteries results. Hardening of the arteries is a natural result of age and also a consequence of high arterial pressure, but hardening from these causes comes after middle life. The changes from syphilis may come early in life; by causing premature hardening of the vessels, it shortens life.

The most distressing consequences of syphilis occur when the late destructive action of the spirochetes is centered on the nervous system. The tissue of the brain and spinal cord is destroyed and replaced with scars. It can no longer function normally. If the brain is involved insanity results; in its most pronounced form this insanity is called paresis. Paresis may not develop until many years have passed after the syphilitic infection. It comes at a time when all other symptoms of the disease have long since passed. A man suffering from paresis is slowly cut off from the surrounding world. He loses his appreciation of the reality of occurrences about him and to replace these realities he fabricates a world of his own. In this fanciful world his ego has full sway and runs to expansive delusions. One day he is a multimillionaire; the next he becomes divine. Eventually paralysis intervenes. His mind deteriorates until he lives merely a vegetative existence in hopeless imbecility.

In locomotor ataxia the syphilitic changes in the nervous system occur in the spinal cord. The symptoms develop slowly as more and more of the spinal cord is destroyed. The feet lose their sensation of position; the gait becomes awkward. The abdomen is stabbed with darting pains. The legs become paralyzed. Finally the man is helplessly bed-ridden but his mind remains clear; he appreciates his suffering and is fully aware of his dismal plight. There are treatments by which both paresis and locomotor ataxia can be arrested, but any damage to the nervous system that occurs before the treatment is instituted is irremediable.

Syphilis is often spoken of as a hereditary disease, but in reality it is not hereditary. Syphilis can be transmitted to the child during pregnancy if the mother has syphilis. That is not hereditary. It is contact infection. To be hereditary the characteristic thus designated must be a part of the germ plasm and be carried in the sperm of the male or the ovum of the female. Syphilis is not transmitted in that manner. Children with syphilis are born only of mothers who themselves have the disease. If a man has syphilis, but before he marries has passed the period during which he can transmit the disease, his children will not "inherit" syphilis from him. A child may acquire smallpox from its mother if she has the disease during her pregnancy. Under such circumstances the child dies before it is born. It is not called hereditary small-pox even if the woman acquired the disease from the child's father. Moral conceptions have colored the ideas of syphilitic transmission until many people believe that a "taint" of syphilis is passed "even to the third generation"—which it is not.

A child which acquires syphilis from its mother during the early stages of her pregnancy frequently dies before birth. Syphilis is one of the greatest causes of miscarriages and of stillborn children of which there are at least 100,000 annually in the United States. But the child does not always die. It is then born with syphilis. The spirochetes of syphilis find in the tender tissues of the baby a medium in which they can grow luxuriantly. They wreak their havoc without stint. Most babies born in the active stage of the disease die within a few weeks after birth. They add their pathetic appeal—a futile human sacrifice—for the propitiation of a disease in which the moralists see a punishment for sin. Such moralists retard the advance of our civilization. Those children who do not die soon after birth from their syphilis can be treated and frequently cured. If they are not treated the effects of their infection appear in deformity of their bodies. Misshapen bones, blindness, deafness, and idiocy may be their lot. Surely the moralists are difficult to satisfy. Even nature intervenes. The man and woman with syphilis acquired from their mothers do not give it to their offspring. Syphilis is not transmitted to the third generation.

The origin of gonorrhea is lost in antiquity. There is about this disease none of the glamour of historical association that there is about syphilis with its relatively recent rise and spread. So far as records go into the past, gonorrhea has been as much of an associate of the human race as has decay of the teeth. At times both of these conditions have been almost equal in their prevalence. Gonorrhea is a disease which has been handed down without a break through countless generations of human beings. The germ which causes it is even more frail and delicate than the spirochete of syphilis; under ordinary conditions it cannot exist outside of the body for more than a few minutes. No animal other than man can acquire the disease. Among adult humans it is transmitted by sexual contact. Like syphilis, it strikes at infants—and blinds them.

Gonorrhea, unlike syphilis, is an acute disease, and moreover it is largely a local disease. Only occasionally does it spread to the blood and cause a generalized infection with rheumatism and heart disease. Formerly it was believed to be more severe in males than in females. During the acute stages of the disease there are evident and painful symptoms in the male. In the female the immediate symptoms of the infection may be so mild as to escape detection, but the subsequent effects are serious. It is only in the last few years, since surgical operations of the abdomen have become common, that the havoc that the infection works on the organs of women has been realized. For women gonorrhea ranks with cancer as a cause for operations and invalidism.

The bacterium which causes gonorrhea was discovered in 1879 by Albert Neisser. It belongs to that large group of germs known as cocci because of their round or oval shape. The different species of cocci cause many diseases. The staphylococcus is so regularly an inhabitant of the human skin that it may almost be spoken of as normal to that locality. It is the pus-forming organism and one which causes boils and most superficial infections. Its near relative, the streptococcus, does not cause formation of pus, but is the common cause of blood-poisoning. The gonococcus, which causes gonorrhea, is shaped like a coffee bean and two germs are usually found together, their flattened sides in apposition. The gonococci occur in vast numbers in the pus which arises from the area which they infect. They are carried in this pus during their transmission.

Gonorrhea, unlike syphilis, cannot infect the skin, but only mucous membrane. The mucous membrane of the genital organs and that of the conjunctiva of the eye are the two localities where it effects its entrance. Brought on to either of these surfaces, the gonococci burrow into the deeper layers of tissue. An acute local infection results in two to five days. Pus streams from the infected surface and carries with it enormous numbers of the cocci. In the male the infection occurs in the urethra, the passage leading to the bladder. The raw and inflamed surface gives rise to intense pain during urination, but aside from this the disease causes little illness. The infection travels up along the walls of the urethra. In favorable cases it does not extend beyond the lower part of the urethra. Often, however, it extends into the generative apparatus, infecting the seminal vesicles, prostate gland, and epididymis; it may also travel into the bladder and even up to the kidneys. In two or three weeks the acute infection subsides. In some cases the disease has eradicated itself or has been eradicated by proper treatment. In other cases foci of the gonococci remain in glands or deep in the mucous membrane. Centered there they cause but little inflammation, but may persist for a long time. The best medical care is required to eradicate them. As no noticeable effects result from these foci of infection, many men remain ignorant of their presence or, in the absence of any discomfort from the disease, refuse to undergo the medical treatment necessary to cure this chronic stage. Such men, without themselves suffering any symptoms of the disease, may nevertheless transmit it.

In women the acute stages of the gonorrheal infection often pass without the occurrence of any symptoms by which the disease can at once be identified. The infection starts in the vagina and from there it extends to the uterus. It spreads further and passes into the Fallopian tubes and through them to the peritoneum lining the abdominal cavity. The inflammation of the tubes often causes them to be closed by the formation of scars; sterility results. If both ends of a tube are thus closed, pus cannot drain from it and the tube becomes distended from the collection of pus. A "pus tube" is thus formed and must be removed by surgical operation. The inflammation causes the organs in the pelvic part of the abdomen to become adherent to each other; they are distorted in shape. These changes are a common cause of invalidism which can be corrected only by surgical operation.

Gonorrhea, like syphilis, may be transmitted from the mother to the baby. The transmission is effected only during the birth of the child. As the baby passes down through the vagina the infected pus is forced into its eyes. On the third or fourth day after birth the lids of the baby's eyes become swollen. The lids and eyeballs are covered with a thick creamy pus. If untreated, the intense inflammation irritates the transparent cornea of the eye and erodes it. The cornea loses its transparency. In such cases the disease runs a course of several weeks; inflammation subsides gradually and the lids open again, but over scarred and sightless eyes.

At one time about a quarter of the blindness throughout the world resulted from gonorrheal infection. Blindness was then much more prevalent than it is today. There is a prophylactic treatment by which gonorrhea of the eyes can be prevented. Most states in this country require by law that this prophylactic treatment shall be given as a routine part of post-natal care; during the last twenty years there has resulted, in consequence, a reduction of nearly 70 per cent in the occurrence of gonorrheal infection of the eyes. This prophylactic measure is not motivated merely by humanitarian interests. The blind are in most cases dependent upon the state for support. The laws designed to prevent venereal blindness are enacted for economic reasons. It is unfortunate that the economics of all venereal infection is not so self-evident as is the blindness of infants.

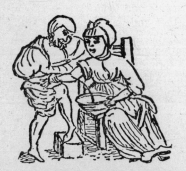

THE BENEFITS OF BLEEDING
A woodcut from the medical poem of
Salerno:
"To bleed doth cheer the pensive, and remove
The raging fires bred by burning love."

# CHAPTER XI

## THE MEDICAL THREAD IN THE MORAL SNARL

rostitution has always been held responsible for the maintenance and spread of venereal diseases. The writings of Moses in the Old Testament refer to prostitution in connection with a venereal disease, probably gonorrhea, which is designated as an "issue." The epidemic spread of syphilis in the fifteenth and sixteenth centuries served to emphasize anew the importance of prostitution in the spread of venereal diseases. Bernard Mandeville, under the pseudonym of "The Late Colonel Harry Mordaunt," wrote in 1740: "The greatest evil that attends this Vice, or could befall Mankind, is the Propagation of that infectious Disease, called *French Pox*, which in two Centuries, has made such indescribable Havoc all over Europe. In these Kingdoms it so seldom failed to attend whoring, now a days mistaken for Gallantry and Politeness, that a hale, robust, Constitution is estem'd a Mark of Ungentility; and a healthy Fellow is look'd upon with the Same View, as if he had spent his life in a Cottage. Our Gentlemen of the Army, whose unsettled life makes it inconvenient for them to marry, are hereby very much weaken'd and enervated; and render'd unfit to undergo such Hardships as are necessary for defending and supporting the Honour of this Country."

Prostitution is not alone responsible for the spread of venereal disease. It is merely the most obvious form of promiscuous sex relations. To persist beyond one generation the venereal diseases must be spread continually to new individuals. This spread can be effected only through sexual promiscuity. The occasional or non-professional prostitute, using the term prostitute in the broadest possible sense, is as much a cause for the spread of the disease among her small circle of intimates as is the habitual prostitute among her larger circle of patrons. The non-professional prostitute is

A

Modeſt Defence

OF

*Publick* STEWS:

OR, AN

ESSAY

UPON

WHORING.

As it is now practis'd in these Kingdoms.

Certainly ſome Kind of Incontinency may be neceſſary
to preſerve Chaſtity, as one Fire is extinguiſhed
by another.
Seneca

Not only Man's Imperial Race, but they
That wing the liquid Air, or ſwim the Sea,
Or haunt the Deſart, ruſh into the Flame,
For Love is Lord of All, and is in All the ſame.
Dryden's Virg.

By the late Colonel HARRY MORDAUNT.

LONDON:

Printed for T. READ, in Dogwell-Court White-
Fryars, Fleet-ſtreet. MDCCXL.
(Price 1 s.)

TITLE PAGE OF BERNARD MANDEVILLE'S SATIRICAL
DEFENSE OF REGULATED PROSTITUTION

even more difficult to control and to eradicate than is her professional sister. The distinction between the two is made in no uncertain words in a pamphlet printed in London for

Francis Pye in 1675. Its author calls the occasional prostitute an "exchange-wench." The title of his pamphlet is: *The Ape-Gentlewoman or the Character of an Exchange-wench*. In the broad language of his time he says: "A Town crack that Kisses for her Bread is a Saint t'her [the Exchange-wench]. Both her [the prostitute's] habitation and her apparel like two friendly Sea Marks, forwarn us of our Ship wreck if we sail in that Channel: But an Exchange-wench like a fatal Rock hid under mild superficies, Ruins a man before he can say *Lord have mercy upon us*."

Bernard Mandeville, quoted in a previous paragraph, satirically suggested a legalized and organized form of prostitution which, by eradicating the exchange-wench and bringing prostitution under medical supervision would result in the elimination of syphilis. His pamphlet is entitled: *A Modest Defence of Publick Stews*. Stews were houses of prostitution. His plan had all the ready virtues of the impossible. The prostitutes were to be organized and controlled with an almost military discipline. There was to be a colony of them. This colony was to include, besides the luxurious houses, a home for "Bastard orphans and superannuated Courtezans." There was to be a hospital attached also where venereal diseases would be treated. Medical examination of the women was to be made at regular intervals and a woman too frequently infected was to be honorably discharged. In this last connection he says: "Three Claps, shall be reckon'd equivalent to one Pox." The small fees collected by the women were to be supplemented from funds obtained by public taxation, and the whole organization was to be supported in such luxury that there could be no competition by exchange-wenches. Mandeville, certain that medical supervision would control venereal infection once the prostitutes were under regulation, concludes: "As the Disease has its Spring and Source entirely from public Whoring, and from thence creeps into private Families. When the source is once dry'd up, the Nation will naturally recover its pristine Health and Vigour."

Mandeville brings out one point that is pertinent in relation to the medical treatment of venereal disease. He says that men who are infected have no incentive for spreading the disease, but that women so infected "have an Inclination." The prostitute must raise the money for her medical treatment by plying her trade with increased activity.

The suggestion made by Mandeville that the infected women be treated at a hospital supported by the revenue from their houses had been tried previously in the city of Toulouse. In the late Middle Ages a public house of prostitution was established there under a royal charter. It was called the Abbaye. The city and the university shared equally in the profits of the enterprise. The inmates of the Abbaye were required to wear white scarfs and white ribbons on their arms as badges of their calling. The prostitutes objected to this costume. When Charles VI visited the city they met him in a body and petitioned for permission to dispense with these insignia; and the king granted the petition. The people of Toulouse were enraged that there was to be no way of distinguishing their wives and daughters from the prostitutes, and assaulted those prostitutes who availed themselves of the new privilege. In retaliation the prostitutes organized a strike. The university soon felt the effects in its curtailed income. An appeal was made to the king to arbitrate the matter. He signified his disapproval of the actions of the town people by placing his own royal *fleurs de lis* over the door of the Abbaye. This sign of royal favor was without effect upon the people. The assaults on the Abbaye became more numerous and it was finally vacated. It was replaced by the *Château vert;* the profits accrued to the city. In the middle of the sixteenth century some moral scruples arose as to the propriety of financing the city administration on the profits of a house of prostitution. In consequence the revenue was ceded to the hospital, but with the condition that the hospital should treat all females with venereal disease free of cost. Syphilis had become prevalent. The plan was tried for six years, but was abandoned because the cost of treating the women was greater than the revenue they yielded.

An institution similar to the Abbaye in Toulouse was

established in the papal city of Avignon. The regulations for this house were drawn up in 1347 under Jane I, "Queen of both the Sicilies, and Countess of Province." The queen was

# THE

## Ape-Gentle-vvoman,

### OR THE

# CHARACTER

### OF AN

# Exchange-wench.

*London, Printed for Francis Pye. 1675.*

TITLE PAGE OF AN ANONYMOUS PAMPHLET ON
PROSTITUTION

at the time twenty-three years of age. The statutes are given here in full, for they throw light upon the customs of the time and show that medical as well as legal regulation of prostitution was attempted even in the Middle Ages.

# THE OLD STATUTES OF THE STEWS OF AVIGNON

(1) On the 8th of August, in the Year 1347, our good Queen Jane gave Leave that a publick Brothel should be set up at Avignon, and ordered that the Wenches, who play'd there, should not walk the Streets, but keep themselves confined within the Brothel, and by Way of Distinction wear a red knot upon their left shoulders.

(2) If any Girl has thus offended and persists in her Offence, that then the Claviger, or Chief of the Beadles, shall lead her through the city by Beat of Drum, a red knot hanging at her Shoulder, back to the Brothel, and shall prohibit her from walking about any more, under the Penalty of being lash'd privately for the first Offence, and of being whipp'd publicly and turned out of the House for the second.

(3) Our good Queen orders that this Brothel shall be erected in Brokenbridge-street, near the Convent of the Augustin Friars as far as to Peter's-gate, and that the Entrance shall be toward the Street, and the Door locked, that no youth may have admittance to the Wenches without Leave from the Abbess or Governess, who is to be chosen every Year by the Directors. The Abbess is to keep the Key and advise the young Men she admits to make no Disturbances, nor frighten the Wenches, and to let them know that in Case of Misdemeanour they will not be suffered to go off securely, but be laid under Confinement by the Beadles.

(4) The Queen commands that on every Saturday the Women in the House be singly examined by the Abbess and a Surgeon appointed by the Directors, and if any of them has contracted any Illness by their Whoring, that they be separated from the rest, and not suffered to prostitute themselves, for fear the Youth who have to do with them should catch their Distempers.

(5) If any of the Wenches in the Brothel proves with Child, let the Abbess take care to prevent a Miscarriage, and give Notice to the Directors to make Provision for the Child.

(6) Let the Abbess diligently take care not to give Admittance to any Person into the Brothel on the Friday and Saturday in Passion-Week, nor on the Holy-day of Easter, under the penalty of being dismissed and whipped.

(7) The Queen orders that the Wenches admitted into the Brothel abstain from Strife and Envying, from Brawling and

Thieving, and that they live lovingly together like Sisters; and in case any Difference arises among them, that they refer it to the Abbess, and stand to her Judgment.

(8) If any Theft be committed, let the Abbess amicably procure Restitution to be made of such things as are stolen. And if the guilty Person refuses to do it, let her be first lashed by the Beadle in private; and if she fall a second time into the same Fault, let her be whipped thro' the City by the common Hangman.

(9) Let the Abbess admit no Jews into the Brothel; and if any one finds means by Stealth to gain Admittance, and lye with any of the Wenches, let him be imprisoned for this Offence, and whipped publickly thro' the streets of the City.

The discrimination against Jews indicated in the ninth article of these statutes is expressive of the general attitude toward these people at the time. By order of St. Louis in 1269 the Jews were forced to "wear the Figure of a Wheel cut out of purple Woolen Cloth, sewed on the upper Part of their Garments on the Breast, and between the shoulders. . . . " In Avignon in 1498 a Jew was publicly whipped for entering the brothel of that city. In spite of general injunctions to the contrary, the high officials of the Church and nobles often called in Jewish physicians to treat them because of their superior skill and attainments. Charlemagne retained two Jewish physicians as his personal attendants.

The distinguishing badge for the professional prostitute, either by legal requirement or from convention, was not confined to Toulouse and Avignon. The story of Judah in the Old Testament refers to the costume of the prostitute. Tamar, the daughter-in-law of Judah, desired to have children in spite of her widowhood. Accordingly she "put her widow garments off from her, and covered her with a veil, and wrapped herself and sat in an open place. . . . When Judah saw her he thought her a harlot, for she had covered her face." The consequent dealings between Tamar and Judah, who failed to recognize her because of the face covering, throw a light on the double standard of sex behavior at that time. Tamar, to keep up her disguise, demanded of her father-in-law a kid as recompense for her favors. He gave her his "signet, and his bracelets, and his staff," as pledges for the kid. Apparently there was no dishonor to a man's reputation in having commerce with a prostitute, for Judah subsequently sent a friend to redeem his pledges. The failure to

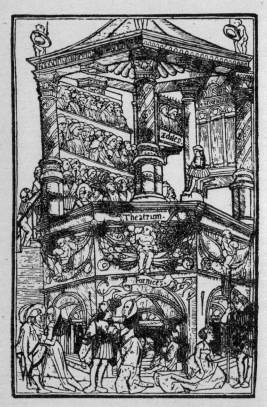

A MEDIEVAL HOUSE OF PROSTITUTION

The open-air theater occupies the second story of the "Fornices." The inmates of the latter are shown soliciting on the street before their quarters.

keep an agreement was dishonorable and when Judah found that the prostitute had left he was alarmed "lest we be shamed" for not having paid the stipulated price. The double standard of behavior appears in Judah's reaction when he discovers that his daughter-in-law is pregnant. He orders her burned for having "played the harlot," but is confounded when she exhibits the pledges he had given her.

Moses attacked the problem of venereal infection, gonorrhea, with strong injunctions against immorality. His attention seems to have been centered on the morals of the Jewish women, for he tolerated an invasion of foreign prostitutes from the Moabites and Syrians. Although these "strange women" were not allowed in the larger cities until the time of Solomon, they nevertheless set up their booths and tents along the highways. There they combined their profession with shopkeeping. These women, for all their Biblical setting, were no doubt as degraded mentally, as filthy in their persons, and as avaricious in their natures as is the modern prostitute. During Solomon's reign Jerusalem was overrun with prostitutes. Samson chose the house of a prostitute for his residence at Gaza; and his fatal acquaintance with another prostitute, Delilah, is an outstanding feature of his story.

Among the Greeks the law designated flowered robes as the costume of the courtesans, but was modified to prevent them from wearing scarlet or purple or jewels. It was the fashion among the courtesans to dye their hair blond or use flaxen wigs. At a late period in Greek history this fashion was followed by women who were not courtesans. All through the ages fashions have originated with courtesans. In Rome it is said that prostitutes could be distinguished from virtuous matrons only by the superior elegance of their dress and the swarm of admirers who surrounded them. As late as the sixteenth century a general Church council at Milan designated the costume which prostitutes were to wear.

Among the Greeks during their later period prostitution became a social institution. The Greek wives were expected to live at home. They were not allowed to appear at the games or theater; in public they veiled their faces. They were uneducated and supplied no intellectual companionship to their husbands; they merely bore legitimate children. The Greek men turned to the courtesans for social relaxation. The better class of these women were trained entertainers. Their participation in banquets and the lascivious scenes which resulted cannot be judged from our present standards of morality. It was open and respectable. The only women who rose to distinction among the Greeks were courtesans. Socrates had no compunction in visiting Aspasia who had migrated from Milesia and established a house of prostitution in Athens. He even gave her sound philosophical advice for running her establishment. Subsequently Aspasia exercised such an influence over Pericles that he divorced his wife. He was accused of allowing Aspasia to govern Athens through her influence over him. Popular feeling rose high against her. The power of Pericles declined. Aspasia was accused of impiety and tried. Pericles appeared as her advocate, but in court his eloquence failed him; he could only clasp Aspasia to his breast and weep. She was acquitted, deserted Pericles, and married a wealthy grain merchant.

The high position attained by some Greek courtesans does not spread virtue on the profession as a whole. The average prostitute there, as everywhere and always, was mean and filthy. Aspasia and others of her type bore the same relative position to their less favored sisters as Madame Du Barry, the mistress of Louis XV, did to the prostitutes of a later period.

Among the Greeks there was nothing dishonorable in having commerce with a prostitute; at Rome, on the contrary, such an act was adultery and subject to serious penalties. Until late in the period of the Roman decline no man of standing entered a house of ill fame without hiding his face; even the degenerate Caligula did so. In spite of the laws, prostitution grew in Rome. Its toleration condoned the crime of adultery. The flouting of the laws by even the emperors themselves contributed to lower the morale of the populace. The laws and customs that had maintained a semblance of chastity and respect for the marriage contract decayed. Sexual promiscuity in Greece was held by custom to be a male privilege; in Rome, with the degeneration of the laws and customs, sexual promiscuity became a practice of both sexes. Among the Greeks a prostitute might rise to a high position, as did Aspasia; among the Romans a matron of

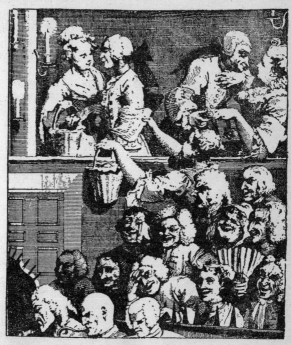

### ORANGE GIRLS

Hogarth's "Laughing Audience," a less obvious representation of the former relation between the theater and prostitution than that shown in the preceding figure. The orange girls sold their favors along with their oranges. Nell Gwynne, mistress of Charles II, who was applauded for her public statement of her profession, was at one time an orange girl and later an actress in the Drury Lane theater.

high station might descend to the lowest levels of degradation. The name of Messalina, the wife of Emperor Claudius,
has come down through the ages to be used today as an
epithet of feminine lasciviousness.

The license of the Romans became in time so monumental
as to inspire a certain awe. Their banquets were gorgeous,
extravagant and sensual. In their public baths of unsurpassed
architecture the sexes mingled intimately. But in the midst
of all this glorified vice the common prostitute remained
what she had been through all ages. Still she was the drab
bearer of venereal disease. The common prostitute of Rome
took refuge under the low arches that covered the dark area-
ways along the sides of the public buildings and larger private
houses. Comments on the stench that arose from these pits
were common in the literature of the time. The arched pits
themselves were called fornices, and we have borrowed from
this term for our generic word fornication.

Out of the mire of Roman depravity the Christian religion
grew up. Its first growth was not deformed by theology. Its
earlier followers exemplified the cardinal virtues of charity
and the brotherhood of all men. The pagan philosophers had
taught virtue and extolled beauty. They had exhorted men
to follow reason; but to them virtue, beauty, and reason were
intellectual qualities. They were to be sought for as men seek
intellectual development in education. But few men are
capable of the appreciation of intellectual qualities; the
masses are left untouched. The Christian religion taught virtue based on love. That quality is not alone of the intellect;
it is an emotion in every human being. The religion grew,
but during the first two and a half centuries retained much
of its original purity. The Christians were persecuted, but
this persecution merely increased the fervor of their religious
enthusiasm. At the end of three centuries Christianity was
the accepted religion of the Roman Empire, but in becoming
accepted had itself accepted much that was Roman.

Under Christianity chastity was a religious virtue. During
the first two hundred and fifty years of the religion there were
men and women of that faith who, with the view to spiritual

perfection, abstained from marriage and lived lives not only of chastity, but also celibacy with rigorous self-denial. These early Christians practiced the virtues of their religion; conflicts were few at first, and they did not bore their fellowmen into indifference or evasion with exasperating disputes over the subtleties of theology. But their concept of chastity was to prove too idealistic and impracticable for men to follow. In the enthusiasm of their great religious work they underrated the normal power of the sexual instinct.

The sexual instinct cannot be eradicated. It is as fundamental as the instinct of self-preservation; perhaps it is even more fundamental. It is part of the fiber of the human character. Attempts at its suppression result in its distortion; it cannot be eradicated. On the other hand, it can be converted from its natural channels and made to appear as creative work. Great reforms and great endeavors in any field are not accomplished by the emasculated. Such endeavors are the result of the conversion or sublimation of a strong sexual instinct. A certain combativeness is necessary for the saint who goes to martyrdom, and his courage has its roots in sex. The early Christians sublimated their sexual instinct into an enthusiasm for the propagation of their religion. At a later date this enthusiasm lost its original fervor. The sexual instinct remained, and so also did the conception of religious chastity which confused it with celibacy. The pressure of the repressed instinct centered attention on celibacy. As chastity became harder to defend, greater efforts were called for its defense. Under the deforming influence of theological interpretation the cardinal virtue of the religion became chastity. All morality was centered in sex. The ideal of chastity became not the purity of the undefiled relations of marriage, but the complete suppression of the whole sexual side of man's nature. The business of religion became the eradication of a natural appetite. Unless outlets are provided for the sexual instinct, either through its natural channels or through sublimation, it makes its own outlets and appears in strange manifestations in the characters of men. The repression exerted on the instinct, like a finger pressed on the globule of mercury, does not destroy it, but simply forces it from its original shape.

One of the strangest manifestations of the repressed sexual instinct among the Christians appeared in the saints of the desert. Men and women left their homes, deserted their wives or husbands and parents, to adopt the useless life of anchorites. Many of the early Christians had lived a life of celibacy, but they had lived in the midst of society, doing their share for its unity and preservation. The saints of the desert, under sway of ascetic frenzy, tortured by an instinct they sought to repress, renounced the world and undertook a solitary existence. In hiding they fought the battle with their instinct. They inflicted silly tortures upon themselves in an effort to assuage the lascivious visions which their minds called up. These visions throve on idleness; the anchorites called them temptations. These poor creatures, victims of an instinct that mocked their efforts, carried their renouncement of worldly things to an extent which precluded bathing and shaving. Cleanliness of the body was regarded as a pollution of the soul. The attitude was expressed by Jerome in the words "Does your skin roughen without bath? Who is once washed in the blood of Christ need not wash again." St. Anthony was never guilty of washing his feet. These hideous, sordid, and emaciated egotists, without knowledge, without patriotism, without natural affection, passing their lives in a long routine of useless and atrocious self-torture, became saints of the Christian religion. They were examples of a false conception of chastity and a perversion of the sex instinct. These men and women, covered with hideous masses of clotted filth, driven into a corner in desperation by an instinct that mastered their lives, were held up as examples to be followed by men and women. This chastity was represented as preferable to marriage. Out of their dreams of some compensation came their hopes of salvation and reward in another world.

St. Simeon Stylites furnishes a most remarkable picture of the desert anchorite. He bound a rope around his body so tightly that it became imbedded in the flesh, which putrefied around it. Worms found their way into the corrupt flesh of ulcers that covered his leg. For a year during which he stood on one foot he had an associate by his side who picked up the worms which fell from his body to replace them in the sores, the saint saying to the worms, "Eat what God has given you." At his death he was pronounced to be the highest model of a Christian saint and an example for the imitation of other anchorites.

The life of one of the anchorites of the desert, St. Mary of Egypt, throws light on the attitude of the early Christians toward prostitutes. The prostitute could atone for her past sins and become a Christian; Christ had forgiven Magdalene. Egyptian Mary was a prostitute, but she became penitent. She confessed to Zosimus that she had practiced her profession for seventeen years at Alexandria. Once converted, she took a boat for Jerusalem and paid her passage by exercising her calling on board. She expiated her sins by a life of penance in the woods. For forty-seven years she wandered, black with filth and covered only with her white hair; but she spoke to no man. To such acts of piety does perversion of sex lead.

A Christian conception of chastity that placed its emphasis upon early and undefiled marriage would have made for the social conquest of venereal diseases. It might have saved the civilization of the Roman Empire and have spared the world the long horror of the Middle Ages. But the chastity sought for was an impossibility for human nature, built as it is around and on a basis of sex. The perversions that resulted from the attempts to suppress sex demoralized society. Theology sought for a way out of the dilemma. The theological conception of morality continued to center in sex. Celibacy was represented as preferable to marriage. All sex relations other than for the immediate purpose of bearing children were sinful. But sins could be forgiven. Forgivable sin was preferable to the demoralization that appeared when the repression of the sexual instinct was forced beyond human endurance. Theological reasoning began to find an excuse for prostitution. St. Augustine said: "Suppress prostitution and capricious lust will overthrow society." Thus according to St. Augustine the prostitute was to be a safeguard of morals.

In the Middle Ages another fallacious belief, probably of Arabic origin, was implanted in the ready soil. According to this belief disease resulted from continence. The fear that "corruption of the flesh" would follow from continence was used to rationalize and condone the behavior of many medieval clerics. Under the belief that continence was harmful the prostitute was regarded as an animated prophylactic against corruption of the flesh. The housekeepers of the medieval clergy were kept, it is said, "not as a source of pleasure, but that superabundant substance might not fall into corruption whereby evil disease would doubtless be increased among the honorable clergy." This conception of the physical unhealthfulness of continence has been maintained in a somewhat modified form even to modern times. That earnest disciple of moderation, Benjamin Franklin, upheld these views. Present knowledge has shown the fallacy of this medieval belief, but it has not changed the fundamental character of the sexual instinct any more than the Christian religion has. If early marriage is impossible, the prevention of promiscuous sexual activity or the perversion of the repressed instinct can be prevented only by furnishing outlets for its sublimation. Our schools and colleges are coming more and more to recognize the importance of emulation in study and athletics in furnishing such outlets.

About the eleventh or twelfth century the prostitutes organized first into such loosely governed bodies as that of the "itinerant wives and maidens," which specialized in fairs and religious councils and finally into the somewhat more respectable brothel system. This system was originated by the famous lawgiver Solon at Athens in 594 B.C., but had fallen into disuse after the sixth century after Christ. The reëstablished brothel houses of European cities were sometimes under ecclesiastical control and were often taxed one-tenth of their earnings. This control did not indicate an approval of prostitution, but was an attempt to supervise and regulate what was then considered a necessary evil. As late as 1321 an

English cardinal purchased a brothel as an investment for sacerdotal funds.

With the change of time and custom the clergy ceased to

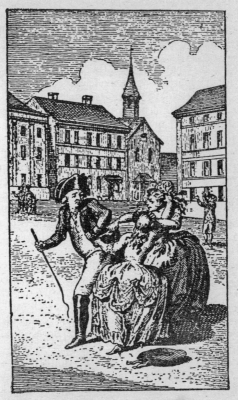

STREET PROSTITUTES

exert any regulation over prostitution. Eventually they came to demand that there should be no regulation, legal or otherwise, and in fact no recognition of the profession. But neither failure to regulate nor denial of existence is effective in end-

ing a subject. It must be added, however, that legal control,
segregation, and medical supervision likewise have been far
from a success in controlling prostitution and this source of
venereal diseases. Prostitution has been attacked by all conceivable means, but since it is part and parcel of the great
sex problem of civilization it will probably continue until
civilization has advanced considerably beyond its present
stage.

In Christian countries the attacks on prostitution have
varied with the moral tone of the leaders of the time. Prostitution has survived all of the vicissitudes to which it has been
subjected. In the fifth century the Emperor Justinian sought
to abolish the system of public prostitution; the penalty
against procurers and brothel-keepers was heavy, but the
prostitute herself was treated with indulgence. He permitted
the marriage of citizens with prostitutes and encouraged it
by his own example. His wife, the Empress Theodora, is said
to have been a prostitute; she was a brilliant and capable
woman. From her we have the example of a reformed prostitute attempting to reform prostitutes. Her process of reformation was as impracticable as all other methods have been.
She built a magnificent palace-prison on the south shore of
the Bosphorus and in one night caused five hundred prostitutes in Constantinople to be seized and incarcerated in this
prison. The women were treated kindly; with one exception,
their every wish was granted. No man was allowed to enter
their asylum. Most of the women committed suicide in their
despair, and the remainder soon died of boredom and vexation.

In the thirteenth century Louis IX of France issued an
edict stating that all prostitutes and all persons making a
living out of prostitution were to be exiled from the kingdom.
A large number of women were seized and imprisoned or
sent across the frontier. A panic seized the customers of the
brothels and for a month the measure appeared to be a success. But by the end of that time the places of the former
prostitutes were filled with recruits who carried on a clandestine traffic. The decree was repealed. Prostitution was

reëstablished under police regulation. As is frequently the case when legislation handles a dirty subject, its officers became soiled. The officials were corrupted and public morals were in no way improved. In 1635 the law abolishing prostitution was enacted again with an even greater severity. All men profiting from the "traffic of prostitution" were to be condemned to the galleys for life, and all prostitutes were to be "whipped, their heads shaved, and banished for life without formal trial." The law served the purposes of private malice; men who wished to revenge themselves on their mistresses accused them of being prostitutes. But the supply of prostitutes was not abated by the rigor of the law. The ordinance prohibiting prostitution remained in effect until the eighteenth century and was the basis for the high-handed measures by which the colonies of Canada were first supplied with wives by forcible emigration from the dregs of Paris.

It serves no purpose here to trace the futile efforts that have been made to suppress prostitution. The sequence of events is typical; official supervision, medical examination, and segregation offend the moralists and fail through their efforts, but are at once replaced by clandestine prostitution. No measure ever applied has abolished prostitution for more than a short time. There is no "solution" ever yet suggested but has failed in practice. It is today as much a problem as it ever was. An entire section of the League of Nations is devoted to the study of this problem.

There can be no question about the part played by prostitution in the spread of venereal diseases. Various estimates based on extensive medical examinations indicate that 85 per cent of all prostitutes are syphilitic. It does not follow directly from these estimates that all of these prostitutes spread the disease, for after they have had it for three or four years the danger of their doing so becomes less. It resolves simply into the fact that the younger third of the prostitutes are the most potent source of contagion; which in turn does not help matters. The status of the prostitute in regard to the venereal diseases is much like the status of the house fly in regard to some other transmissible diseases. Syphilis does not spring up spontaneously in the prostitute any more than does the typhoid germ on the foot of the fly. Both acquire the infection which they carry from contact with a source of the disease; both transmit the disease. Unfortunately, it is easier to exterminate the fly and destroy the filth in which it breeds than it is to reform the prostitute and abolish the social and economic conditions which produce her. The prostitute is blamed, and rightly so, for the spread of venereal disease, but she should not bear all of the blame. It is one of those gruesome facts which strike too hard for tears and find their only relief in brutal cynicism, that between the despised prostitute on the left hand and the honored wife and mother on the right hand there is a connecting link—the man; he carries the disease from one to the other. It is he who makes the prostitute, it is he who infects her, it is he who makes laws against her, and it is he who carries syphilis from her to his wife and children.

There will always be a supply, at a sufficiently high price, of any article, no matter how illicit, whether prostitutes or drugs, for which there is a demand. It would be more logical —and also wiser—to strike at the demand for prostitution rather than at the supply. Such a procedure is the reverse of the usual procedure. It is customary to make allowance for human desire and weakness, but not for cold and calculated action, particularly if it is for gain. The purveyor of drugs is treated more severely by the law than is the purchaser and consumer of the drugs. Presumably this distinction is made on the ground that the purveyor creates and sustains the demand for drugs. Likewise the law strikes primarily at the prostitute and not at the man who is her accomplice in venery, for, by analogy, he is assumed to be acting merely in response to a desire created by the prostitute. There is a distinction, however, between the unnatural and created desire for drugs and the natural and spontaneous desire of sex. There is in the whole situation a faint suggestion, to say the least, that man has shifted the blame on to the prostitute to cover up his own hypocrisy. He has done so in order that he may represent himself as a martyr to the wiles of the Circe who transforms him into the companion of the swineherder, Syphilos.

Early marriage has been suggested as a means of counteracting prostitution and syphilis. Most cases of syphilis are acquired by the male between the ages of twenty and twenty-six years; the maximum rate of acquisition falls at twenty-three years. In the whole population the infection is two to three times as prevalent among males as among females. Syphilis is, therefore, a disease primarily acquired by the young unmarried male; for him the prostitute is the source of infection. Where early marriage has existed as a nearly universal custom there has been little prostitution and consequently little syphilis. For economic, educational, and social reasons, the tendency in most countries today is away from early marriage. There results a prolongation of the danger period for syphilitic infection.

According to the best opinion it would appear at present to be impossible to eradicate prostitution. The failure of the social method of attacking the venereal disease does not prevent an attempt to treat the problem of the venereal diseases as independent from the problem of prostitution—an attempt to unravel the medical thread from the moral snarl. The first great step in this direction is to see it for what it is—not a question of morals, but a problem in sanitation and public health. For venereal disease medicine offers what it can offer for very few diseases indeed—both a prevention and a cure.

BOOKS PUBLISHED BY J. CALLOW.

11—DIRECTIONS FOR LEARNING TO SWIM; by attending to which, a person who has never been in the water may escape being drowned, By BENJAMIN FRANKLIN, L. L. D.

The authority of the American Bacon is of great weight in medicine, as in every other branch of science, that he touches, and particularly in what respects immersion in water; for doubtless he spent more time in this element than any philosopher of modern days.

## BENJAMIN FRANKLIN ON SWIMMING

From an advertisement for a book of directions written by Franklin.

## Part Five

# THE HEALING ART

## CHAPTER XII

## THE HALT, THE LAME, AND THE BLIND

hile the methods that have been used to treat disease seem at first sight to be numerous and dissimilar, they are all simply variations of three basic measures: First, faith healing; second, hygienic therapy; and third, drug cures.

In the first of these, faith healing, an attempt is made to remove morbid states by means of influences exerted upon the mind. The early and medieval Christians were practicing faith healing when they exorcised the devils that to them seemed to cause disease, and in so doing they followed a principle which had been developed among primitive peoples. The same principle persists today as Christian Science and other modes of religious healing. And also as psychoanalysis and Couéism.

The second means of treatment, hygienic therapy, is founded on the recognition of the fact that the body tends to cure itself and that people recover from disease. The measures of the treatment are thus designed to supply the conditions under which they get well, to assist the body to cure itself, and to minimize the effects of the disease. Such treatment includes rest, sunlight, bathing, fresh air, and diet; but it also includes anti-toxins and curative serums.

The third means of treatment, the use of drugs, is a relic of poison lore. As medicaments, drugs may be used with several different purposes in view. They may be given as an antidote or specific for the disease. In ancient times theriac and mithrodatic were given as universal antidotes and as specifics for all disease; today quinine is used as a specific for malaria and salvarsan as a specific for syphilis. Drugs may also be given to combat the symptoms of disease. Thus opium is used for pain. Again the drugs may be given to stimulate sluggish bodily functions, as calomel used as a physic.

In various stages of civilization at various times each of the three methods of treating disease has had periods of ascendancy. In the lowest grades of civilization faith healing predominates, while in the highest grades of civilization hygienic therapy predominates, but is assisted by a moderate use of drugs. Faith healing is the characteristic medicine of primitive and superstitious people, and until five hundred years before Christ it was the principal method of treating disease. At that time hygienic therapy began among the Greeks, and, somewhat later, drug cures were gradually combined with it. When the Christian religion came in the influence of its mysticism slowly forced out these measures and treatment returned once more to faith healing. For thirteen centuries faith healing maintained its ascendancy. A form of drug treatment persisted, however, and at about the time of the Renaissance its use increased extensively. Religious forms of faith healing were slowly discarded, but hygienic therapy was not at once revived. The drug treatment which thus came in was not a rational treatment. The drugs which were used were for the most part useless and some were actually harmful. The increasing belief in drug treatment and the corresponding diminishing belief in faith healing were correlated to a decline in the respect for religion. But the illogical choice of drugs and the illogical belief in their efficacy were then correlated to the fanaticism from which civilization was slowly emerging as personal liberty was won. As knowledge gradually accumulated and formed what we now call science, hygienic therapy slowly returned and drugs were relegated to a subordinate position. This state of affairs was reached only in the last part of the nineteenth century. In spite of the growth of science, faith healing has persisted and still persists in non-medical cults. Such truth as it contains is now being slowly taken over into modern medicine. Eventually all three methods of treatment

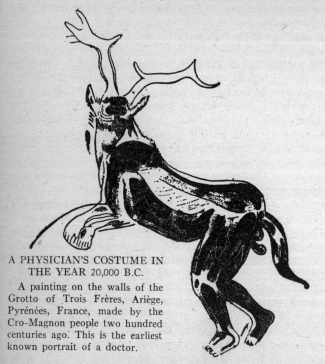

A PHYSICIAN'S COSTUME IN THE YEAR 20,000 B.C.

A painting on the walls of the Grotto of Trois Frères, Ariège, Pyrénées, France, made by the Cro-Magnon people two hundred centuries ago. This is the earliest known portrait of a doctor.

will be combined to produce a rational practice to a common end in treating human disease.

Primitive man sees in diseases the working of supernatural forces. For him disease is caused by a demon; or it is something induced by human enemies through the power of sorcery; or it is caused by the malevolent influence of a spirit, it may be that of a dead man, or an animal, or even of a plant. It was the business of the medicine-man to drive away the demon, outwit the sorcery of the enemy, and placate the dead. To accomplish these ends he distracted the patient's attention from his sufferings; he inspired him with confidence in his recovery; and finally left him with a token to remind him of the efficacy of the cure. To fix the patient's attention on the treatment the medicine-man dressed fantastically. Sometimes he clothed himself in animal skins until he resembled a huge bear standing on its hind legs. He shouted and danced and waved a rattle. After he had completed his personal treatment he provided his patient with an amulet to be worn on his person to ward off the demons. He named some fetish, an object to be avoided or some article to be omitted from the diet, or he specified some act to be performed in order to maintain the medicine. These acts were usually fantastic: to avoid stepping on some object or to carry out a certain procedure in entering or leaving a hut. The amulets, the fetishes, and the grotesque acts served to maintain the confidence of the patient. The method used by the medicine-man in treating disease was essentially the same as that used today by a father of a young child who has bumped its head; thus the father may dangle his watch in front of the child, or he may contort his face, or behave grotesquely to make the child forget the pain.

Faith healing that is practiced today among civilized peoples differs only in form from the faith healing of the most primitive peoples. The howling medicine-man of former times and the quiet Christian Science healer of today use the same essential principles in their treatments. These essentials are to attract the patient's attention, to gain his confidence, and to inspire him with faith in his recovery even to the extent of denying the existence of his disease. It must be frankly recognized that some diseases can be cured in this manner, and the symptoms of many others can be relieved temporarily. In such cases the patient is inspired to make his own cure or to relieve his symptoms as the child forgets its pain in watching the antics of its father. The central element of faith healing is to inspire confidence in the patient; the patient must have sincere belief. No faith cure ever worked on an unconscious man, an animal, or an idiot, and only the crudest kinds work on children. The extent to which faith in faith cures may go is shown by the fact that St. Hilarion, of the fourth century, is said to have courageously confronted and relieved a possessed camel. A bishop of Lusanne once excommunicated all the May-bugs in his diocese.

Faith healing has many names. Its opponents call it superstition; its supporters call it psychic healing, the laying on of hands, chiropractic treatment, psychoanalysis, or Christian Science. To the list might be added also the "confidence in the doctor" inspired by the old family practitioner of two generations ago. Most of his medicines served as an amulet or fetish to remind the patient of the confidence he inspired. Regardless of their names, all forms of faith healing are alike in essence, and all had their beginnings in the medicine of the primitive savage.

Faith healing is not to be dismissed lightly. It has its dangers, but it also makes its cures. The dangers come when it is tried with fanatical persistence for those diseases which it does not benefit, and which, if not treated positively, result in disablement or death. When used with intelligent discretion—as it rarely is—faith healing is a useful form of treatment. The basis of faith healing lies in the influence of the mind on the activity of the body. The mind is a function of the brain and through the brain is in constant communication with every part of the body by means of the nerves which extend to and from the brain. The activity of every organ of the body is controlled by the nervous system. The movement of an arm or a leg, the secretion of saliva, the variation in the flow of blood to an organ, the movements of breathing, the rate of the heartbeat, the temperature of the body, are all controlled by the nervous system. Diseases are manifested as disturbances in bodily functions. The temperature rises; but fever is merely a symptom of disease. It appears because the portion of the brain which regulates the size of the blood vessels in the skin causes these vessels to constrict and thus lessens the loss of heat from the body.

Due to the constriction of the vessels, the skin becomes cold; there is first chilliness and shivering. Later the vessels in the skin relax, the skin becomes warm, and the sensations of fever occur. The brain and nervous system, acted upon by toxins of disease, produce the symptoms of chill and fever in the same manner as the brain, influenced by mild fear, causes blanching of the face. The chill of disease is the same as the chill which comes with stronger fear; in both cases "goose flesh" results as the minute cutaneous muscles cause the hairs to stand on end in an effort to diminish the loss of heat from the body. In man the erection of the hairs is less evident than it is in animals such as the cat; man instead of bristling has goose flesh. In fever the heart beats rapidly; by counting the pulse the physician can estimate the severity of the fever. The heart also beats rapidly in emotion.

Paralysis of a limb may be a sign of serious disease, but a man may be paralyzed with fear and he may be struck dumb or blind with terror. Diarrhea also is a symptom of disease, but it is likewise often a complication of emotion. King James I of England was prone to diarrhea from the emotion aroused by distressing matters of state. The excessive secretion of saliva, called salivation, may occur in disease, while in fever the mouth may dry out and become parched. The saliva is also secreted excessively when a savory food is merely thought of; and the mouth dries out with fear. This last is shown by the glass of water put before the public speaker; he drinks before he speaks because he is frightened and afterward because he has dried his mouth by talking. The dry mouth of fear was one of the early legal tests, a form of "ordeal." The mouth of the defendant was filled with flour; if he was innocent and felt no fear, his saliva flowed and he was able to swallow the flour; if he was guilty his fear kept his mouth dry and he choked. Vomiting may come from illness and it may also come from fear or the smell of some disgusting substance. The pressure of the blood in the artery rises slowly as the kidneys harden with age, but it also rises even from the emotion caused by having a physician apply the apparatus to determine its height. The blood of a man with diabetes contains an abnormal amount of sugar and some of it finds its way into his urine; strong emotions suffered in restraint may temporarily cause both of these symptoms, as in the football substitute sitting on the side lines or the student faced with a difficult examination.

Most of the symptoms of disease can be counterfeited by the influence of the nervous system upon bodily functions. Mental irritation or depression can produce dyspepsia, jaundice, or a general decline. Fright may produce palpitation of the heart, and heart failure has resulted from business reverses. After cities are destroyed by earthquakes men and women are found dead who show no signs of injury. The modern surgeon is worried by the patient who faces an operation with the conviction that he will die. The man with incurable cancer cheers up and gains weight on taking a new patent medicine; he writes a testimonial of his cure; later he declines and dies of cancer. There are on record a number of cases of persons mentally depressed, but not otherwise unwell, who have accurately predicted the time of their death. Thus Dr. John Billings mentions the case of an officer who had sustained a slight flesh wound at the battle of Gettysburg. The man, although unusually robust, became depressed mentally and declared at the start that he would die, which he did on the fourth day. A post-mortem examination showed that every organ was healthy and the wound was too trivial to cause death.

Pain, which is the supreme subjective phenomenon of disease, is almost wholly mental. A man during rage feels no pain from injury until after his anger has cooled; the same man waiting in the anteroom of the dentist may suffer agony in anticipation. The early Christians, while being burned alive, signaled to their friends who waited for the ordeal, by raising their seared arms in the flames to signfy that they felt no pain. Religious enthusiasm was their anesthetic, as it has been for many fanatics who have voluntarily mutilated their bodies.

The gravest disturbances of the body are seen in a disease of the imagination called hysteria. Hysteros in Greek

means uterus, and the Greeks in naming hysteria conceived
of the uterus as the center of the disease. They thus anticipated Freud's views on sex repression and its neuroses by
twenty-five hundred years. The classical examples of hysteria
are afforded by the female saints who were subject to so-
called demoniacal obsession. In France during the Middle
Ages there was an epidemic of incubuses. An incubus was
a male demon who assailed the chastity of girls; similarly,
a succubus was a female demon who robbed boys of their
innocence. The male demons were far more numerous and
enterprising than the female demons. For one boy who con-

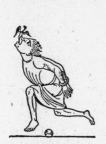 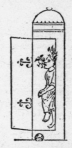 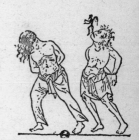

POSSESSION BY DEVILS
Miniatures by de Landsberg.

fessed that a succubus had attacked him in his sleep there
were a score of girls who showed evidence that they had been
violated and who were satisfied that it could have been none
other than the devil that had done so. Pope Innocent VIII
issued a bull to provide the faithful with an efficacious
formula for exorcising incubuses. Numerous women, most of
whom were nuns, confessed that they had been subject to
scandalous abuses by the devil, who visited them, and that
neither fasting nor prayer nor spiritual exercise could release
them from this plague. In the year 1637 a formal public
discussion took place in Paris on the subject of whether
incubuses could procreate their species. The point pertinent
here is that some of the women who believed themselves

attacked by demons and who were not trying simply to cloak a more worldly alliance showed definite marks of the devil's ruthlessness. Bruises appeared on their breasts clearly outlined in the shape of a hoof, to mark where the devil had trod on them. These bruises seemed to afford, then, convincing evidence that force had been applied to these women, but such bruises can even now occur on girls suffering with major hysteria. Hysterical persons involuntarily counterfeit the symptoms of physical disease as a means of attracting attention to themselves, of attaining sympathy, and of avoiding disagreeable situations.

Paralysis of a limb and lameness are common symptoms of hysteria; the limb may be drawn up in a deforming contracture, or palsied. Persons with hysteria may become mute or blind, their sensations may be perverted, they may vomit obstinately or lose their appetite and waste away. Hysterical women may believe themselves pregnant and show all the signs of that condition, suppression of the menses, colostrum in the breast, morning sickness, and swelling of the abdomen. This may continue until the time for delivery has long passed and their minds have turned to some other manifestation. Bloody Mary of England, daughter of Henry VIII and sister of Queen Elizabeth, is said to have had such a pseudopregnancy. Even in women who are not hysterical the fear of pregnancy will often delay the menses for a short time. Pseudo-hydrophobia is a disease that sometimes occurs in highly imaginative people. True hydrophobia is a disease which is acquired by infection from the virus found in the saliva of rabid animals. When the disease develops it is inevitably fatal; and in some persons fear of the disease is very great. If they are bitten by an animal their imagination may be so active that they develop the symptoms of rabies without having the disease. They may even exaggerate the symptoms and go into a frenzy, barking and snapping like a dog even though such symptoms do not appear in true rabies. True rabies cannot be cured by any known means, but pseudo-rabies responds readily to faith healing. A guilty conscience is sometimes responsible for the symptoms of gonorrhea, and only a microscopic examination can tell whether the sufferer needs the injections of a genito-urinary specialist or the confessional to relieve the symptoms.

Hysterical patients are numerous; and it is the hysterical patients among the halt, the lame, and the blind who pass from one medical man to another unrelieved, but who readily become the shining examples of the faith healer's skill. Thereafter they sing his praises. Only recently has the medical profession studied particularly this group of patients, for whom pills and elixirs, diet and physical hygiene are of no benefit. The treatment of the soldier suffering from shell shock was a notable example of mental healing carried out under medical methods. Under psychological study, faith healing is being salvaged from the hands of the charlatan and the fanatic. It is becoming a rudimentary science.

Not all men and women who have responded to faith cures are hysterical. There are numerous cases of bedridden invalids crippled by rheumatism and unable for years to put a foot on the ground, who nevertheless under some great stress, such as the house burning down around them, have shown remarkable returns of activity. The rheumatism which had crippled them had been real in the beginning, but during a long illness they had got into the habit of believing themselves crippled even after they were well. They had lost confidence in themselves. Some years ago minor railroad accidents often resulted in some of the passengers developing stiff backs. The condition was called "railroad-spine." It was invariably cured when the railroad paid damages; nothing else could aid it. Finally the imaginary origin of the disease was recognized, damages were no longer paid, and the disease no longer occurred. People who become dyspeptic, bilious, or melancholy from worry and frustrated desires are cured when their worries cease or their desires are realized. Homesickness and lovesickness are real diseases, and no medicine is so good for one as a trip home, while marriage is a permanent cure for the other.

In the body nearly every action involves a reaction. The brain affects the activity of the body, and the activity of the body in turn affects the brain. A melancholy state of mind may cause a bilious attack and a bilious attack may cause a melancholy state of mind. Disease may originate in the mind or it may originate in the body. The two are connected so closely that it is sometimes difficult to distinguish which one of them is the real seat of the distemper. The faith healer believes that all disease is mental and he carries his

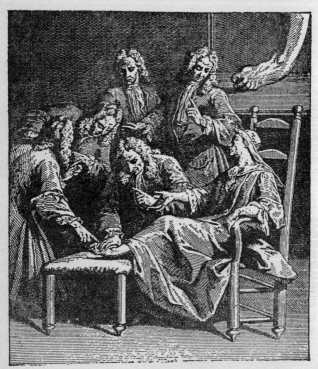

CLUBFOOT RESULTING FROM HYSTERIA

This deformity was examined by five surgeons, who declared that it was incurable (in the eighteenth century such deformities could not be corrected by surgery). The foot was restored to the normal shape when the woman recovered from her hysteria.

belief to fanatical extremes. The physician is sometimes equally convinced that all disease is physical and he looks with contempt upon imaginary ailments which are none the less real to the sufferers.

The chief difficulty in the matter arises from the fact that an arbitrary distinction has been drawn between the body and the mind. The two are not separate entities. The brain is an organ of the body just as is the liver or heart. The brain, like the liver, depends upon the rest of the body for warmth and nourishment. The liver when stimulated secretes bile, the heart when stimulated pumps blood, and the brain when stimulated secretes thoughts. The brain and nervous system, because of their action in coördinating the activity of all parts of the body, appear to have a more important corporeal function than other organs of the body. Such is not the case. Its function, the mind, is dependent upon the working of the brain quite as much as the function of any other organ is upon its living physico-chemical processes.

It is an ancient and fallacious practice to impute metaphysical qualities to certain organs. The heroes of the Homeric poems had their souls in their livers, the heroines of romantic literature concealed theirs in their hearts, orthodox people of the present time have theirs in their brains. As recently as Shakespeare's time the sexual passions were supposed to be centered in the liver: when Ford asks Pistol, "Love my wife?" Pistol replies, "With liver burning hot." In literature of today the heart is still the seat of "tender emotions." Thus there is the broken heart, the sweetheart, the sacred heart, and all the imagery of St. Valentine. In spite of its allegorical elevation the heart quite automatically pumps blood and does nothing more.

The blood itself has a peculiar significance in the minds of many people. It is regarded as the real and final link in "persons of the same blood." Blood also has its significance in the popular fallacy of the disease, as "bad blood." In reality the only peculiarity of the blood lies in the fact that it is a liquid tissue and one of the least alive in the body. It is merely a pabulum which carries gas and food from one part of the body to another. The peculiar virtues formerly attributed to the blood are shown by the comments occasioned during the early attempts of transfusion from one person to another. Bayle was anxious to know whether it would change the temperament of the man receiving the blood and whether transfusion of sheep's blood to a dog would ultimately convert the dog to a sheep. A German surgeon proposed to use transfusion to reconcile the parties of unhappy marriages; the incompatible pair were to be reciprocally transfused and thus, by sharing the same blood,

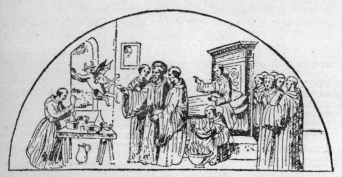

ST. GUALBERT FREEING A SICK MONK OF HIS DEVIL

would consequently have the same traits and the same interests in life.

Even the secretions of the body do not escape allegorical significance. The sweat of the brow is noble and that of the feet ignoble. Tears and saliva are essentially the same sort of secretion, but one is shed for tender emotions and the other is spat in derision.

None of the parts of the body is superlative or independent; they are all dependent and correlated. Each organ of the body when disordered manifests a characteristic disturbance, and this disturbance involves all of the parts of the body which are dependent upon the functioning of that organ. When the heart is damaged by disease there is shortness of breath and the legs swell with dropsy; the blood supply to the brain fails and unconsciousness follows. No one of these symptoms points directly to the heart as the seat of the trouble. Unconsciousness, shortness of breath, and swelling of the legs might be caused by a disturbance centered entirely in the brain. The distinction must be made by a trained observer. He studies the heart; he listens to its action and determines its size and notes its regularity. If he finds the abnormality in the heart he treats that organ. On the other hand the patient may believe his heart is diseased when in reality his symptoms arise from a gastric disturbance. In such cases his overwrought imagination may fabricate additional symptoms. The trained observer after making an examination can tell the patient that there is nothing wrong with his heart. If the patient has confidence in the physician his symptoms may disappear. Medical diagnosis may thus serve as an end in treating disease. More often, however, the patient retains his conviction that his heart is disordered. This conviction is increased rather than decreased when he consults other physicians and finds none to agree with him. Finally he falls into the hands of a faith healer or joins a healing cult. His "heart disease" is then cured.

Diseases may be divided into three classes: first, those which are entirely mental; second, those which are physical but tend to cure themselves; third, those which are physical but do not tend to cure themselves. Eighty to ninety per cent of all diseases belong to the first two classes. A man with a paralysis of his leg of mental origin, with a head cold, with lumbago, or with a stomach-ache from overeating gets well under the attention of a faith healer, a chiropractor, or even by taking patent medicine, and all but the paralytic will get well if nothing were done. On the other hand, such diseases as diphtheria, malaria, syphilis, cancer, diabetes, tuberculosis, and pernicious anemia do not get well with faith healing, chiropractic treatment, or psychoanalysis. If they are to be cured, the best medical attention is essential. The trained physician picks out from his patients the 10 or 20 per cent for whom his treatment may be life-saving. Under the ministrations of a faith healer these patients would die. But even if they did, the faith healer's result would be still 80 or 90 per cent effective. Furthermore, there is a tendency for the followers of faith cures to backslide and call the physician when they are seriously ill or in pain.

The belief in faith cures rests upon testimony. There is no form of reasoning more fallacious than that which leads to the testimony of the untrained observer. Such an observer invariably falls into that great fallacy of *post hoc ergo propter hoc:* the argument that he was sick, he was treated, he is now well, and therefore the treatment cured him. Eighty to ninety per cent of all ailments get well of themselves under fair conditions, but most people imagine that such recoveries are positive cures. The cure is invariably attributed to whatever procedure was used as a treatment. One of the greatest benefits of medical science lies in diagnosis; it picks out from the one hundred patients the ten or twenty who would die soon without proper treatment. The quack and the faith healer may receive the benefit for the cures of the remaining eighty or ninety cases in every hundred; in fact, the body has simply to heal itself.

There was one form of faith healing, now extinct, which was preceded by a sort of medical examination. It was the "royal touch" for the "king's evil" and epilepsy. The king's evil was scrofula, or tuberculosis of the glands of the neck, although at the time the royal touch was in practice any swelling of the neck was placed under this general classification and accepted by the royal physician for the king's treatment.

According to tradition the practice of the king's touch originated with Edward the Confessor, in England. The account of its beginning is as follows: "A young woman had married a husband of her own age, but having no issue by the union, the humours collected abundantly about her neck, she contracted a sore disorder, and the glands swelling in a dreadful manner. Admonished in a dream to have the part affected washed by the king, she entered the palace, and the king himself fulfilled this labor of love by rubbing the woman's neck with his fingers dipped in water. Joyous health followed his healing hand; the lurid skin opened, so that worms flowed out with the purulent matter, and the tumor subsided. But as the orifice of the ulcer was large and unsightly, he commanded her to be supported at royal expense until she should be perfectly cured. However, before a week had expired, a fair new skin returned, and hid the scars so completely that nothing of the original wound could be discovered; and within a year, becoming the mother of twins, she increased the admiration of Edward's holiness." In other words, she gave a testimony of her cure.

This miraculous ability to effect cures by the laying on of hands was thought to be inherited by the successors of Edward, but later it was included as part of the divine right of kings. The practice of touching for the king's evil developed into an elaborate ceremony. The assembled patients were examined by the king's physician and those considered unsuited for treatment were turned away. Those chosen for treatment were required to submit a certificate that they had never before been touched for the disease—a significant fact in relation to the permanency of the cures. The sufferers submitted to the king were blessed, their sores were touched, and a gold piece was hung about the neck of each. The gold piece was analogous to the amulet of the savage and was probably a potent factor in keeping up the practice. The outlay of coins sometimes rose to a figure as high as $50,000 annually, and after the time of Elizabeth the size of the coin was reduced.

Not all of the kings believed in the efficacy of their touch. James I wished to drop the practice as a superstition, but was persuaded to continue it for political reasons. William III expressed his sentiments in the whole matter by the words he used when laying on his hands, "May God give you better health and more sense." He finally refused to continue the practice and was in consequence accused of cruelty. Queen Anne was the last of the English royalty to carry on the practice; after her death it was discontinued. Dr. Samuel Johnson was one of the last persons touched; he was at the time four years old, and from Boswell's account it is known that he suffered from scrofula all his life.

The king's touch was not limited to the English royalty, but was practiced also by the kings of France. Louis XIV touched sixteen hundred persons on one Easter Sunday, although an outspoken commentator says that no one was cured. As in England, each patient received payment as part

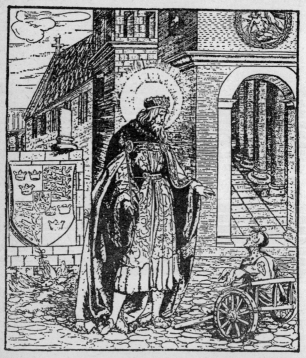

KING EDWARD THE CONFESSOR APPLYING FAITH HEAL-
ING

From a woodcut after a drawing by Hans Burgkmaier. This king is credited with having started the practice of touching for the king's evil, which is scrofula or tuberculosis of the glands of the neck.

of his treatment. The practice of touching for scrofula was terminated in France only a short time before the French Revolution.

The more dissolute the king, the more virtue seemed to be attributed to his touch. Charles II was the busiest of all the healers. Even when he was in exile in the Netherlands he was besieged by patients. On one day in the year 1684 the crowd applying for treatment was so great that six or seven of the sick were trampled to death. It is noteworthy that more people are said to have died of scrofula in the time of Charles II than in any other period of English history.

The kings of England also dispensed "cramp rings" to be used for preventing cramps and fits. Henry VIII, even after his separation from the Church, continued the practice, and there is in existence a letter from Anne Boleyn which tells of their distribution. It reads: "Mr. Stephens, I send you here cramp rings for you and Mr. Gregory and Mr. Peter, praying you to distribute them as you think best—Anne Boleyn." The practice of providing cramp rings was discontinued by Edward VI. Queen Elizabeth had a blessed ring which she wore suspended between her breasts. The ring had "the virtue of expelling infected air." It was analogous to the asafetida bags of later days.

During the Middle Ages faith healing was raised to a greater ascendancy than at any period other than the most primitive. It was the "age of faith," a period made glorious by magnificent cathedrals, but characterized also by domestic squalor, theological bigotry, and pestilential diseases. Christian superstition was at its height. During and after the decline of the Roman Empire the art of treating disease developed by the Greek physicians disintegrated under the influence of Christianity. The Greeks had dispensed with priestly healing, and they had converted the Romans from their dependence upon a multitude of healing gods and home remedies to an acceptance of rational therapy. But under Christian influence rational therapy based on observation at the bedside was replaced by faith healing as crude and superstitious as that of primitive peoples.

The early and medieval Christians accepted the doctrine of the power of demons in the lives of men; they saw this power particularly in the demoniac production of disease. They believed in miracles and especially in the miraculous healing of diseases. The demonological belief of the Christians was inherited from the doctrine of the Jews, who were firm believers in demons and the "possession by devils." Thus the logical cure of disease consisted in the exorcism of devils. Jesus himself cured by casting out devils. Following His example, Christians everywhere became exorcists. Jewish demonology was continued among Christian converts and the belief in supernatural interpositions in human affairs was widely accepted. Nothing has retarded the growth of scientific medicine during the past two thousand years so much as the iron grip of theology in maintaining practices based on belief in this supernatural origin of disease.

Christian theology retarded the development of means to cure the sick, but at the same time the Christian religion partially compensated for this detriment by introducing an entirely new attitude toward the sick. Formerly the destitute sick rarely received charitable aid, and certainly they received no personal ministrations during their sickness. Foundlings were deserted on the temple steps, to be adopted or to die, as chance dictated. Under the precepts of Jesus the sick and the weak were to be cared for by the strong and healthy. Charity hospitals were founded. For centuries these institutions were simply refuges for the destitute sick. Medical care was not given. It is only in recent times, since modern medical treatment has been developed, that hospitals supply proper care as well as refuge for the sick. Nevertheless, the modern charity hospitals, foundling homes, and the municipal care of the sick and infirm have originated in the Christian religion and have developed from their predecessors of early Christian days.

The whole conception of disease, under the early Christian religion, can be summed up in the words of St. Augustine in the fifth century: "All diseases of Christians are to be ascribed to demons, chiefly do they torment the fresh baptized, yea, even the guiltless new-born infant." For the sixth century Gregory the Great was a broad-minded man, yet even he solemnly relates that a·nun, having eaten some lettuce without making the sign of the cross, swallowed a devil, and that when the devil was commanded to come forth by a holy man it did so and said: "How am I to blame? I was sitting on the lettuce, and this woman, not having made the sign of the cross, ate me along with it."

Men who cast out devils were very careful to keep their mouths closed while carrying out their exorcism, lest the devil should jump from the mouth of the patient into their own mouths. Nowadays the droplets of saliva blown about in sneezing have taken the place of devils in the transmission of disease. According to medieval belief the devils of disease were also prone to enter the mouths of human beings during sleep. As late as the seventeenth century King Charles II of Spain had his confessor and two friars sit beside his bed while he slept to keep away the devils. Until recent times it was believed that night air caused disease and bedroom windows were closed tightly at night. This belief in the harmfulness of night air was a remnant of the ancient belief in wandering devils as the cause of disease.

Under the belief that possession by devils causes disease, the sick were treated by prayers, by exorcism of the devils, by the laying on of hands, and by the contact of holy relics. They were encouraged to greater faith. All cures were attributed to the method of treatment. And since, as stated above, 80 to 90 per cent of all illness gets well of itself, there were naturally many cures attributed to this treatment. Cures lead to testimonials and testimonials are enlarged in tradition. If the patient stubbornly retained his illness, it was assumed that he personally refused to get well and he was treated accordingly. During epidemics of pestilential diseases such stubborn sufferers were sometimes carried to churches, a dozen at a time, securely bound together. They were thrown upon the floor of the church and lay there until they died or until, their faith returning, their devil was expelled, and with it their illness. Recoveries were not frequent under this treatment, but the patient and not the treatment was blamed.

The power by which some of the saints effected miraculous cures was supposed to persist and emanate from their relics and from articles they had consecrated. Sacred pools where sufferers were bathed, shrines where they prayed, and relics

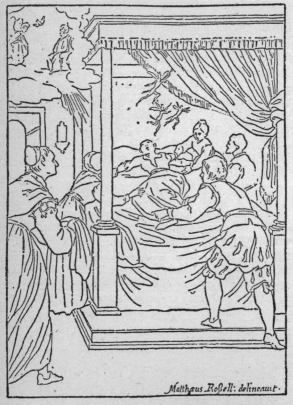

*Matthæus Roßell: delineauit.*

**A WOMAN DELIVERED OF THREE DEVILS**
From the work of Matteo Rosselli in a church at Florence.

which they touched became the means of effecting cures. The demand for relics led to a business in supplying them; it developed in the Holy Land and flourished profitably. The fact that most of the relics which were purchased by the

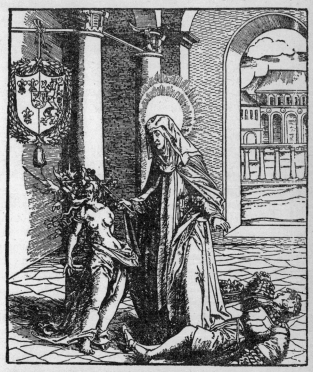

ST. RADEGONDE, QUEEN OF FRANCE, EXORCISING A DEVIL
From a woodcut after a drawing of Hans Burgkmaier.

crusaders and pilgrims and brought back to Europe were of contemporaneous manufacture did not interfere in the least with their healing virtue.

The most cherished curative relic was the wood of the true cross, and if the pieces of it scattered throughout Europe had been collected in one spot there would have been enough for many crosses. Tears of the Saviour, the Virgin Mary, and St. Peter were brought back from the Holy Land centuries after their deaths, and so also was the blood of Jesus and the milk of Mary. The unscrupulous ecclesiastics of the Holy Land carried on a flourishing business in selling parings from their own toenails, which they represented to the pilgrims who annually visited Palestine as coming from the nails of dead saints. The parings from the nails of St. Peter were unusually prolific, and an amazing quantity of them found their way into Europe. One monastery in Jerusalem even offered for sale what was represented to the gullible as the finger of the Holy Ghost, and another monastery had a feather from the same source.

There was rivalry between the different monasteries and churches to possess the most attractive and efficacious relics. This rivalry was partly a matter of profit, for the sick who were benefited at the church made payments, and in some cases great fortunes were amassed from these donations. In the twelfth century the shrine at the cathedral at Cologne obtained the skulls of the Three Wise Men of the East who brought gifts to the Infant Jesus. In competition the church of St. Gereon produced the relics of St. Gereon and his whole band of martyrs. The competitive spirit spread to the church of St. Ursula, and a whole cemetery was despoiled to cover the interior walls of the monastery with the relics of St. Ursula and her eleven thousand virgin martyrs. The fact that many of these bones were unquestionably those of men did not affect their curative value. The supplicants believed that the relics were real and they believed also that they possessed a supernatural curative value. So far as real cures resulted, they were effected entirely through the minds of the sufferers, as is always the case with faith cures.

In modern times the most famous healing shrines are those of Lourdes in France (vividly described in Zola's novel, *Lourdes*) and St. Anne de Beaupré in Canada. Relics and shrines cure today as they did in medieval times. Modern physicians even have sent some of their patients to be thus treated. All diseases due to hysteria or to melancholy states of mind are susceptible to such cures. Even men and women suffering from incurable diseases are temporarily improved by the hope that is inspired in them.

Many of the Christian saints personally practiced the healing art either by exorcism of devils or by the laying on of hands. They carried on the medicine of primitive man. They took up the practice where it had been left by the priests of Æsculapius five hundred years before Christ, when for a few hundred years rational medicine replaced faith healing. The cures of the saints were carried on with gradually diminishing zeal; the practice then fell into the hands of the kings of England and France in the royal touch. After royalty had ceased to practice faith healing the art passed through the hands of such charlatans as Valentine Greatrakes, Cagliostro, Mesmer, and Andrew Jackson Davis, and so into the hands of Dowie, Eddy, and Coué. From the primitive medicine-man to the Christian Science "reader" the method of treatment has differed only in detail. The strength of all such healers lies in the faith of their disciples; so long as confidence is supreme, treatment brings peace and security even though death results.

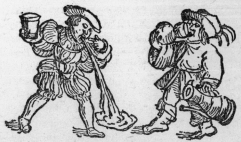

"A KIND OF MEDICINE"
A woodcut from the medical poem of **Salerno.**
"If wine have overnight a surfet brought,
   A thing we wish to you should happen feeld:
Then early in the morning drinke a draught,
   And that a kind of remedie shall yield."

# CHAPTER XIII

## WHITE MAGIC AND BLACK

aith healing cults of today are the revivals of primitive, early Christian, and medieval practices. The healer still finds a fanatical following. But such cults are now short-lived, usually rising and passing away during one or two generations. To obtain the desired impression upon the patients, bizarre surroundings, weird procedures, strange philosophies, or a glorified and even semi-divine showman, are necessary. These drapings of the faith cure must be frequently changed; the bizarre effects that impress one generation become amusing in the greater sophistication of the next. Philosophies pass out of date and must be rewritten. The fountainhead of the faith dies and his followers disperse, or he commits some worldly act and the illusion is destroyed. One of the most successful charlatans of faith healing was Cagliostro, who lived in the time of Louis XVI. Dumas has used him for a central character in his *Memoirs of a Physician* and its sequel. Cagliostro used mysticism and alchemy as the trappings for his cures. He treated nobles all over Europe for diseases that the physicians of those days could not cure; he sold beds that provided painless childbirth, chairs that cured rheumatism, and, for those who could afford it, he supplied an elixir of life.

In the eighteenth century James Graham, of London, revived the miraculous beds of Cagliostro, but along with another line of approach. In 1779 he opened a Temple of Health in London and there among other pieces of quackery exploited a "celestial bed" the use of which, at a price, assured conception to the occupants. To quote from an article written at the time and reprinted in the *British Medical Journal* for 1911: "A sumptuous bed in brocaded damask supported by four crystal pillars of spiral shape

festooned with garlands of flowers in gilded metal is its
essential feature; and for a fee of fifty guineas Dr. Graham
offers couples, old and young, the means of getting offspring.
On whatever side one gets into this bed, which is called

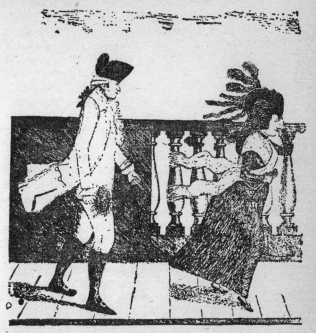

JAMES GRAHAM, THE PROPRIETOR OF A "CELESTIAL BED"

A quack of the eighteenth century who developed a treatment guaranteed to maintain life to the age of one hundred years, but who
nevertheless died while still quite young.

'Celestial,' one hears an organ played in unison with three
others, which make agreeable music consisting of varied airs
which carry the happy couple into the arms of Morpheus.
For nearly an hour that the concert lasts one sees in the bed
streams of light which play especially over the pillows. When

the time for getting up has come, the magician comes to feel the pulse of the faithful, gives them breakfast, and sends them away full of hope, not forgetting to recommend them to send him other clients." One of Graham's assistants in the Temple of Health was Emma Lyon, afterward Lady Hamilton, whose name is associated with that of Nelson. The Temple of Health failed after a few years and Graham developed a fasting cure, something on the order of that later preached by Upton Sinclair and others as a new revelation. Graham's cure was to assure life for a century, but he died before he was fifty.

A less mercenary figure in the field of faith healing in the past was Valentine Greatrakes, the stroker. At the outbreak of the Irish Rebellion in 1641 he joined Cromwell's army. Cromwell drove out King Charles, but Cromwell refused to accept either the throne or the practice of the royal touch. Valentine Greatrakes came forward to fill the need for a toucher. He was inspired to do so by a dream, and by successive dreams he was inspired to extend his curative touch to almost every known malady. Many men of education and high position testified to the cures made by Greatrakes; even Robert Boyle, one of the fathers of modern chemistry, joined in the praise. In spite of their initial success Greatrake's cures did not persist. Fewer and fewer patients came to visit him, his curative power ceased to be talked of, and finally he retired. The people required some other novelty to catch their attention and effect their cures.

Personal healers who cure by the laying on of hands, by prayer, or by a species of exorcism were still common in the nineteenth century and are so even now. Many of these healers attracted attention only locally. The late Earl of Sandwich, for instance, conceived that he had a "gift" for healing. He practiced upon his servants with some success and later extended his efforts farther afield. Some of his patients failed to respond to his curative touch; but according to the earl it was the fault of the patient. Others of his patients got well after treatments which at the time had brought no results. These cases the earl counted as cures.

Thus only death or permanent disability could be counted as a failure; his method of reasoning was the same as that of religious healers of medieval time. The earl speaks naïvely of the reaction of his friends toward his gift for healing: "Old friends so disliked the idea that they began by shunning all allusion to the subject and now avoid my society." It is probable that the enthusiasm in his new acquisition made the earl something of a bore. The leader of a cult of mental healing usually becomes self-centered, intolerant, and selfish; and he usually feels driven to make converts to his belief. To a less degree the same qualities appear in the devotees of the cult.

It is an extraordinary fact that many faith healers arose in the United States during the nineteenth and twentieth centuries. They found here a following such as could be obtained nowhere else at this time. These healers established cults based on theories of a religious or metaphysical nature. In the 'forties of the nineteenth century Andrew Jackson Davis, a cobbler of Poughkeepsie, New York, advanced a metaphysical doctrine of life, health, and the cure of disease. His book setting forth his views was entitled *The Principles of Nature, Her Divine Revelations and a Voice to Mankind*. This book had a large sale, quite as large as Mrs. Eddy's on Christian Science. At the time of its appearance it was pronounced by a professor in a college of New York City to be "one of the most finished specimens of philosophical argument in the English language." Editions of the book were published as late as the Civil War, but this "finished specimen of philosophical argument" is now merely a curiosity. Without the publicity which Davis created by reports of his marvelous cures the book now seems filled with the shallowest and wordiest twaddle. Yet Davis's following before the Civil War formed quite as large a body as do the Christian Scientists of today. Like the founder of Christian Science, Davis made a fortune. He lacked, however, Mrs. Eddy's organizing ability, and his cult died out even during his lifetime. At the height of his success, however, Davis appeared before the United States Senate in the effort to have his methods officially sanctioned and financially supported by the government. This is not the only instance in which the United States Senate has seriously considered an official recognition for faith healing; a few states have in fact afforded chiropractic treatment such recognition. In 1854 the Senate was petitioned to bestow its official sanction upon spiritualism and to make it a national institution. The matter was discussed in the Senate but was finally rejected.

The theories which Davis expounded were the direct antithesis of those which Mrs. Eddy supported. In his metaphysical conception there was no mind, but only matter and power, while in Mrs. Eddy's metaphysics there is no matter, but only mind. Nevertheless, Davis's followers were as cheerfully free of disease as are the followers of Mrs. Eddy.

Although many healing cults started in the United States in the nineteenth century, only a few of them attracted more than passing attention and most have now died out and are forgotten. In the middle of the nineteenth century George O. Barnes, the Mountain Evangelist, obtained a large following, mostly in Kentucky. He believed that the devil caused disease and he cured by anointing with oil and with religious invocations. Similarly, the leader of the Mormons, Joseph Smith, Jr., performed faith healing. One of the elders of the church advertised to "set bones through faith in Christ" and made this statement regarding the treatment: "While commanding the bones, they come together, making a noise like the crushing of an old basket." Smith failed as a spiritual healer when Asiatic cholera broke out among his followers.

Another faith healer who attracted wide attention was Francis Schlatter. In 1893 he left Denver, Colorado, and wandered as far as New Mexico, bareheaded and barefooted, over the mountains and plains, led, as he asserted, by divine inspiration. He returned to Denver as a faith healer, and his fame grew until he was visited by patients from all over the United States. Each day a line of four or five thousand people formed before his house, where he stood behind a picket fence to touch each sufferer that filed past him. Schlatter attempted to extend his curative work to those who could not come to him, by sending blessed handkerchiefs through the mail. The government took a hand in the matter at this stage and denied him the use of the mails on the ground of fraud, and Schlatter's following diminished and finally ceased altogether.

One of the most eminent faith healers of recent times was John Alexander Dowie, whose work has extended well into the twentieth century. For some years he was connected with the Divine Healing Association, but eventually he broke away from this organization and established the Christian Catholic Church which after 1901 was centered at Zion City, a suburb of Chicago. Dowie maintained that disease was the work of the devil and that prayer and the laying on of hands was a cure for it—a revival of early Christian and medieval beliefs. His disbelief in the methods of modern medicine is evident from the title of one of his pamphlets: *Doctors, Drugs and Devils*. In a previous chapter a quotation was given from this work, in which is set forth Dowie's ideas of anatomical dissection.

The outstanding faith healer of the nineteenth century was Phineas Quimby, of Maine. His importance comes not so much from his own work as from the influence he exerted in the origin of New Thought and Christian Science. Quimby began faith healing with the use of hypnotism, which was then called animal magnetism. This type of cure was extensively and profitably exploited by Mesmer in the eighteenth century. Mesmer called his practice animal magnetism, but it was more generally known as mesmerism and later as hypnotism. In the middle of the nineteenth century this revival of animal magnetism attracted much attention, and vast power was imputed to those who practiced hypnotism. For a time it was believed that persons under the influence of hypnotism could be made to commit crimes, even murder. The story of Trilby, the servant girl with a croaking voice, and the hypnotist Svengali, who made of her an operatic prima donna, is illustrative of the belief current about hypnotism. It is true that the mind while in the hypnotic state is abnormally susceptible to suggestion—in fact, only an abnormally suggestible person can be hypnotized—

but such persons can do nothing during the hypnotic state which is contrary to their natural characteristics or ability. Hypnotism persists today as an occasional practice in dealing with drug addicts and neurotics and in acts on the vaudeville stage.

During his early days as a practitioner of faith healing Quimby's method of treatment consisted in sitting beside his patient—usually a woman—putting his left hand on her bare abdomen, and with the other hand rubbing her head. He told the patient that in so doing animal magnetism flowed out of his body into hers and that the animal magnetism thus acquired would cure her. After a time Quimby discovered that he could obtain just as good cures without laying on his hands. All he had to do then was to sit beside his patient, look into her eyes, and have her tell him her troubles and all her thoughts. The procedure was a sort of psychoanalysis without the pseudo-scientific trimmings of that practice. After having listened sympathetically to his patients' troubles for a few years Quimby found that he could cure without enduring protracted dissertations covering lack of sympathy, unrequited love, and all the other grievances of the "misunderstood woman." He developed a metaphysical cure. He taught that there is no evil in the world. Evil exists only in the mind. Illness results from evil thoughts, and when the evil thoughts are expelled from the mind disease disappears. Health-giving forces from God are everywhere about people, but many people withhold these forces by the fear of disease. To avoid disease it is necessary to keep thoughts of disease out of the mind; to think only good and not evil. These principles have continued as the basis of the New Thought. It is an optimistic philosophy that has prevented much suffering and made life happier for many people. It is what William James called the religion of "healthymindedness." Unhappiness and suffering do indeed exist only in mind; but unfortunately disease has an objective existence. New Thought is a sort of mental prophylaxis against disease, but the mortality among its adherents is just as high as among non-adherents; but perhaps they die happier.

Quimby's metaphysical conception of disease led directly to the founding of Christian Science. Its organizer, Mrs. Mary A. Morse Baker Glover Patterson Eddy, was born in Bow, New Hampshire, about 1821; she counted among her ancestors Sir John McNeill[1] of Scotland, and the poetess Hannah More. As a child she was said to be neurotic and subject to fits of nervousness which interfered with her schooling,[2] a fact which may account for the numerous ungrammatical passages in her later writings. At the age of twenty-two she married George Washington Glover, a stone mason, who died six months later and before the birth of her only child. During ten years of widowhood she stayed with relatives and had long periods of illness of a hysterical character. A psychoanalyst would, no doubt, have discovered many interesting repressions and complexes in her personality during this time. She experimented with various meth-

---

[1] This statement is made by Mary Eddy in her autobiography *Retrospection and Introspection,* and appears in an article published with her sanction in the *Ladies' Home Journal* for November, 1903. A member of the McNeill family promptly published a denial of this imputed relationship (*London Truth,* 1904). Mary Eddy, however, continued to use the McNeill coat-of-arms on her stationery and defended her action in a statement widely published in 1907. She says: "The facts regarding the McNeill coat-of-arms are as follows: Fannie McNeill, President Pierce's niece, afterwards Mrs. Judge Potter, presented to me my coat-of-arms saying that it was taken in connection with her own family coat-of-arms. I never doubted the veracity of the gift." The coat-of-arms included the motto of the Bath, which was given to Sir John McNeill for use only during his lifetime. The incident is typical of many of Mary Eddy's actions.

[2] Mary Eddy in *Retrospection and Introspection* states that she was kept out of school much of the time because her father "was taught to believe" that her brain was too large for her body; she says that her brother Albert taught her Greek, Latin, and Hebrew. Her definition of the significance of Adam's name is a commentary on her knowledge of Hebrew. In *Science and Health,* second edition, this statement appears: "Divide the name Adam into two syllables, and it reads *A dam,* or obstruction." Adam, the first mortal man, was thus "a dam" to spiritual life.

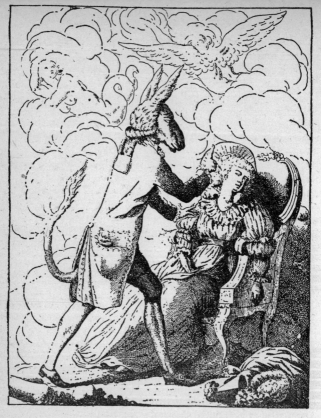

**ANIMAL MAGNETISM**
A caricature of the procedure made popular by Mesmer.

ods of treatment, trying the Graham system of diet,[1] homeopathy, spiritualism, and mesmerism. In 1853 she married

---

[1] *Science and Health,* 1875 edition. Graham was the originator of Graham bread. Mary Eddy, like most hypochondriacs, seemed to turn to each new health fad that appeared, but it was not until she met Quimby that she discovered how profitable these fads might be for their backers. She made a large fortune out of Christian Science.

Daniel Patterson, an itinerant dentist, who deserted her in 1862[1] and from whom she subsequently obtained a divorce.

Her nervous disorders persisted in spite of—or because of—this unsatisfactory marriage, and she turned to Quimby for help. Under his ministrations her health improved, thus clearly showing the neurotic origin of her affliction. She studied Quimby's methods and, later, dates her discovery of the principle of Christian Science from the year of his death, 1866.[2] For the next few years she wandered about from town to town in the vicinity of Boston in straitened circumstances, teaching what she then called Quimby's Science, healing, and endeavoring to obtain a following. In 1875 she succeeded in gathering a small group of disciples, and in the same year published her book, *Science and Health*. From its small beginning the cult of Christian Science has grown to include many thousands of people.

During the early days of Christian Science the affairs of the organization were frequently in disorder, and its contro-

---

[1] Mary Eddy's statement of this desertion is as follows (letter to the *Boston Post*, March 7, 1883): ". . . My husband had eloped with a married woman from one of the wealthy families of this city, leaving no trace save his last letter to us wherein he wrote: 'I hope sometime to be worthy of so good a wife!'" Even on reading the entire statement, it is impossible to determine what city is meant by "this city"; the antecedent of "so good a wife" is likewise ambiguous and it is difficult to tell whether he refers to his legitimate wife or to the wife with whom he is thus said to have eloped. The truth of the matter is there is no ground for Mary Eddy's imputation against her husband's character; he was a long-suffering man who finally left an uncongenial wife, went alone, and continued for some time to contribute to her support.

[2] *Science and Health*, 1898 edition: "In the year 1866, I discovered the Science of Metaphysical Healing, and named it Christian Science." Quimby, however, in a manuscript written in 1863 and entitled *Aristocracy and Democracy*, had also called his healing Christian Science; usually, however, Quimby referred to his theory as the "Science of Health and Happiness." For a number of years Mary Eddy used and taught Quimby's practice of rubbing the head of the patient under treatment, but subsequently she disclaimed this procedure (Eddy, *Science of Man*, 1876).

versies were aired in law courts and newspapers. Mary Eddy never quite succeeded in getting away from some of the ideas of animal magnetism which she had obtained from Quimby. Her cures had nothing to do directly with this belief, but she developed what would appear to be delusions of persecution and felt that malicious animal magnetism emanating from her enemies was producing many ills and had caused the death of her third husband, Asa Eddy.[1] She even instigated a suit to enjoin her enemies from exerting this influence and to have them punished for doing so.

Malicious animal magnetism is obviously merely another name for witchcraft. It is, in fact, the exact opposite of faith healing; instead of inspiring health by faith, witchcraft inspires disease. Witchcraft was the black magic of the Middle Ages. The persecution of witches, which caused the deaths of thousands of innocent children and old women, developed on an enormous scale in Europe in the fifteenth century. It was undertaken under an interpretation of a bull issued by Pope Innocent VIII directed against heretics. Its real authority, however, was the Bible. Exodus xxii: 18, two chapters after the Ten Commandments, reads, "Thou shalt not suffer a witch to live." The rack and other methods of torture were used to obtain confession of witchcraft. Men were employed to hunt out witches and paid for each one they detected. The witches were usually burned, and one executioner in Germany during his term of office burned alive seven hundred of these old women. Queen Elizabeth made witchcraft a capital offense in England, and King James I wrote a book on the subject and lent his personal support to the persecution. Witch-hunting reached America in 1684 and a shrewish old woman in Pennsylvania was tried that year before William Penn and a jury of Quakers. The verdict of these sensible people was: "The prisoner is guilty of the common fame of being a witch but not guilty

---

[1] Mary Eddy in an interview in the *Boston Post*, June 5, 1882, says, "My husband's death was caused by malicious animal magnetism." She had married Asa Eddy, a sewing-machine agent, in 1876. The marriage license recorded her age as forty years, but she was then fifty-five.

as she stands indicted." In New England, however, the superstition found supporters in two ministers, the Rev. Cotton Mather and Samuel Parris, the one an alumnus and the other a student of Harvard College. At their instigation twenty people were put to death and fifty-five others tortured or frightened into confessions. For a time the jails of Salem were filled with the accused and suspected. The panic over witchcraft was, however, short-lived in New England;

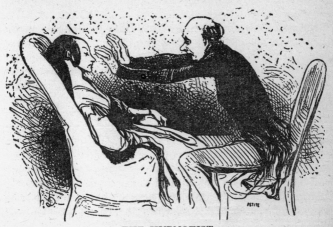

THE HYPNOTIST
An etching by Daumier.

the common sense of the people soon asserted itself and the prisoners were liberated.

Thus when Mary Eddy assigned hysterical ailments to malicious animal magnetism and asked the courts of Salem, in 1878, to punish alleged persecutors, she was attempting to revive witchcraft and the punishment of witches. But along with this black magic she introduced white magic. The absent treatment she advocated was a phase of beneficial animal magnetism, that is white magic in contrast to the harmful black magic or witchcraft.

After organizing her church Mrs. Eddy disclaimed any connection with Quimby's teachings, and this connection has been much disputed. The facts of the matter are that neither Mary Baker Eddy nor Phineas Quimby discovered the basis of Christian Science. All the forms of healing Christianity which developed in the nineteenth century were plagiarisms, compounded in varying degrees from existing religious conceptions, occult medicine, and bizarre metaphysics. The leaders of the various cults all acquired their metaphysical materials from the same sources.

The principle advocated by Mrs. Eddy for the prevention and treatment of disease was based upon the ancient metaphysical conception that as matter is known only through the senses, it has no existence except in mind. Matter is merely an illusion. In applying this theory to disease Mary Eddy says:[1] "Mind is all and matter naught . . . man is never sick; for mind is not sick; and matter cannot be. False belief is both the tempter and the tempted, the sin and the sinner, the disease and its cure. . . . The cure of disease is effected by making the disease appear to be—what it really is—an illusion." Similar ideas were advocated in the seventeenth century by the illustrious English philosopher, Bishop Berkeley. He advocated also the use of tar water as a cure for the afflictions to which the (non-existent) flesh is heir.

Some of the precepts laid down in Mrs. Eddy's *Science and Health* are repellent to fastidious people. But when Mary Eddy wrote her book she was apparently in a dilemma. According to the hypothesis that she advocated, the body existed only as a mental illusion and such an hypothesis carried to its logical conclusion precludes the necessity of bathing. Mrs. Eddy was raised during a time when frequent bathing was not a cardinal virtue even among cultured people, and it may be imagined that she herself was not fastidious in her person, for she says:[2] ". . . Washing should be only to keep the body clean, and this can be done

---

[1] *Science and Health,* edition of 1875.

[2] *Ibid.*

with less than daily scrubbing the whole surface." Again, in dealing with the care of infants, she says:[1] "The daily ablution of an infant is no more natural or necessary than to take a fish out of water and cover it with dirt once a day that it may thrive better in its natural element."

The caution toward water shown by Mary Eddy was not original with her; it was maintained generally and wholeheartedly in the Middle Ages. Frederick the Great rarely washed even his face, and in the nineteenth century the thesis of dirtiness had supporters who were much more outspoken than Mary Eddy. Thus Thomas Walker, of England, in 1835 experimented in improving his health by ceasing to wash, and after a time he found that washing was indeed superfluous. He discovered that under such circumstances there was a free and constant exhalation from the skin. A French physician has pointed out that in his country even today the workingmen, clerks, and small tradesmen look upon bathing not so much as a luxury as an eccentricity. A famous surgeon is quoted as saying in effect that in French hospital practice clean knees are an index of moral frailty.

On the care of infants Mary Eddy gives this advice[2] (she did not raise her own child): "The condition of the stomach, bowels, food, clothing, etc., is of no serious importance to your child. Your views regarding them will produce the only result they can have on the health of your child." A statement simply of white magic.

The disadvantages of magic—even white magic—appear when a follower of Christian Science is affected with cancer and treats the disease with the "science of metaphysical healing"; her friends, even her husband, wait with optimism as the disease passes without interference into the inoperable stage, and then watch her waste away to death. But such magic or religion is criminal when a child with diphtheria in a Christian Science family is refused antitoxin. In deaths under such circumstances the law has sometimes found the parents guilty of criminal neglect.

---

[1] *Ibid.*

[2] *Ibid.*

The best feature of Christian Science is the optimism it teaches to its followers; it teaches them not to brood over the ills of life. Its fallacy is its metaphysics, which teaches that all ills are mental. Christian Science, like the innumerable forms of faith healing which have preceded it and those which will follow it, will probably not be of long duration. All forms of faith healing during their maturity have shown a vigor which is no indication of duration. Many of them have attracted even greater followings than has Christian Science, but after reaching their maturity they have slowly decayed and have served only to enrich new forms of faith healing.

Most of the followers of Christian Science are educated but rather sentimental people. As a whole they are not well read, for the teachings of Mrs. Eddy discouraged the reading of any books other than her *Science and Health* from the numerous editions of which she received large royalties. There is no other accredited book on Christian Science, for Mrs. Eddy thoroughly suppressed any efforts of her followers to compete with her in the literary field. Christian Science makes no appeal to people who are poor. And no metaphysical forms of faith healing ever attract the ignorant or the young. For them some conception of a stronger and more impressive nature is required. Chiropractic manipulation furnishes such a robust form of treatment.

Chiropractic treatment is an old form of faith cure under a new name; its forerunner was osteopathy, and the forerunner of osteopathy was the bone manipulation practiced by "joint-adjusters" or "bone-setters." The practice of "bonesetting" has come down from antiquity; its practioners have claimed that the malposition of the bones interferes with the flow of vital forces. These joint-adjusters claim, moreover, that they can recognize dislocations and subluxations which escape the ordinary physician. Formerly this ability to recognize and correct bony malposition was supposed to be hereditary. But the alleged art is now taught in a number of schools, all of which are in America. Bone-setters have always made remarkable cures, but so did the relics from the

Holy Land and so have a horde of healers of all cults. A statement frequently repeated in previous chapters is that 80 to 90 per cent of all patients get well under any treatment, or none, and that when one of these patients gets well his case is invariably attributed to the virtues of the "treatment."

The most famous bone-setter was Mrs. Mapp, who lived in the eighteenth century and was a contemporary of the quacks "Spot" Ward and Chevalier Taylor. She was the daughter of an English bone-setter and her sister was the celebrated "Polly Peecham," who married the Duke of Bolton. Mrs. Mapp settled in Epsom; her fame became widespread and many of the nobility were among her patients. The *Gentleman's Magazine* for 1736 says: ". . . The attention of the public has been taken off from the wonder working of Mr. Ward to a strolling woman now at Epsom who calls herself 'crazy Sal'; and had performed cures in bone-setting to admiration, and occasioned so great a resort that the town offered her 100 guineas to continue there a year." Mrs. Mapp became a national character and attracted public attention wherever she appeared. A story is told of her which is reminiscent of one told of Nell Gwynne. One day, in driving in her carriage and four through London, she was mistaken for one of the king's German mistresses, who were very unpopular. A mob gathered and stopped her carriage. Mrs. Mapp put her head out of the window and cried: "Damn your bloods, don't you know me? I am Mrs. Mapp the bone-setter." The crowd cheered her as she drove away.

Hogarth drew an unflattering caricature of "Crazy Sal," and if one may judge from the drawing, cross-eyed Sal. On one side of her is "Spot" Ward and on the other Chevalier Taylor (see pages 52, 53). The two men hold gold-headed canes, distinctive of the medical profession of that period, while Mrs. Mapp brandishes a bone. The title of the drawing is "The Undertaker's Arms." A statement concerning Mrs. Mapp is made by Percival Pott, a famous English surgeon of the eighteenth century. He says: "We all remember that even the absurdities and impracticability of her own promises and engagement were by no means equal to the expectations and credulity of those who ran after her; that is of all ranks and degrees of people from the lowest laborer or mechanic up to those of the most exalted rank and station; several of whom not only did not hesitate to believe implicitly the most extravagant assertions of an ignorant, illiberal, drunken, female savage, but even solicited her company; at least seemed to enjoy her society."

Bone-setting was given a new name by Andrew Still, of Kansas. He called it osteopathy. His first patient was a young lady suffering from "nervous prostration"; all of the local doctors had tried to cure her, but had failed. Andrew Still saw her and without even an examination informed her that she had a partial dislocation of the neck. He lifted her head, pulled her neck, and told her she would get well, which she eventually did. On the basis of this case Still built up a whole theory. According to this theory all disease is due to partial dislocation of the spine; the misplaced vertebræ press upon the nerves emerging from the spine and disease results from this obstruction to the "flow of life forces through the nerves." To cure disease it is therefore only necessary to manipulate the spine, twist the neck, and pull the head. The whole procedure is merely the "laying on of hands," but a laying on with impressive force. Osteopaths and chiropractors are not allowed to practice in England, and America is now the happy hunting-ground for all cults, as Europe was in the Middle Ages. The *British Medical Journal* in commenting on osteopathy and chiropractic said: "It appears to observers at a distance that osteopathy and chiropractic are little more than terminological adaptations of 'bone-setting,' with the site of the operation cleverly transferred from the knee or ankle, where results, if any, can at least be seen, to the backbone, where they cannot."

The founder of osteopathy had a mystical turn of mind and, like most faith healers, carried a religious element into his practice. As to the origin of osteopathy he said: "God is the Father of osteopathy and I am not ashamed of the child of His mind." Unlike osteopathy, the founders of chiropractic did not use the religious element; they substituted a publicity agent and a belief in the power of advertising. Osteopathy, chiropractic, and bone-setting are all essentially the same things under different names.

There is no ground for the theory that disease is caused by dislocated vertebræ pressing on nerves. In the first place, most of the vertebræ are so constructed and overlapped that they can get out of position only when the bone is broken. When a man breaks his back and the nerves are thus pressed upon, paralysis results, but no other symptoms of disease. Again, tuberculosis of the spine in producing hunchback destroys the bone, so that the vertebræ crush together. But hunchback people may be healthy.

The accessories of faith cures are of almost endless variety; whatever holds the public attention can be made into a faith cure. Faith healing is applied to diet. The warriors of some primitive peoples believed that by eating the raw heart of their slain enemies or the heart of the lion they could absorb bravery. Since bravery is wholly a mental quality, beneficial results no doubt follow this practice. Such beliefs do not stop with primitive peoples, for a Greek monk of the eleventh century records the fact that the physician who performed the autopsy on the divine Cyril cut out and ate his liver. He thus obtained the virtues of the subject he was dissecting. It is said that a sorcerer and itinerant physician sought to cure a nervous disease of Pope Innocent VIII by having him drink the blood of three small children. The belief that fish is peculiarly a food for the brain still persists; it was a fallacious application of a fallacious discovery that the flesh of fish was particularly rich in substances found in the brain. An equally illogical application has followed the interest aroused by the discovery of vitamines. These substances in various prepared forms are exploited as a means of increasing vigor. The fact is that vitamines are found more abundantly in such commonplace articles as tomatoes than in the prepared compounds; but tomatoes lack the alluring qualities of pills and cakes of yeast; that humble vegetable lacks particularly testimonials. It is the faith in yeast that obtains any results that cannot be obtained equally as well with fruits and vegetables.

Still another form of faith healing is the "appliance cure." Among historical examples are the "childbirth bed" and "rheumatism chair" of Cagliostro and the cramp rings of Henry VIII, but especially Perkins's "tractors," which had their vogue soon after the Revolutionary War. The originator of the tractors was Dr. Elisha Perkins, of Norwich, Connecticut, a graduate of Yale College. Dr. Perkins appears to have been a man of strict principle, for his biographer says that, contrary to the custom of the time, he undertook an arduous medical practice "without the aid of artificial stimulants, never making use of ardent spirits." In those days a gallon of Jamaica rum could be purchased for a few pence and every household had its stock. Charlatans were not common in America during the eighteenth century, although there were many men practicing medicine who had not obtained university degrees; they studied with older practitioners and were good physicians according to the standards of the time. Europe during the same period was overrun with charlatans and quacks of the most blatant type. That there were some in America also is shown by an extract from the *Constitutional Gazette* of 1776: "New York, March 9. The famous Doctor DuBuke, a Frenchman who was branded here last January term for stealing indigo, etc., departed last Thursday from the city in the Amboy stage boat to visit Philadelphia and the southern Colonies. He professes himself a dentist and has practiced in the colonies under various names."

In 1796 Dr. Perkins patented his "tractors." They consisted of two short metallic rods. For the treatment of disease the rods were placed in contact and drawn over the skin. The popular information of the time was well suited to a cure suggestive of electric current. Galvani had shown that the legs of a frog twitched when touched by different metals brought in contact. Benjamin Franklin had then recently discovered that lightning was electricity, and Volta was experimenting with his voltaic pile, the forerunner of the electric battery. Perkins's tractors excited interest and were sold throughout this country and abroad. A Perkins Institute was established in London. After some years the cure died out; it was demonstrated that patients recovered just as well when stroked with two pieces of wood as with the metallic tractors, provided they were told that it was the Perkins tractors that were being applied.

Appliance cures more than any other variety of faith cure have to be altered to suit the times. In the middle of the nineteenth century blue window glass was a novelty and was widely sold to cure disease. The patient was directed to lie in the sun under a screen made of the blue glass. Blue glass ceased to cure when it became common. Later, a blue electric-light bulb of curious shape was used: it was, and still is, called the "violet-light treatment" (not ultra-violet). One of the latest appliance cures in an electromagnet shaped like a life-preserver; it is put around the body and attached to a lighting socket. The iron of the blood is supposed to respond to the flow of magnetism. As it does not, the whole affair is simply the old magnetic battery of Mesmer with modern improvements. It is sold to people who have heard that there is iron in the blood and know that a magnet attracts iron, but who have never heard of Mesmer or Elisha Perkins.

Faith healing, both past and present, has assumed innumerable forms and there will probably be many more in the future as old methods are revived, renamed, and adjusted to the latest scientific fad. The medical profession generally avoids faith cures, for the "mumbo jumbo" necessary to impress the patient approaches the method of the quack and charlatan too nearly to be compatible with medical ethics. Even those physicians who have attempted to practice faith healing scientifically, as for instance by psychoanalysis, resort to procedures which impress most physicians as fantastic.

Physicians a few generations ago employed faith healing much more than do modern physicians. They were more intimately acquainted with their patients than is usual now, but they were less thoroughly grounded in the science of medicine. Bread or sugar pills found a place in their prescriptions, and their bitterest medicines were sometimes dispensed for the most imaginary ailments. Modern specialization in the branches of medicine, and particularly the extension of hospital service, have lessened the use of these placeboes for imaginary ills. Their place has not, however, been filled by an increased "confidence in the physician" which with the old family practitioner was a potent factor in the treatment of disease. The modern physician can treat serious diseases much more successfully than could the physician of a few generations ago, but in many instances his attention is less attracted by the minor ills of mankind. It is possible that the present vogue for faith cures conducted by religious sects or by medical charlatans is an expression of the unsympathetic attitude of the medical profession toward minor and imaginary ailments.

CLAIRVOYANT, Magnetic and Electric Physicians, have recently furnished a house on Quincy avenue, in QUINCY, MASS., where they are still Healing the Sick with good success. Board and treatment reasonable. Address, QUINCY, MASS. 6w*—June 6.

ANY PERSON desiring to learn how to heal the sick can receive of the undersigned instruction that will enable them to commence healing on a principle of science with a success far beyond any of the present modes. No medicine, electricity, physiology or hygiene required for un paralleled success in the most difficult cases No pay is required unless this skill is obtained. Address, MRS. MARY B. GLOVER, Amesbury, Mass., Box 61 tf†—June 20.

MRS. MARY LEWIS, by sending their autograph, or lock of hair, will give psychometrical delineations of character, answer questions, &c Terms $1 00 and red stamp.

## AN ADVERTISEMENT BY MARY BAKER EDDY

Then Mrs. Glover, offering to teach Christian Science. This advertisement appeared in 1868 in the *Banner of Light*, the official organ of the New England Spiritualists.

# CHAPTER XIV

## A DRUG ON THE MARKET

here is a close connection between drug cures and faith healing. An immense number of substances have been used to treat disease, but only a few of these substances have any direct influence on the symptoms of disease, and some are actually harmful in their effects. Most of the substances that have been used as remedies depend upon their appeal to the imagination for the healing virtues they are believed to possess. Holy relics were formerly applied to the outside of the body, and for the same reason "medicines" with no more healing properties than holy relics were, and sometimes still are, applied to the inside of the body. Aside from a small number of drugs which are indispensable to modern medicine, the medicaments applied internally and the holy relics applied externally have the same action, and the relics are both more effective psychologically and safer toxicologically.

The history of most medicaments is implied in the two definitions given in the dictionary for the word "drug." One of these definitions is, "a simple medicinal substance." The other definition is, "a thing no longer in demand—a drug on the market." Curative properties have been attributed to nearly every substance when it was new, unusual, or difficult to obtain and which can be forced into the human system. When the novelty of these substances wears off they cease to be used as medicaments. The potato when first introduced into Europe was a novelty and sold for a high price, and was not used as a food, but as a "medicine." It was supposed to be, and under the circumstances probably was, an aphrodisiac useful in curing impotence or as an ingredient of love philters. Gold dissolved in acid, "potable gold," was once a sovereign remedy for nearly every ill that flesh is heir to; Roger Bacon was one of its advocates. The search for the acids to dissolve the gold resulted in notable advances in chemistry. Pearls, musk and crocodile dung, unicorn's horn, Egyptian mummy and sarsaparilla, have all had their vogue as drug cures, as have also several thousand other substances of a merit equally dubious. The prescription for the drugs used in the treatment of Sir Unton, ambassador from Queen Elizabeth to the court of Henry IV, is extant in a letter dated March 21, 1595, which states that "the king's physicians gave him Confectio Alcarmas compounded of musk, amber, gold, pearl, and unicorn's horn, with a pidgeon applied to his side, and all other means that art could devise." Sir Unton died, probably of pneumonia or appendicitis, but it cannot be said that the treatment harmed him, for every ingredient of the confectio was pharmacologically inert.

The belief is still widely held that drugs in some mysterious way are a necessary part of the treatment of all diseases. Ignorant and superstitious people are dissatisfied with any treatment by a physician unless it includes a bottle of some vile-tasting concoction or a box of colored pills. For such people the "medicine" has an essentially thaumaturgic value; it is a sort of amulet worn internally by which they are periodically nauseated, griped, or otherwise forcibly reminded that they are getting well. To many people all drugs that they can swallow are indiscriminately "good for sickness." In this connection Oliver Wendell Holmes tells the story of a man who applied to a Boston physician for relief from abdominal pain and a persistent metallic taste in his mouth. The physician's inquiries disclosed the fact that the man had been swallowing pills from a box he had found on the street. His idea was that since pills were good in case of sickness, they would probably do him some good, even though he was not sick at the time. The pills contained mercury and he had poisoned himself. But the belief in the necessity of drugs in treating disease is not confined to ignorant people. James Walsh records the following incident in regard to the English philosopher, Carlyle, who is considered by some people to be one of the deepest thinkers of the nine-teenth century. Carlyle heard that his friend Henry Taylor was ill and immediately went to see him, bringing what was left of some medicine that had helped Mrs. Carlyle when she was ill. Carlyle did not know what was the matter with his friend and he had forgotten for what complaint Mrs. Carlyle had used the medicine. But the medicine had benefited her and therefore it should benefit his friend. He did not stop to think of all the things that might have been the matter with his wife which, from the very nature of things, could not have been wrong with Henry Taylor.

The part played by superstition in choosing drugs to treat disease is illustrated by the use of such substances as Egyptian mummy. The mummy found in the European market resembled rosin and had no more physiological effect than rosin. Nevertheless, powdered mummy was a prominent ingredient of medieval and Renaissance prescriptions. Most of the mummy used was adulterated or counterfeited, and Paré said that mummy was sometimes "made in our France" from bodies stolen from the gallows; but adds: "Nevertheless, I believe that they are as good as those brought from Egypt; because they are none of them of any value." Mummy was used as an almost universal remedy among those people who could afford to purchase it, as is shown by the following incident. In 1580 Monsieur Christophe des Ursins was thrown from his horse and Paré was called to attend him. Although seventy years of age, Paré promptly mounted his horse and rode into the country where the wounded man lay. When the patient recovered consciousness he asked Paré why he had not applied mummy to the wound, a question which prompted Paré to proclaim his disbelief in this remedy, which was held in high esteem by physicians of the time; in fact, his statements excited the violent opposition of the whole Paris Faculty of Medicine. Although Paré was singularly free from medical superstition, considering the time in which he lived, nevertheless his book on monsters gives amazing reasons for bodily malformations. The stories scattered through his writings of a girl turned suddenly, and much to her surprise, into a boy, and of a frog found in the center of a rock, recall the fact that he is of the sixteenth century.

Unicorn's horn was another highly prized remedy of the medieval period and Renaissance. The horn was supposedly derived from the mythical unicorn, possibly the narwhal, but was in reality nothing but ivory. Unicorn's horn was sold for an enormous price; a specimen in Dresden was estimated in the sixteenth century to be worth $75,000. It was valued as a remedy despite the fact that the identical substance is in every tooth and is therefore in the mouth of everyone who has any teeth. The cost of unicorn's horn confined its use to the nobility. When the Dauphin (later Henry II) married Catherine de' Medici, the bride's uncle, Pope Clement VII, presented Francis I, the bridegroom's father, with a piece of unicorn's horn. It was said to possess the power of destroying poison mixed with food—a valuable dietary precaution for kings and popes of that age. When Elizabeth, daughter of Henry II, had smallpox, the constable, Anne de Montmorenci, sent a piece of unicorn's horn for her treatment. Paré tried unsuccessfully to abolish the custom prevailing in the French court of dipping a piece of unicorn's horn in the king's cup before he drank, as a precaution against poisoning. Instead of abolishing the custom Paré precipitated an attack against himself for his skepticism, on the ground that the king had refused to part with his horn for a hundred thousand crowns, and that fact in itself was proof that the horn must be useful. In England the belief in unicorn's horn as an antidote for poison lasted until the reign of Charles II, when the Royal Society was requested to investigate the properties of a cup made from rhinoceros horn. The society reported that the cup was useless as an antidote. Unicorn's horn was not exclusively a European remedy, for Governor Endicott loaned Governor John Winthrop a horn for use in his medical practice.

Another famous antidote for poison was the bezoar stone, which was supposed to prevent melancholia and all kinds of poisoning, including snake bite. These stones were concretions formed in the intestines of some animals, usually goats; these were often gallstones. Medical properties were attributed to them by the Arabs, who had many superstitions centered about stones of one kind or another. The belief in bezoars was carried into Europe, and men who could afford

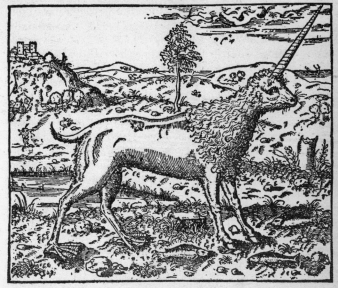

### THE UNICORN

The horn of this fabled animal was supposed to possess miraculous properties of neutralizing poisons. The pieces of horn in commerce in the fifteenth and sixteenth centuries were from either the narwhal or the elephant.

to purchase them carried them as universal antidotes. Charles IX of France was presented with a bezoar of which he was very proud. Paré told him that there was no universal antidote, but the king was firm in his convictions as to the value of his bezoar. He consented, however, to experiment with the stone on a condemned criminal. He accordingly sent for his provost and asked if he had on hand any prisoner who merited hanging. Paré says: "He told him that he had in his prison a cook who had stolen two silver plates from his master, and that the next day he was to be hung up and strangled. The king told him he wished to experiment with a stone which they said was good against all poison, and that he should ask the cook after his condemnation if he would take a certain poison, and that they would at once give him an antidote; to which the cook very willingly agreed, saying that he liked much better to die of poison in the prison, than to be strangled in view of the people. An apothecary gave him a certain poison in a drink and at once the bezoar stone. Having these two good drugs in his stomach, he took to vomiting and purging, saying that he was burning inside, and called for water to drink, which was not denied him. An hour later, having been told that the cook had taken this good drug, I prayed the provost to let me see him, which he accorded, accompanied by three of his archers, and I found the poor cook on all-fours, going like an animal, his tongue hanging out from his mouth, his eyes and face red, retching and in cold sweat, bleeding from his ears, nose, and mouth. I made him drink oil, thinking to aid him and save his life, but it was no use because it was too late, and he died miserably, crying it would have been better to have died on the gibbet. He lived about seven hours." Paré performed an autopsy on the cook and found that the apothecary had administered bichloride of mercury. The king, it is said, caused the bezoar stone to be burned after Paré had demonstrated its worthlessness. Possibly he thought that he had been cheated, for bezoar stones were often counterfeited by substituting pebbles. In fact, during the reign of King James I of England considerable attention was attracted by legal action brought against a goldsmith for having sold a hundred pounds' worth of counterfeit bezoar stones. In any event, the use of the stone did not cease at once, for the records show that Governor John Winthrop, desiring a bezoar to use in his practice, was supplied by Governor Endicott who had obtained the stone from a Mr. Humphry.

Mummy, unicorn's horn, and bezoars appealed to the imagination because of their unusual character, but even the most commonplace substances might develop supposedly medicinal virtues if they had unusual or gruesome associations. Usnea was a substance of this nature. It was moss; not ordinary moss, but moss scraped from the skull of a criminal who had been hung in chains. Usnea was an official drug in the pharmacopeia until the nineteenth century; it was carried by all apothecary shops, and the first edition of the Encyclopedia Britannica devoted a section to its curative properties. Usnea was present in the prescriptions of the best physicians over a period extending from the Middle Ages until well after the American Revolution. There were many testimonials to the relief that it had brought to patients with nervous or wasting diseases. The counterpart of Usnea for external application was a piece of the rope with which a man had been hanged. The rope was the property of the hangman; he cut it into as many pieces as possible and auctioned them off to the highest bidders. Cures could be obtained by stroking the skin with the rope quite as effectively as by the use of Perkins's tractors.

Disgusting substances formerly were used as drugs, largely because of the impression they make on the sufferer. Such substances were extensively employed because they were cheaper than mummy, unicorn's horn, bezoars, pearls, and potable gold, which were the remedies of the nobility. Cotton Mather used crushed sow bugs in his practice and crushed body lice, and incinerated toads have also had their place in medicine. When Robert Boyle expurgated the pharmacopeia of its most dubious remedies he nevertheless included in the revised list the sole of an old shoe "worn by some man that walked much," which was to be ground up and taken internally for dysentery. Insects, toads, and old shoes were the least objectionable of the many remedies of that age. In the late Middle Ages the apothecaries of Europe complained that most of the crocodile dung they received from Egypt was adulterated by dishonest traders. Excrement and urine have had a notable place in medicine, and Pliny in his

*Natural History* speaks highly of the medicinal virtues of menstrual blood. This last substance, in addition to its effect on disease, would kill insect pests at a distance and even quell storms at sea. The physicians of the sixteenth and seventeenth centuries apparently tried to make the deaths of their patients as unpleasant as possible; when Cardinal Richelieu was on his death-bed a female charlatan prescribed for him a mixture of horse dung in white wine, and the cardinal drank it. In the eighteenth century Fauchard, a Frenchman who made notable contributions to dentistry, advised his patients to use their own urine as a mouthwash in case of toothache. Urine was an old remedy, but subject to occasional revival; Madame de Sévigné recommended it highly in the seventeenth century.

Madame de Sévigné had numerous medical foibles and she thought the "sympathetic powder" of Sir Kenelme Digby "a perfectly divine remedy." This sympathetic powder was a revival of the weapon ointment. Weapon ointment was used for healing wounds, but, instead of being applied to them, the injured part was washed and bandaged and the weapon with which the wound was inflicted was carefully anointed with the ointment. This treatment was mostly used by empiric and ignorant barbers during the late Middle Ages, but it was advocated by Paracelsus and used by some of the respectable members of the medical profession. The ointment was usually composed of materials which appeal strongly to the imagination, such as human blood, eunuch's fat, and moss from a criminal's skull. The treatment was often successful; in fact it was a better form of wound treatment than that current among the medical profession at the time. A wound washed, bandaged, and let alone heals more quickly and with less infection than one to which is applied such healing ointments as were then used.

Sir Kenelme Digby's sympathetic powder was an outgrowth of the weapon ointment. It had an advantage over the ointment in that it was not applied to the weapon inflicting the wound, an accessory often difficult to obtain, but instead

# A LATE
# DISCOURSE

Made in a Solemne Assembly
of Nobles and Learned
Men at *Montpellier*
in *France*;

By Sr. *Kenelme Digby*, Knight, &c.

Touching the Cure of W o u n d s
by the *Powder of Sympathy*; With
Instructions how to make the
said Powder; whereby many
other Secrets of Nature
are unfolded.

*Fœlix qui potuit Rerum cognoscere
causas.*

Rendred faithfully out of French
into English

By R. *White, Gent.*

London, Printed for R. *Lownes*, and
*T Davies*, and are to be sold at their shops in
Sr. Pauls Church yard, at the sign of the *White
Lion*, and at the *Bible* over against the little
North Door of St. Pauls Church, 1658.

---

TITLE PAGE TO KENELME DIGBY'S BOOK ON THE POWDER
OF SYMPATHY

This book detailed the procedure for treating wounds by dipping
the blood-stained garment in copper sulphate, but applying no treatment to the wound itself. The practice was a variation of that in
which the weapon causing the wound was anointed with ointment instead of the wound. The method sponsored by Digby had an advantage over that of "weapon salve," for the weapon was sometimes
difficult to obtain. Wounds usually healed with less infection under
these forms of absent treatment than they did under the dirty plasters
and poultices of the sixteenth-century surgeons.

to the clothes soiled with blood from the wound. The sympathetic powder was originally introduced into Europe in the seventeenth century by a friar who obtained it in the East. The Grand Duke of Florence tried to obtain the friar's secret but failed to do so. Digby was fortunate enough to do the friar a favor and received in return the recipe for the sympathetic powder. Sir Kenelme was an Englishman who at different periods of his life was an admiral, a theologian, a critic, a metaphysician, and a disciple of alchemy. He interested himself in quasi-medical fads, and the gossip of the time says he killed his wife by feeding her too much viper's flesh to improve her complexion. Digby performed remarkable cures with his sympathetic powder applied to the bloody clothes of his wounded friends. According to the Dictionnaire des Sciences Medicales, "King James First, his son Charles the First, the Duke of Buckingham, then Prime Minister, and all the principal personages of the time were cognizant of this fact; and James himself, being curious to know the secret of this remedy, asked it of Sir Kenelme, who revealed it to him and his Majesty had the opportunity of making several trials of its efficacy, which all succeeded in a surprising manner." The wonderful sympathetic powder was copper sulphate or blue vitriol, a caustic substance now occasionally used in eye ointments to treat trachoma and extensively employed in sprays to kill fungous growth on trees.

Faith healing by means of drugs is now largely exploited by the manufacturers of patent or proprietary medicines. These substances are not generally prescribed by physicians; they are taken by people who, with the aid of a newspaper advertisement, make their own diagnosis, or none, and pick out their own drugs. Disgusting remedies are no longer needed to impress people, for the necessary impression can now be obtained with printers' ink.

Drug cures and faith healing have produced similar results because both are evaluated by the same fallacious test. Sick men touched holy relics and they afterward got well; therefore they assumed that they were cured by the relics. Similarly, sick men took drugs and afterward got well;

therefore they assumed that they were cured by the drugs. As a result of this type of reasoning almost every conceivable substance that could be taken internally has been used in the

( 104 )

of Mothers work upon the bodies of their children, while they are yet big with them, therefore I will relate unto you some of them ; and so I told her sundry stories upon this subject, as that of the Queen of *Ethiopia*, who was delivered of a white boy, which was attributed to a Picture of the Blessed Virgin, which she had alwaies neat the Teaster of her bed, whereunto she bore great devotion. I urged another of a woman who was brought to bed of a child all hairy, because of a portrait of Saint John Baptist in the Wildernesse, where he wore a Coat of Cammels hair. I related unto her also the strange antipathy which the late King *James* had to a naked sword, whereof the cause was ascribed, in regard some *Scotch* Lords had entred once violently into the bed-chamber of the Queen his mother, while she was with child of him, where her Secretary, an *Italian*, was dispatching some letters for her, whom they hacked, and killed with naked swords before her

( 105 )

her face, and threw him at her feet; and they grew so barbarous, that there wanted but little but that they had hurt the Queen her self, who endeavouring to save her Secretary, by interposing herself, had her skin rased in divers places; which *Buchanan* himself makes mention of. Hence it came that her son King *James* had such an aversion all his life-time after to a naked sword, that he could not see one without a great emotion of his spirits; although otherwise couragious enough, yet he could never overmaster his passions in this particular, I remember when he dubbed me Knight, in the ceremony of puting the point of a naked sword upon my shoulder, he could not endure to look upon it, but turned his face another way, insomuch, that in lieu of touching my shoulder, he had almost thrust the point into my eyes, had not the Duke of *Buckingham* guided his hand aright.

### KENELME DIGBY ON PRENATAL INFLUENCE

Pages 104 and 105 from Digby's *Discourse* on the powder of sympathy. The text here is more concerned with the power of sympathy. The belief in maternal impression still persists as a popular superstition.

treatment of disease. Formerly the only essential for the introduction of a drug was its recommendation by someone who had used it or heard of its use. Consequently, travel, conquest of new lands, and extension of commerce resulted in continual additions to the remedies in use. During the Middle Ages and Renaissance drugs were introduced into Europe from Egyptian, Greek, Roman, Arabian, and Indian sources and, after it was discovered, from America as well.

The drugs used so extensively in European medicine were brought from every part of the world. In order to obtain these exotic substances it was necessary to maintain commerce with distant countries. The search for a short route to India to obtain spices led to exploration and the discovery of America. The spices that were sought were used in medicine rather than as condiments. The European taste did not demand aloes, opium, pepper, sandalwood, Persian rhubarb, and camphor for its table; the spice trade was in reality the drug trade. From the ninth to the fifteenth century it was largely controlled by the Venetian Republic, for after they had defeated their competitors, the Genoese, the Venetians held the supremacy of the seas until the Portuguese entered the drug trade. The fall of Constantinople in 1453 disrupted the Eastern trade and the price of drugs rose to such a height that the Portuguese and Spaniards entered into the trade. The Portuguese, led by Vasco da Gama, doubled the Cape and sailed into Calicut. The Venetian sea supremacy was ended. The news that the Portuguese ships, loaded with spice, had arrived in the harbor of Lisbon threw the merchants of the Rialto into a panic. During the next hundred years Portugal was the center of the drug trade. Like Vasco da Gama, Columbus sought to find a direct route to India and instead landed in America. The drug trade belonged to whatever nation held the supremacy of the seas. In the seventeenth century the Dutch superseded the Portuguese and were in turn displaced by the English.

The Dutch made an effort to monopolize the drug trade. They destroyed the plants and trees bearing spices on islands which were not under their control and introduced them into their possessions. To monopolize the plant from which mace and nutmeg are obtained they immersed the kernels in milk of lime for three months to prevent their germination in case they were planted in other lands; they kept the entire nutmeg

crop in stock at Amsterdam for sixteen years. The Connecticut Yankees, who were accused of manufacturing wooden
nutmegs, were not sophisticating a spice, but instead a drug
which at the time was thought to be necessary in treating

*The effigies of a maid all hairie, and an infant that was black by the imagination of their Parents.*

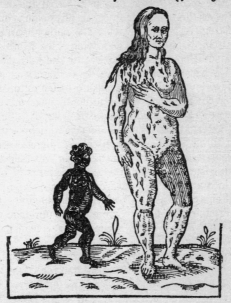

### THE EFFECTS OF PRENATAL INFLUENCE

An example supplied by Paré. These "effigies" were made to supply
illustrations for a "history" he had heard; he himself had seen neither
the "maid" nor the "infant."

disease and which brought a very high price. In the period
during which the Dutch controlled the drug trade the English
were forced to obtain their supplies by the capture of Dutch
and Portuguese vessels. In the battle to control the drug
trade "torrents of blood were shed for the apparently inof-

fensive clove." Yet none of these spices so valued in the medicine of two and three hundred years ago are used today in treating disease.

Some idea of the nature and number of the drug substances used in the medicine of the past may be obtained from the records of the treatment given King Charles II at the time of his death. These records are extant in the writings of a Dr. Scarburgh, one of the twelve or fourteen physicians called in to treat the king. At eight o'clock on Monday morning of February 2, 1685, King Charles was being shaved in his bedroom. With a sudden cry he fell backward and had a violent convulsion. He became unconscious, rallied once or twice, and after a few days died. Seventeenth-century autopsy records are far from complete, but one could hazard a guess that the king suffered with an embolism—that is, a floating blood clot which had plugged up an artery and deprived some portion of his brain of blood—or else his kidneys were diseased. As the first step in treatment the king was bled to the extent of a pint from a vein in his right arm. Next his shoulder was cut into and the incised area "cupped" to suck out an additional eight ounces of blood. After this homicidal onslaught the drugging began. An emetic and purgative were administered, and soon after a second purgative. This was followed by an enema containing antimony, sacred bitters, rock salt, mallow leaves, violets, beet roots, camomile flowers, fennel seed, linseed, cinnamon cardamon seed, saphron, cochineal, and aloes. The enema was repeated in two hours and a purgative given. The king's head was shaved and a blister raised on his scalp. A sneezing powder of hellebore root was administered, and also a powder of cowslip flowers "to strengthen his brain." The cathartics were repeated at frequent intervals and interspersed with a soothing drink composed of barley water, licorice and sweet almond. Likewise white wine, absinthe and anise were given, as also were extracts of thistle leaves, mint, rue, and angelica. For external treatment a plaster of Burgundy pitch and pigeon dung was applied to the king's feet. The bleeding and purging continued, and to the medicaments were added melon seeds, manna, slippery elm, black cherry water, an extract of flowers of lime, lily-of-the-valley, peony, lavender, and dissolved pearls. Later came gentian root, nutmeg, quinine, and cloves. The king's condition did not improve, indeed it grew worse, and in the emergency forty drops of extract of human skull were administered to allay convulsions. A rallying dose of Raleigh's antidote was forced down the king's throat; this antidote contained an enormous number of herbs and animal extracts. Finally bezoar stone was given. Then says Scarburgh: "Alas! after an ill-fated night his serene majesty's strength seemed exhausted to such a degree that the whole assembly of physicians lost all hope and became despondent: still so as not to appear to fail in doing their duty in any detail, they brought into play the most active cordial." As a sort of grand summary to this pharmaceutical debauch a mixture of Raleigh's antidote, pearl julep, and ammonia was forced down the throat of the dying king.

King Charles was helpless before the drugging of his physicians, who wished "to leave no stones unturned in his treatment." But King James I was more resistant; he took physic only once and refused to be bled. It has been said that James's life, "owing partly to constitutional causes and partly to his excess in food and drink and other indulgences, was one long disease." He was unable to walk until he was six years old, a weakness explained by Mayenne as due to the bad milk of a drunken wet nurse. He had catarrh, probably due to enlarged adenoids and tonsils, was troubled with indigestion and frequently had colic, but ate and drank excessively. His teeth decayed and he was forced to bolt his food. A diarrhea affected him when he was worried, and he had hemorrhoids that bled annoyingly. He developed rheumatism of the joints and in consequence frequently fell from his horse. He had gout and malaria, but he died bravely resisting medical treatment. The Duke of Buckingham was accused of poisoning him, but was freed of the charge.

In the seventeenth century there was more exact knowledge of poisons than of medicinal drugs. The medicinal properties of drugs could not be correctly estimated until scientific methods were developed in the eighteenth and nineteenth centuries. Prior to that time experiments were conducted only on poisons, for with poisons the results are certain and immediate. Modern pharmacology, the study of the action of drugs, developed out of this early study of the action of poisons. The ancient lore of poisons was concerned largely with snake venom. In all civilizations the choice of medicinal substances and poisons has shown a similar course. Poisonous animal substances were used first. The venoms from the viper, the asp, and the water snake were employed to poison arrows. The earliest pharmacological experiments were conducted with snake venoms administered to slaves or prisoners of war. The well-known tale of Cleopatra testing the poison of her asp on her slaves before she applied it to herself is typical of the pharmocological methods of that time. Cleopatra was apparently no novice in medical matters, for she was the alleged author of several works dealing with diseases peculiar to women and with venereal diseases. Her experiments with the asp were similar to the research conducted centuries later by Paré and Charles IX with the bezoar stone, except that a mineral poison was substituted for the animal poison.

One of the most energetic of the early pharmacologists was Mithridates, king of Pontus, in the second century before Christ. His pharmacological studies were made possible by the influence of Greek learning on Egyptian civilization. The early Egyptian physicians made considerable use of drugs. Their drugs were of the kind usually found in early civilizations: a few effective remedies lost in a mass of substances of purely superstitious origin. They used opium, squill, and other vegetable substances, but also excrement and urine. It is said that the urine of a faithful wife was with them effective in the treatment of sore eyes. The tale concerning the difficulty in obtaining this remedy (or the ineffectiveness of its cures) has come down with variations through folk tales. For many centuries the medical system of the Egyptians was not subject to foreign influence, for the early

Egyptians punished with death every stranger who entered their country. About 500 B.C., however, they began to tolerate foreigners. Greek physicians came to Egypt and under their influence Egyptian medicine declined and was replaced by Greek medicine. By the time that Alexandria was founded, by Alexander the Great, nothing was left of Egyptian medicine but a miserable sort of alchemy and magic. During the Middle Ages all Egyptian knowledge was regarded as sorcery.

Mithridates was versed in the Greek medicine of Egypt and undertook his pharmacological experiments to find a universal antidote against poison. His attention centered largely upon snake venoms, but he employed men to search throughout the known world to find poisonous substances of all kinds. These he administered to slaves, studying the effects and trying to find an antidote. After his death his recipe was discovered. This compound was known as mithradaticum and with some variations in the hands of later physicians was developed into theriac. In subsequent times theriac was more extensively employed than any other medicinal remedy. It contained from thirty-seven to sixty-three ingredients, all of which are worthless as remedies. The main ingredient of the compound was the flesh of vipers. The viper is a poisonous snake, but, like all snakes, it has immunity to its own venom; therefore, by the process of early medical reasoning, it was supposed to confer this immunity upon people who took it as a drug. Theriac was used as a cure-all even up to a hundred years ago. It was taken internally in the treatment of all diseases, and applied externally in the treatment of all wounds. During the Renaissance the preparation of theriac was an elaborate official affair carried out under the supervision of city officials to prevent adulteration. Eventually theriac became known as treacle, and when theriac was discarded as a remedy the term treacle was applied to molasses. The sulphur and treacle administered to all young people a generation or two ago as a spring tonic was derived from the old belief in theriac.

Greek medical practice, as established by Hippocrates five hundred years before Christ, did not include an extensive use of drugs. At the great University of Alexandria, however, a more extensive use of drugs was grafted upon Greek medical learning. After the fall of Corinth Greek physicians migrated to Rome. The Romans used many drugs. The combined influence of Greek, Alexandrian, and Roman medicine brought in an extensive use of drugs.

The increasing importance of drugs led Dioscorides to compile a list of drugs, the first extensive *materia medica*. Dioscorides was a surgeon in the army of Nero. In the second century after Christ he traveled from country to country with the army and in his spare time collected information concerning the remedies in use in each country. The substances which he described formed the remedies used in Europe during the Middle Ages and, with some additions from Arabic sources and from America, the remedies used in the Renaissance. His book was the source from which the Herbals were all derived. These Herbals described the cultivation, collection, and properties of herbs. They were the popular books of medical knowledge during the medieval period; the people of those days dosed themselves according to directions of the Herbals, just as people of a few years ago dosed themselves with the remedies described in almanacs, and as they do today with the drugs described in newspaper advertisements.

The substances listed in Dioscorides's book were worked into a system by Galen. This system was the medical religion of the Christian era up to the seventeenth century. It has left its mark on medicine even to this day, for efforts are still being made to rid the pharmacopeias of the compounds containing a dozen or more worthless herbs. Such compounds are called vegetable simples, or galenicals.

Galen was born in Pergamum in Asia Minor in 131 A.D. He undertook the study of medicine at an early age, and then for eight years wandered from city to city, adding to his store of medical knowledge. He returned to Pergamum when he was twenty-eight, and with the influence of the temple officials obtained a political appointment as physician to the gladiators. Within a few years, however, a riot broke out in Pergamum and he was forced to leave the city and start on his travels again. He stopped for a while at Rome, and there rose rapidly in favor among his patients, but again he left, this time either because he feared injury from professional rivals, or, as his enemies said, because an epidemic of the plague was imminent. He returned to Pergamum for a short time, but was summoned by the Emperor Marcus Aurelius to join the Roman army. The plague overtook the army and forced it to return to Rome. Galen was back again in the city he had so recently left, but this time he was private physician to the emperor. In this situation he found ample time for research and writing.

Galen was an energetic experimenter, but his method was faulty in that he insisted on having a theory for every phenomenon, whether or not it had any basis in fact. His superficial theories displaced the less showy and more laborious methods of Hippocrates, which were based upon direct observations and logical interpretation. Galen developed an elaborate theory of disease and its treatment based on the prevalent metaphysical conceptions of the nature of the body. According to this theory, the body, like the universe, was composed of four elements—fire, air, water, and earth. These elements represented the qualities of the body: fire was hot, air was dry, water was wet, and earth was cold. Health consisted in preserving each of these qualities in its proper proportions in the body. In health heat and cold were balanced, and so also were dryness and moisture. Disease resulted when the balance between the four qualities was disturbed; and disease was to be cured by administering drugs to restore the proper balance. The various drugs had the four fundamental qualities of the body; some were cooling, others were heating or moistening or drying. A disease with fever was to be treated with cooling drugs, and a disease with chills was to be treated with heating drugs. The selection of the proper heating, cooling, moistening, or drying drugs was determined by the character and intensity of the disease. Drugs possessed these fundamental qualities in different degrees. Thus bitter almond was heating to the first degree and drying to the second degree, while pepper

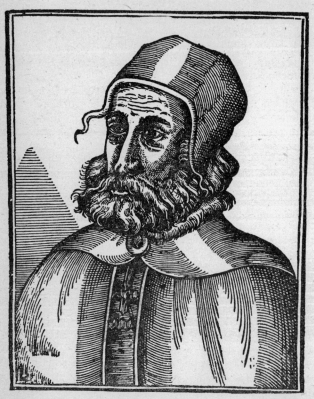

"GALEN, PRINCE OF PHYSICIANS NEXT TO HIPPOCRATES"
From Paré's *Surgery*.

was heating to the fourth degree and cucumber seeds were cooling to a similar degree. The common expression "cool as a cucumber" is derived from the therapeutic theory of Galen.

Galen administered elaborate mixtures of herbs in order to restore the proper balance of qualities in the body. His disciples in the following centuries carried this practice to extremes. Even after the Galenical system was dropped by physicians it persisted as the use of herbs for home remedies: sassafras tea to cool the blood. It persisted also in proprietary medicines, as is exampled by "Lydia Pinkham's Vegetable Compound," and it is carried on even today in the practice of uneducated "herb doctors."

Several thousand drugs were necessary for the Galenic system of therapeutics. A hundred or more drugs might be included in a single prescription. To gather, prepare, and store the necessary herbs was a laborious task. In Roman times the physicians themselves collected their drugs and prepared their own medicine. But there were also dealers in drugs who sold their wares to people unable to afford the services of a physician. The apothecaries' trade was then in the hands of a low class of men and retired prostitutes. In addition to selling herbs they treated venereal diseases which reputable physicians usually refused.

For many centuries after the Roman times physicians continued to dispense their own medicines. In fact, it is only in recent years that the majority have ceased to do so. Moreover, the Roman attitude toward venereal diseases continued and the treatment of venereal diseases has only recently been wrested from the hands of quacks and charlatans. As late as the eighteenth century the hospital at Vienna twice a year appointed a man who was not a physician to treat the cases of syphilis which had collected during six months.

The apothecaries of Europe during the Middle Ages were drug-peddlers who attended fairs and (like the apothecary in *Romeo and Juliet*) sold poisons and love philters as well as medicinal herbs. Old women and midwives carried on a similar trade. The first apothecary shops in Europe were grocery stores where herbs and other medicinal supplies were carried as a sideline. In the fourteenth century, however, the taste in cosmetics and medicaments grew more fastidious, and apothecaries' shops were organized to supply the refinement that had been lacking in the grocery store. A bill sent to Queen Elizabeth by her apothecary indicates the elaborate compounds which these shops were called upon to supply. It includes: "A confection made like mannas Christi, with bezoar stone and unicorn's horn; a royal sweet meat made with incised rhubarb; rose water for the King of Navarre's ambassador; a conserve of barberries with preserved Damascene plums and other things for Mr. Raleigh [presumably later Sir Walter Raleigh]; and sweet scent to be used at the christening of Sir Richard Knightley's son. . . ." The supplies dispensed by the apothecaries were not all of this regal character, however, for in a bill to Edward Nicholas in 1633, the following items appear:

A dose of purgative pills........................2s6d
A purge for your son..........................3s
A purge for your Worship......................3s6d
A glass of chalybeat wine.....................4s
A dose of pills for Mrs. Nicholas.............1s
A purge potion ..............................3s6d
A powder to fume the bed clothes..............4s

The prevalence of purgatives in the medicinal supplies of Mr. Nicholas is not surprising. In those days few Englishmen ate vegetables in any quantity; meat and pastry were the staple articles of diet. The lack of green vegetables in the diet of those times is seen in Pepys's *Diary;* meals are recorded with six or seven kinds of meat, with pastry and wine, but there is rarely a reference to vegetables. In consequence of this rich diet constipation was very prevalent and energetic purgatives were taken at intervals of about a fortnight. The taker, then, in the terms of the time, "retired for physic." The administration of enemas was originally a regular and profitable part of the apothecary's business and was practiced either by the apothecary himself or by his assistant. Subsequently, this duty passed from the apothecaries to the barbers.

The belief in the ill effects of constipation and the necessity of purging in health as well as in illness is one of extreme antiquity. The ancient Egyptians took emetics and purgatives three times a month on the principle that all diseases arise from food and are to be prevented in this way.

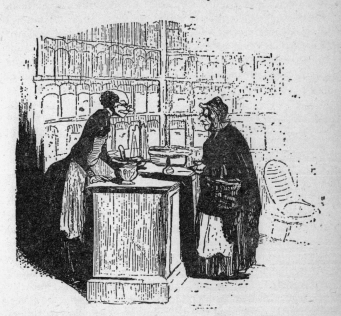

"THE APOTHECARY"
An etching by Daumier.

It was in effect the theory now called "autointoxication." The belief in the necessity of regular purging has persisted down to modern times. Until recently physicians gave purgatives as the first step in treating nearly all diseases, and often the purgatives were either the powerful salts of antimony or mercury (calomel). Throughout the ages people have been subject to an appalling amount of unnecessary purging. The number thus hastened to their end was probably nearly as large as the number of those who died as a result of the withdrawal of blood for the treatment of disease. Dr. Sangrado of *Gil Blas* symbolized the intensive blood-letting common in the seventeenth century. The medical profession now rarely practices bleeding and fortunately the laity do not perform therapeutic venesection on themselves. They can and do purge themselves, however, and many persons still hold to the old belief that constipation is in itself a disease and not merely a symptom. It is, in fact, usually a symptom that the diet is improper or that the intestine has been habituated to purgative drugs as the result of frequent purging. In the nineteenth century the ancient belief in purging for purging's sake lost ground and the outlook is now bright for an era in which the intestine will be left to its duty undisturbed.

The purgative drugs that people use today are purchased from apothecaries, usually without a prescription from a physician. Formerly the apothecaries not only supplied drugs, but also advised as to the drugs to be used. They diagnosed the diseases of their customers and supplied them with the medicaments for treatment. This practice was looked upon by the physicians as unfair, and in France and England during the sixteenth and seventeenth centuries there were continual disputes between them and the apothecaries. In France the argument was settled in the seventeenth century in favor of the physicians, and the apothecaries, supposedly at least, ceased to practice medicine. In England, however, the decision was against the physicians. Public sentiment there in the seventeenth century was strongly in favor of the apothecaries. They had remained at their posts during the epidemic of plague after most of the physicians had fled. In the early part of the eighteenth century an apothecary who had prescribed medicine was arrested and tried as a test case. The trial aroused considerable partisanship. The physicians were supported by some of the prominent literary men of the time. Dr. Samuel Johnson said he was "on the side of charity against intrigues of interest, and of regular learning against licentious usurpation of medical authority."

The "interest" referred to was the apothecaries. Pope commented on the apothecaries with:

> Modern pothecaries taught the art
> By doctor's bills to play the doctor's part
> Bold in the practice of mistaken rules.

The apothecaries won out in the trial and were allowed to carry on a quasi-medical practice until 1866, when the law was changed to require a medical education as a prerequisite to the prescription of drugs.

DEATH'S HEAD FROM ONE OF
DEKKER'S PLAGUE PAMPHLETS

# CHAPTER XV

# THE TURNING-POINT

he prescription of medicaments by apothecaries unversed in medicine, and by ignorant old women, was not particularly dangerous to their patients so long as the system of Galen was followed. The vile-tasting mixtures of herbs did not help cure disease, but neither did they do the patient much harm. Physicians used the same drugs. Conditions changed, however, when such poisonous drugs as mercury and antimony were introduced. The use of these powerful substances was due largely to Theophrastus von Hohenheim, better known as Paracelsus, one of the most striking figures in medicine. He not only founded a system of therapy, but also dabbled extensively in mysticism. Modern mystics claim that he belonged to their field rather than to that of medicine—and physicians on the whole are content to allow the claim. Paracelsus is by no means the only physician who has gone off on a tangent of mysticism; Emanuel Swedenborg was a physician and in his early days published an anatomical and physiological work much valued in the eighteenth century.

Paracelsus was born in 1493 in Switzerland. It was the century of great reformers—Luther in religion, Vesalius in anatomy, Paré in surgery, and Paracelsus in therapy. Paracelsus spent most of his life in wandering from country to country, imbibing the medical opinions of physicians, barbers, bath-keepers, executioners, and old women, as he said, "in order to understand the wonders of nature." During his travels he learned a great deal about medical practice, low company, and mysticism.

Paracelsus acquired a reputation as a successful practitioner of medicine and at the age of thirty-two was appointed

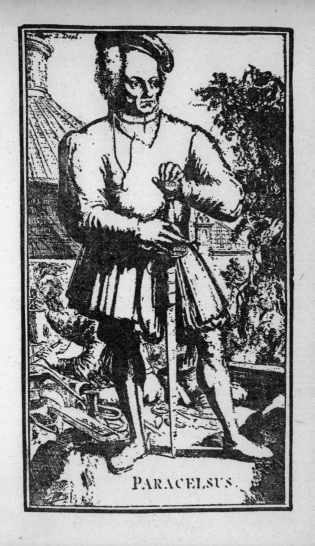

PARACELSUS.

AUREOLUS THEOPHRASTUS BOMBASTUS VON HOHENHEIM,
better known as Paracelsus.

professor of medicine at the University of Basel. His first
official act at the university was to build a bonfire in his
lecture-room to burn the works of Galen. He lectured to his
students in German instead of the customary Latin, an innovation which drew many students to his classes but outraged
the faculty of the university. The substance of his lectures
outraged them still more and finally bored his students. He
openly vaunted himself as a second Hippocrates and stormed
against the principles then prevalent in medicine. His charges
against medicine were justified, but the manner in which he
made them was tyrannical and vulgar. His character was
fundamentally that of an intellectual bully, and it had not
improved under the company he had frequented during
his wanderings. He defined his position, in regard both to
his university colleagues and to his students, by the statement
that "all the universities have less experience than my beard,
and that the down on my neck is more learned than my
auditors." Paracelsus brought the manner of the tavern wine-
room into his lecture-room. Many of his sallies, it is said,
drifted "from the obscene into the incomprehensible."

Within a year after his arrival at Basel he was in conflict
with the city authorities and was brought to trial. After
abusing the court roundly he fled from the city to avoid the
consequences of his impudence. He resumed his wanderings,
and in September, 1541, died as the result of an injury received in a drunken brawl at Salzburg.

Paracelsus was popular among the common people whom
he treated, but was reviled by medical men of the times.
Perhaps the judgment of the people was the truer measure
of his real character; Paré was beloved by the soldiers, but
detested by the medical faculty of Paris. The charges against
Paracelsus may not all be well founded. One of them was
that he was a drunkard, but drunkards were common in the
sixteenth century. The character of Luther bears no stigma
on this score, yet his habits were in some respects no better
than those of Paracelsus. There was one charge which was
never made against Paracelsus—he was never accused of
lasciviousness. His enemies, unable to make this charge,

spread the story that in his childhood he had been castrated by a hog.

The medical teachings of Paracelsus are overlaid by a nonsensical mass of astrology, mysticism, and alchemy. He had traveled in the Orient, and there, as in every country that he visited, he had acquired a smattering of current metaphysics. The ideas that Paracelsus held on medical subjects were far in advance of his time. There were then no words in any language with which he could express his thoughts precisely, and he could present them only in the vague language of mysticism. One consequence has been that Paracelsus's mysticism was subsequently emphasized as a contribution to theosophy, and, apart from his more solid contributions to medicine, the writings of Paracelsus thus became one of the principal sources drawn on by mystical sects and particularly the secret society of the Rosicrucians. Yet this element of mysticism was in reality only the husk of his work, for in spite of his mysticism Paracelsus did not believe in demoniacal possession and the supernatural origin of disease. He made positive contributions to medicine. He ridiculed the absurd mixtures of herbs that Galen had advocated, and substituted for them simple but powerful medicaments. His interests centered in chemistry, then called alchemy, and most of the remedies he chose were mineral substances. Among them was mercury.

Paracelsus believed that there was a specific remedy for each disease if only the remedy could be found. In fact, however, from among all the specifics he advocated only one came very near being a true specific. That one was mercury for the treatment of syphilis. Paracelsus not only supplied a remedy for syphilis, but was the first physician to describe the stages of the disease and its transmission to children.

Syphilis was then a new disease in Europe. Its occurrence was a factor in breaking the hold of the Galenic therapy. Galen was unacquainted with the disease, and, as he had made no provision for its treatment, many physicians refused at first to treat syphilis. A physician of Mentz, writing in 1532, said: "At first the poor people, who were infected with this distemper, were expelled from human society, like a putrid carcass, and being forsaken by the physician (who would neither give their advice about them nor visit them) they dwelt in the fields and woods." Numerous herb remedies were tried, but failed to have any influence upon the disease. Unlike acute infections in which the patients die quickly or get well, syphilis progresses slowly. The failures were therefore obvious. Guaiacum, or hollywood, was the remedy used by the natives of Haiti, and for that reason it was imported into Europe and used extensively. Sarsaparilla and sassafras were also tried, but to no better effect. While physicians were trying their herbs or refusing to treat syphilis, vagabond quacks undertook to cure with mercury. Their success forced the physicians also to use mercury in treating syphilis. This form of treatment did much to popularize the mineral medicaments which Paracelsus advocated.

These mineral substances are powerful poisons, and except in the treatment of syphilis their adoption was in reality disadvantageous. Nevertheless, once the physicians began the use of mineral drugs they employed them extensively and in large doses. Patients with syphilis were dosed with mercury internally and rubbed with it externally until the saliva flowed from their mouths in a steady stream, their teeth were loosened, and their health permanently impaired by mercury poisoning. Calomel replaced the milder vegetable purgative and was given by the teaspoonful. The salt of antimony, tartar emetic, was introduced into medical practice as an emetic and purgative.

Paracelsus had used antimony under the name of stibium, but later the name was changed and the drug popularized by a medical book published in 1604 and entitled *The Triumphant Chariot of Antimony*. The author's name was given as Basile Valentine, a monk, but it is doubtful if such a person existed, and it is believed that an alchemist wrote the book. The origin of the name antimony as given in this book is as follows: The author alleges that he had observed that some pigs which had eaten food containing antimony became very fat. He was led by this observation to try what effect it would have on some monks who had become emaciated as a result of prolonged fasting. He tried the experiment; the monks all died. Hence the name stibium was replaced by antimony, meaning antagonist to monks.

At first the remedy was widely used by the medical profession, but it was soon found that it was indeed a virulent poison. The reaction against the use of antimony was very strong in some quarters, and the medical profession was divided in a controversy as to whether antimony is a remedy or simply a poison. The controversy was particularly heated in Paris and the physicians opposed to the use of antimony were ably assisted by the satire of Molière. The great dramatist cherished a grudge against the medical profession partly because they could do nothing for his own malady, consumption, and partly because he believed they had killed his only son with antimony. The argument over antimony had just been settled in favor of discarding the substance when King Louis XIV became ill with typhoid fever. After he had been ill for about two weeks a quack who promised relief was allowed to treat him. He gave the king a dose of antimony and soon afterward the king recovered from the typhoid fever. In consequence of this royal recovery antimony was again popularized and its use continued until the nineteenth century.

When Napoleon was a prisoner on the island of St. Helena he was stricken with a disease of the stomach, either cancer or ulcer, and his physician dosed him with tartar emetic in a glass of lemonade. Napoleon was made violently ill by the emetic and in consequence became distrustful of his physician. The next time the paroxysms of pain seized him and his cries of *"Oh, mon pylore!"* brought his physician to his side with a glass of tartar emetic, Napoleon passed it surreptitiously on to his attendant, Montholan. A few minutes later that hero was violently ill, and during the remaining few months of his life Napoleon dispensed with the services of his physician.

The revival of the use of antimony on the basis of the recovery of Louis XIV from typhoid fever is typical of the reasoning of that time in medical matters. It ran thus: The king was sick, he took antimony, he is now well; therefore antimony cured him. Most of the reasoning applied to medical treatment was of this kind over a period extending from the beginning of the Christian era to the nineteenth century. It was only within the nineteenth century that the development of science, particularly in chemistry and physics, began to have an influence upon medicine. This influence taught the physician to ask some such question as: "Would King Louis XIV have got well without antimony?" Science demands a certain type of evidence which is afforded only by what are called "control" observations. Controlled observations in medicine require that the improvement in health occurs only when treatment is given. Scientifically, the fact that the patient got well under the treatment proves nothing, for he might have done so without it or even in spite of it. The proof which science requires is logically very simple, however difficult to carry out in practice. All that it is necessary to do to prove whether antimony is or is not a cure for typhoid fever is to administer the drug to a hundred patients with typhoid fever and keep a record of the number who recover; and as a "control" to keep a record of the number of recoveries among a hundred patients with typhoid who are not treated with antimony. A comparison of the number of recoveries under the two conditions would at once demonstrate whether antimony is simply useless, or beneficial, or definitely harmful.

This simple method for determining the curative value of drugs did not come into use until the nineteenth century. When it was finally applied, the mass of useless remedies that had been collected over many centuries was slowly discarded, and only the few that were of real value were retained. The scientific principle now seems obvious. But if the reader will ask himself what are his beliefs in politics, economics, religion, ethics, and a host of other matters on which he acts with confidence, and will then demand of himself by what "control" observations each belief is buttressed, he will find how short is the distance to which the scientific method has as yet penetrated even in modern thought. So true is this that even a scientific economist may be a faddist in medical matters; and many skillful physicians make bad investments.

The development of the scientific method involved a complete revision of medicine. It was necessary to alter the instruction given in the schools of medicine and to develop a new generation of physicians. This change proceeded slowly, and at the same time that the scientific method was being introduced there grew up beside it a form of treatment which embodied the most mystical elements in the works of Paracelsus. This treatment was the homeopathy of Hahnemann. Its theory was based upon two conceptions—the claim that "like cures like" (*similia similibus curantur*)—and the belief in the "signature" of drugs. The therapy of Galen was based on the principle of opposites; that is, if fever results (or is supposed to result) from the administration of a drug, then that drug is (according to Galen) suited for treating chills; or if a drug causes purging, then it is suited to treat constipation. Paracelsus maintained that drugs producing an action like the disease might also be useful in its treatment. Thus a drug which produces fever may be suitable for treating a fever, and a purge may be beneficial in treating diarrhea. He did not, however, confine himself to either type of treatment. Hahnemann in the early part of the nineteenth century advocated the doctrine that all diseases should be treated with drugs producing like effects. Moreover, in selecting some of his drugs he employed the principle of so-called "signatures" which he borrowed from Paracelsus. This theory is based on the astrological conception that the stars impress the "signature" of disease upon drugs. It was believed that this "signature" can be recognized from the form and color of the plant from which the drug is obtained. Thus the root of the orchid, because it is shaped like a testicle (in Latin the word *orchid* means testicle), should be used in curing diseases of that organ; and since the black spot in the flower euphrasia—eyebright—resembles the pupil of the eye, that plant should, according to homeopathy, be applied to diseases of the eye. The nutmeg vaguely resembles the brain in appearance; it has, therefore, the signature of the brain and could be used in treating diseases of the brain. If a theory thus palpably based upon superstition were enthusiastically introduced today it would still obtain a following, for modern men and women are no more intelligent than their ancestors; but this following would not now be from among the medical profession. In the early part of the nineteenth century, however, the scientific method of controlled experiments had not been widely developed and most of the medical profession were no more able to judge the merits of a medical theory than the layman uneducated in the essentials of scientific research is now.

Hahnemann was successful in introducing homeopathy, and because of its success it was accepted and practiced by many physicians. The secret of its success lay not in the effects of the drugs that were used, for these drugs were administered in amounts too infinitesimal to have any effect. Homeopathists practically gave no medicine at all, for Hahnemann advanced the belief that the smaller the dose the greater the effect. If he had said, not "the greater the effect," but "the better the results," he would have been right, for then most of the medical profession were giving excessively large doses of potent and often poisonous drugs. They were thus doing positive harm to their patients. The small doses used by the homeopaths did no good, but neither did they do any harm. The patient stayed in bed and, as Paré would have said, "God healed him." The distinction between the homeopaths and allopaths—the name applied to the regular medical practitioners by the homeopaths—has been summed up satirically, thus: The patients of the homeopaths died of the disease and the patients of the allopaths died of the cure.

The vogue of homeopathy was brief; it was soon replaced by scientific medicine, which showed that only a few drugs are of value in treating disease, but that these few are indispensable and must be used in effective amounts. In regard to the use of drugs, Oliver Wendell Holmes said in 1860, when scientific methods were having their first effect on medi-

cine: "Throw out opium, which the Creator himself seems
to prescribe, for we often see the scarlet poppy growing in
the cornfields, as if it were foreseen that wherever there is
hunger to be fed there must also be pain to be soothed;
throw out a few specifics which our art did not discover;
. . . throw out wine, which is a food, and the vapors which
produce the miracle of anesthesia—and I firmly believe that
if the whole *materia medica,* as now used, could be sunk to
the bottom of the sea, it would be all the better for mankind
—and all the worse for the fishes."

Opium and anesthetics relieve pain and the specifics
definitely cure disease or relieve its symptoms. At the time
Holmes wrote, the chief specifics known were quinine for
malaria and mercury for syphilis, with the possible addition
of digitalis for heart disease, colchicum for gout, iodine for
goiter, and ipecac for dysentery. In the quotation above
Holmes says that "our art did not discover these specifics";
and, with the exception of mercury, which was introduced by
Paracelsus, this statement was justified. Prior to the development of scientific medicine most of the really valuable drugs
had been discovered by non-medical people. As Holmes says:
"Medicine . . . appropriates everything from every source
that can be of the slightest use to anybody who is ailing in
any way, or likely to be ailing from any cause. It learned
from a monk how to use antimony, from a Jesuit how to cure
ague, from a friar how to cut for stone, from a soldier how
to treat gout, from a sailor how to keep off scurvy, from a
postmaster how to sound the Eustachian tube, from a dairy
maid how to prevent smallpox, and from an old market
woman how to catch the itch insect. It borrowed acupunc-
ture and the moxa from the Japanese heathen, and was
taught the use of lobelia by the American savage."

Holmes, in speaking of the Jesuit who taught how to cure
ague, refers to the introduction of quinine. Cinchona, as this
drug was called, had long been used by the Peruvian Indians
as a cure for fevers. It was brought into Europe as a secret
remedy by the Jesuits in 1632, and later by Juan del Vego,
physician to the Count of Chinchon. The name cinchona was

given the drug in honor of the countess, who was cured of malaria by its use. Europe at that time was in great need of a drug to cure malaria and had been for centuries, for malaria was one of the most prevalent and dangerous diseases. Alexander the Great died in Babylon of malaria complicated with alcoholism. Louis XIV of France contracted malaria and was cured with quinine. Cromwell, in England, likewise acquired the disease, but did not receive quinine, and died; presumably King James I also died of malaria. Malaria was very prevalent before the mosquito was recognized as the agent of transmission and means thus afforded for controlling the disease. Many fevers, called agues, were of malarial origin. Quinine was extensively and beneficially used to treat them. But even after malaria was controlled in most civilized countries by eradicating the Anopheles mosquito, the tradition that quinine was a remedy for fevers in general continued. It has no remedial value except for malaria; nevertheless, it is still an ingredient of proprietary and home remedies for colds and non-malarial fevers.

At about the same time that quinine was introduced into Europe the near-drugs tobacco, coffee, tea, chocolate, and the vegetable, the potato, came into use. The first coffee-house was established in Constantinople in 1554 and in London in 1652; coffee then cost nearly thirty dollars a pound. Tobacco was less well received, for in 1624 the pope threatened the users of snuff with excommunication, the Turks imposed the death penalty for smoking, and the Emperor of Russia ordered that "tobacco drinkers" should have their noses slit, after which they were to be whipped and then deported to Siberia.

The sailor whom Holmes says taught "how to keep off the scurvy" was Captain Cook, the discoverer of the Hawaiian Islands. Scurvy was formerly very common among sailors who went on long voyages during which they lived on salted food and were deprived of fresh meat and vegetables. Captain Cook discovered the connection between the disease and the diet which causes it. Today scurvy is known to occur from lack of vitamine C, one of the food substances necessary in small amounts for health and proper growth. In recent years other vitamines have been discovered. There is one called A, without which children cannot grow and in adults the eyes become sore; B, in the absence of which a form of neuritis called beri-beri develops; another without which reproduction cannot take place; and still another which acts like sunlight in preventing rickets. The administration of vitamines cures the diseases which result from their deficiency in the diet, but they cannot strictly be called specific remedies any more than food can be called a specific for starvation or iron a cure for anemia, iodine for simple goiter, or salt for heat cramps. These conditions result from dietary deficiencies which are made good by foods—not by drugs in the true sense. These diseases are merely manifestations of the fact that the body cannot operate normally unless it is supplied with all the materials necessary for its operation.

In recent years much scientific attention has been given to the needs of the body; in consequence the treatment of disease is now centered on supplying these needs rather than the extensive use of drugs. For centuries past the attention of physicians has been directed almost exclusively toward efforts to drive out disease with drugs as rats are exterminated from a house with poison. Modern methods of treatment, however, are returning to the ancient form used by Hippocrates—sunlight, baths, fresh air, and a supply of those things by which the body makes its own recoveries from diseases. One of the greatest advances under modern medical investigation has been the discovery of the substances which the body requires for its normal operation, and the diseases which result when these substances are lacking. Vitamines, iron, sunlight, and iodine are only one aspect of the problem, for other substances which are needed arise in the body itself and their deficiency results in disease.

It has been discovered that the thyroid gland in the neck produces a secretion which can be formed only when iodine is present in the diet. Iodine is therefore one of the substances necessary to maintain health. But it has also been discovered that the thyroid gland of some people will not form its secretion even when the supply of iodine is adequate. In consequence of this failure of the gland children develop a disease known as cretinism. The child fails to grow; its body is dwarfed and distorted in shape; mentally it is an imbecile. There were once many institutions where cretins were cared for, but this is no longer the case, for it is now known that the deficient secretion of the gland can be made up by feeding an extract from the thyroid gland of sheep. When this treatment is started early in life the misshapen bodies of the children straighten out and grow normally and imbecility gives place to normal-mindedness. The administration of thyroid extract must be continued throughout life, however, or the condition of myxedema develops. Myxedema is the adult form of cretinism and it sometimes occurs in persons in whom the thyroid deficiency develops late in life. Persons so affected put on weight, their skin becomes puffy and dry, their hair falls out, and they lose their mental alertness. The feeding of thyroid extract in the exact amount necessary restores them to a normal condition.

Insulin for the treatment of diabetes is another method of supplying deficiency of the body and controlling the disease which results from the deficiency. In diabetes the body is unable to utilize sugar as a food. This inability results because an insufficient amount of insulin is secreted in the pancreas and circulated in the blood. Insulin which is now supplied as a medicament is the secretion obtained from the pancreas of sheep. When administered in proper amounts to persons suffering from diabetes the symptoms of the disease are relieved, just as the symptoms of cretinism are relieved by thyroid extract or those of scurvy are relieved by fruit juices, and rickets by sunlight. But neither insulin nor thyroid extract is a cure in the sense of specific drugs. They simply supply substances which are deficient in the body; and their administration must be continued indefinitely unless the body corrects its own deficiency in the meantime.

Still another remedy of the same type is liver for the

treatment of pernicious anemia. This disease, like all other forms of anemia, is characterized by a diminution in the amount of red coloring matter in the blood, but, unlike other forms of anemia, it is not remedied by the administration of iron. Instead, paralysis and weakness develop and eventually death results. It has only recently been discovered that eating liver or even taking an extract of liver cures the disease.

The use of animal substances—thyroid glands, pancreatic extract, and liver—as remedies is suggestive of the ancient belief in acquiring bravery by eating the heart of a lion. But the ancient belief had merely superstition to support it; no well-arranged "control" experiment was performed. Scientific methods and controlled experiments would have demonstrated its fallacy just as scientific methods have demonstrated the value of treatment with insulin, thyroid extract, and liver. Even today, however, the popular fancy and even some medical fancy have been caught by the successful use of animal extract. Superstitions have been revived in an effort to rejuvenate old men with extract of the testicle. Superstitions die hard indeed when they are supported by a popular desire; the idea of rejuvenation recurs in many forms. The ancient Jews put their enfeebled patriarchs to bed with young girls, who were supposed to radiate vitality; Mohammed selected two wives, ages, respectively, seven and eight years, to strengthen his failing powers; Ponce de Leon sought for the fountain of youth; some physicians of the seventeenth century advocated a transfusion of blood for rejuvenation; and the alchemist of the Renaissance grew old in the search for the elixir of life.

# CHAPTER XVI

## TOWARD A BETTER CIVILIZATION

reat discoveries are sometimes foreshadowed and their benefits in part anticipated. Thus, before Pasteur had fully demonstrated the principle of bacterial infection, Semmelweis had devised a means of controlling childbed fever and Lister had introduced the antiseptic principle into surgery. Both of these innovations were of inestimable benefit in the fields where they were applied. They were, however, limited to these fields. Semmelweis did not realize that his method of preventing puerperal infection would also prevent surgical infection. When this fact was discovered by Lister he did not extend his ideas of air-borne infection to include the contagious diseases. Neither of these men grasped the full conception of bacterial infection. That was left for Pasteur. He discovered a basic principle and showed its application to all infection and to all contagious diseases. Whereas Lister had revolutionized surgery, Pasteur revolutionized all of medicine.

The subject of bacterial infection has been touched on in previous chapters, but the discovery of the principle of infection is dealt with here more fully because it is an outstanding example of the application of the scientific method in medicine. Pasteur's work was the result of the prolonged and laborious application of these methods, which were then new in the field of medicine. The force which the scientific method has supplied for the advancement of medicine is seen nowhere more clearly than in the change that medicine has undergone since Pasteur's discovery. Pasteur's work was done within the memory of men now living; he died in 1895.

As a result of Pasteur's work, men were able for the first time to contend intelligently against contagious diseases.

Consequently, a wholly new type of medical science has been developed. Preventive medicine has come to the front. Prophylaxis to prevent illness has replaced treatment; treatment now merely attempts to overcome what should have been prevented. The measures for the prevention of infectious diseases are among the strongest weapons for the betterment of mankind now in the hands of civilization. If civilization would allow them to be used to the fullest extent, the treatment of infectious diseases would eventually become unnecessary, for they would cease to exist.

Pasteur was a French chemist and not a physician. His work started with the study of crystals, and the two forms of tartaric acid occurring in wine; it then extended to the diseases of wine, and so, step by step, to the diseases of insects, domestic animals, and finally man. In every stage of his advance he made discoveries, and any one of his contributions to science would have brought him fame. The diseases of wine which first attracted Pasteur's attention were a serious economic problem in France. In healthy wines the grape juice simply fermented to produce alcohol, while sick wines putrefied and became bitter and ropy. Pasteur first studied fermentation and found that it was due to the activity of yeast, which he said was "a living thing just as you are. The yeast eats the sugar just as you eat your food, and then throws out as waste the alcohol and carbonic acid just as your body throws off the waste from food that it cannot use."

His study of fermentation drew him into the controversy of spontaneous generation. This had been a favorite subject of consideration for philosophers and metaphysicians. The question involved was: Do all living things come from seeds or eggs in which life already exists, or can life be created out of non-living matter—that is, generated spontaneously? The prevailing opinion was that spontaneous generation was possible, and that fleas, lice, flies, and other vermin arise spontaneously from decomposing organic matter. With the invention of the microscope it became possible to see bacteria, and these microörganisms also were supposed to be the products of spontaneous generation. Pasteur settled the question of spontaneous generation by the method of controlled experiments. He filled two flasks with a fermentable solution. One of these he boiled to kill all living matter in the solution and covered it to keep out dust. The other flask of fluid, which was his control, he treated precisely the same except in one respect. After boiling it he did not cover it to exclude the dust. The fluid thus exposed fermented, for yeast and other organisms carried in the air as dust settled in it and multiplied. The fluid in the flask from which dust was excluded remained sterile. Life did not develop in it. Pasteur thus established the principle that living organisms do not arise spontaneously. He also showed that organisms causing fermentation or putrefaction must be brought in from some outside source; in other words, infection is necessary before fermentation or putrefaction can occur.

With this idea he returned to the study of spoiled wine. On examining the wine he found bacteria in it. He was then able to tell the wine manufacturers that "these little rod-shaped bodies [bacteria] are the cause of the disease in your wines. They enter it from the air, and when conditions are favorable for their growth they start an unhealthy fermentation, just as the yeast starts a healthy fermentation." Pasteur next demonstrated that the organisms causing the disease in wine could be killed by heating the wine. This process of heating at a temperature sufficiently high to kill germs but not so high as to injure the fluid is called pasteurization. Its most beneficial application today is in the treatment of milk. After it was discovered that human disease is essentially the same as the "unhealthy fermentation" in wine, it was also discovered that milk was often a source of infection with the germs of tuberculosis, typhoid, septic sore throat, and other diseases.

Pasteur's attention was next directed to a disease of silkworms. As in the case of sick wine, the disease of silkworms was a serious economic problem, for raising silk is one of the leading industries of France and has been so from the time of Henry IV. In 1849 an epidemic disease attacked the silk-worms, and in consequence the annual revenue from silk fell from about five million dollars to less than a third of a million. The silk industry of the whole world was threatened with extermination, for the disease spread from France to Spain and then to Turkey, Syria, and China. Pasteur at the request of the government undertook to determine the cause of the disease. For five years he worked on the problem with the laborious and painstaking methods of science. He discovered that the silkworms were suffering from two infectious diseases; he supplied a preventive for both and thus restored prosperity to the silk industry.

During the five years spent in this work he was criticized for his slowness; although ill and discouraged, he worked on. His two daughters died and he himself became partially paralyzed. The French government provided him with a laboratory in which to carry on his work and finally voted him a pension of about five hundred dollars a year. These signs of appreciation encouraged him to keep on, but what was even more satisfactory was a letter from Lister. Lister had introduced antisepsis into surgery and in so doing had revolutionized surgery. He wrote to Pasteur that antisepsis was an application of his discovery of the cause of fermentation and putrefaction of wine. Lister found that infection in wounds arose from the same cause as did the diseases of wine.

It was only in 1875, barely half a century ago, that Pasteur undertook the study of contagious diseases in animals. As in the cases of the wine industry and the silk industry, the incentive was economic. An epidemic of anthrax was spreading among the sheep of France. This disease is caused by the anthrax bacillus, but there was then no way of preventing its spread. Pasteur undertook this problem. While working on it he made the only accidental discovery in his career. It was a discovery of the first importance, for it not only led directly to the control of anthrax, but also opened the way for the use of vaccines in other diseases.

Pasteur was studying chicken cholera, a troublesome epidemic disease. He had isolated the organism of the disease and he grew it in broth. In order to maintain an active growth of the bacilli, it was necessary to renew the broth frequently. If it was not renewed the bacilli poisoned themselves with their own waste products, just as the yeast plant, during fermentation, poisons itself with the alcohol it produces and eventually ceases its activity. Pasteur renewed his cultures of the bacilli by taking a small quantity of the broth containing the organism and putting it in fresh broth. A few drops of the broth containing the germs placed on bread and fed to chickens induced the disease and invariably killed them. In the course of his experiments he chanced to feed chickens with bacilli which had remained for many days in the same broth. Much to his surprise, these chickens did not die; they sickened for a few days and then recovered. It occurred to Pasteur to feed them with virulent bacilli from a fresh culture. The chickens which had received the attenuated bacilli were not even made sick by the bacilli which invariably killed the other chickens. They had acquired an immunity by overcoming the infection from the weakened strain of bacilli. Pasteur repeated the experiments many times and always with the same results. He thus established the principle of bacterial vaccination.

Pasteur then applied this principle of vaccination to the prevention of anthrax in sheep. He grew the anthrax bacilli and then weakened them in the same way that the bacilli of chicken cholera had been weakened. The attenuated bacilli were then injected into sheep. The sheep survived and were thereafter immune from even a virulent strain of anthrax. When Pasteur announced his discovery it met with opposition. He was challenged to a public trial of his method. He accepted the challenge and conducted the test by the method of control experiments.

A flock of fifty sheep was divided into two groups; twenty-five received injections of weakened anthrax culture and twenty-five, as controls, were untreated. Both groups were then infected with anthrax. A comparison of the number of fatalities in each group at once indicated whether the method of prevention was of value. On May 2, 1881, at Pouilly-le-Fort, a large crowd of sheep-raisers, veterinarians and physicians gathered to see Pasteur administer the vaccine to the twenty-five sheep. The vaccine was administered again in larger quantities on May 17th. Two weeks later both groups of sheep were infected with virulent anthrax bacilli. On June 2nd the crowd again gathered to see the outcome of the experiment. All of the sheep which had received the vaccine were alive; all of the sheep which had not received the vaccine were dead.

Pasteur's discoveries had benefited the wine industry, the silk industry, and the sheep industry; and as Huxley, the English biologist, said, the results obtained from these "discoveries alone would suffice to cover the war indemnity of five billions paid by France to Germany in 1870." But Pasteur's work was not yet complete. He had before him the most difficult of his problems—the application of his principles to the control of human diseases. For this effort he chose to study rabies, or hydrophobia. This disease was then much more prevalent among animals than it is now, and human cases were common. Although the loss of life from rabies was less than from some other infectious diseases, rabies was more feared. There was always a chance of recovery from other diseases, but rabies was invariably fatal. After a long series of experiments Pasteur discovered that the virus of rabies was fixed in the nervous system. He did not isolate the organism; in fact, it has not even now been isolated with certainty; hence he could not grow it in broth to obtain a vaccine—*i.e.*, a weakened strain—as he had for the organisms of chicken cholera and anthrax. He did, however, grow it in the nervous system of living rabbits. After the rabbits had died from rabies he removed the spinal cord, and by drying it weakened the virus which it contained. He ground up the spinal cord containing the attenuated virus and injected this material into rabbits. The rabbits so treated were then found to be immune to rabies. When men or animals are infected with rabies the symptoms of the disease do not develop for three weeks or more. The immunity from the vaccine develops in a much shorter time. It is therefore possible to prevent rabies even after infection has taken place.

Pasteur's first human patient was Joseph Meister, an Alsatian boy nine years of age. He had been bitten in fourteen places by a rabid dog. Pasteur hesitated to apply his immunizing vaccine for fear it would harm the boy, but finally he was persuaded to do so, since otherwise it was inevitable that the boy would die of rabies. Pasteur administered the new prophylaxis and rabies did not develop. Soon afterwards a second case was brought to him. A shepherd boy of fourteen, named Berger Gupille, had struggled with a rabid dog to prevent it from biting some younger boys. He had himself been bitten. The vaccine of Pasteur saved him from rabies. In the yard of the Pasteur Institute at Paris there is a statue of this shepherd boy showing him struggling with the rabid dog.

After these two successful cases people who had been bitten by rabid dogs came from all over Europe to receive the vaccine. The first Americans to receive treatment were four children from Newark, New Jersey. They were sent to Paris and treated there in December, 1885, six months after Pasteur had treated Joseph Meister. The following year a supply of the virus was sent to America.

Pasteur applied none of his discoveries to the treatment of disease. They were all directed to preventing disease. The recognition of the cause of infectious diseases made possible the development of preventive medicine. The application of the measures of prevention has made even the most unhealthy quarters of modern cities more healthy than were the palaces of a century ago. Preventive measures applied to the health of communities have influenced civilization more profoundly than any other advancement. Many of these preventive measures are for the individual as well as for the community. Vaccination against typhoid fever, diphtheria, scarlet fever, and recently against tuberculosis, is an example of this personal prophylaxis. Syphilis was among the first of the diseases against which a prophylaxis was developed. In fact, this disease has had more measures provided for its control than any other disease. A prophylaxis against syphilis was developed by the Russian biologist Metchnikoff, who was Pasteur's pupil. In 1906 he announced that syphilis could be prevented by rubbing an ointment containing 33 per cent of calomel over the area of infection, provided that the application was made within a few hours after infection had occurred. Metchnikoff developed his method of prophylaxis by the use of controlled experiments performed on apes and finally on a man who volunteered to be inoculated. But infection was prevented by the use of the prophylaxis. In 1909 Metchnikoff received the Nobel prize.

Application of the principles developed by Pasteur led also to the discovery of diphtheria antitoxin. This antitoxin, although not a drug, is one of the few specifics for the cure of disease. Diphtheria is ordinarily a local infection of the throat. It would be no more serious than a severe sore throat from infection with some other organism if it were not for the fact that the diphtheria bacilli, while living on the surface, produce a poison or toxin which passes into the blood and acts upon the nervous system and heart to produce a serious and often fatal disease. For centuries diphtheria was the most fatal disease of children. Until recent years no treatment was successful against it. Persons who have diphtheria and recover do so because their bodies form an antitoxin which neutralizes the toxin of the bacilli; such persons are thereafter immune to the disease because they retain some of the antitoxin. This antitoxin directly counteracts the effects of the diphtheria toxin; it is literally an antidote. Diphtheria antitoxin can be produced in horses which are injected with gradually increased amounts of diphtheria toxin separated from the living bacilli. The antitoxin formed in the horse is present in its blood. The blood is drawn in small quantities at a time, a serum is separated, and, after some further treatment, this serum furnishes the commercial antitoxin. When this serum is injected into a child with diphtheria the toxin absorbed from the throat is neutralized and the disease is stopped.

Diphtheria antitoxin was placed in the hands of the medical profession in the same year that Pasteur died. In that year, 1895, as in former years, 50 per cent of the children who developed diphtheria died from the disease. Within five years after the introduction of antitoxin the mortality had fallen to 12 per cent. It has diminished steadily ever since as the value of antitoxin has become more fully appreciated and its use correspondingly much more general. Formerly deaths from diphtheria were very common, but now a single death in a city is the subject of adverse comment.

Unfortunately, few bacteria produce toxins which can be neutralized by antitoxins. Many, however, by their action in the body cause slight changes in the blood. In some diseases these changes can be detected by serological tests, so that a method of diagnosing the disease is thus made possible. Such is the case of syphilis. This method of diagnosis for syphilis was developed by Wassermann, and is now known as the Wassermann reaction. It is based on the fact that the blood from patients with syphilis contains a substance which disintegrates the red corpuscles in sheep's blood. This disintegration is not induced by blood from a person free from syphilis. Before this test was developed there was no reliable method by which syphilis could be detected after it had passed beyond the early stages, nor was there any way of telling when the disease was cured. But now there are very few diseases which can be diagnosed with the precision that Wassermann's reaction affords for syphilis. Among the results of the general use of the Wassermann reaction has been the demonstration that syphilis is both much more prevalent and much more persistent than was formerly supposed, and that many cases of illness are due to syphilis which were formerly assigned to other causes. In the late stages of syphilis a form of tumor called a "gumma" may form in various organs of the body and interfere with their activities. The symptoms which result are often not clearly indicative of syphilis; they may simulate cancer and serious surgical operations may appear necessary. In all such cases the Wassermann reaction points to the real cause of the disturbance and to the proper treatment, and operation is avoided.

Diagnosis of disease is probably the most important service that the physician renders to his patient. But many patients fail to see the importance of this service. They are less interested in the name of their disorder than in its cure; they expect either surgical treatment or pills. They fail to realize that unless the physician can diagnose the disease he can furnish no remedy for it. Diagnosis enables the physician to pick out from the many diseases causing somewhat similar symptoms the few for which medicine has remedies; and, what is equally important, it enables him also to pick out diseases in their early stages, for which, even if he has no remedy, he can offer means by which their course can be arrested. There are no drugs, vaccines, or serums for the treatment of tuberculosis, but if the disease is diagnosed in its earliest stages it can usually be arrested. If the disease is allowed to progress the result is invalidism or death.

Similarly, there is no cure for hardening of the arteries, but the heightened arterial pressure which almost invariably precedes the hardening by months or even years can be detected and often relieved. Untimely hardening of the arteries is thus prevented. Cancer is generally curable in its early stages by surgical operation; in its late stages it is fatal. In a large percentage of all cases of cancer, life or death depends upon early diagnosis. Few cancers except those on the surface of the body are detected in their earliest stages. A blood test for cancer as reliable as the Wassermann reaction for syphilis would result in the saving of thousands of lives annually. This saving of life would in itself involve only improvement in diagnosis.

An interesting development of the diagnosis of syphilis

has been the proof that some of the older treatments of syphilis are much less effective than they were thought to be. Some four centuries ago Paracelsus introduced the use of mercury for treating syphilis, and during all the years since it has been assumed to be a treatment that actually cured. John Hunter deliberately inoculated himself with syphilis in order to study it; he was confident that he could cure himself with mercury. He later died of heart disease, and this was undoubtedly, in his case, a late effect of syphilis. When the Wassermann reaction came into use it was found that mercury often fails to effect a complete cure. It lessens the severity of the disease but fails to eradicate all of the spirochetes. The latent effects of the disease develop in spite of the treatment, and these latest effects were formerly attributed to other causes; it is only in recent years that it has become known that paresis, locomotor ataxia, and certain forms of heart disease are due to syphilis. Formerly it was believed that one attack of syphilis conferred immunity against all subsequent infection. After salvarsan came into use for the treatment of syphilis and the disease was really cured, it was found that there was no immunity from the disease, and that in such cured persons a reinfection could occur. The apparent immunity formerly arose from the fact that mercury fails to make a complete cure and so long as the disease remains a fresh infection cannot occur.

The diagnosis of syphilis, made possible by the Wassermann reaction, showed the necessity for a means of treatment more effective than mercury. The Wassermann reaction was introduced in 1907; five years later Ehrlich announced the discovery of salvarsan for the treatment of syphilis. The discovery of salvarsan vindicated in part one of the beliefs of Paracelsus. He had maintained that there was a specific for every disease and that chemistry was the agency for obtaining these specifics. In the twentieth century his belief was revived in scientific form by Ehrlich. He found that certain tissues or parts of tissues have the property of absorbing some dyes and refusing to absorb others.

Such is the case also with bacteria and with animal parasites. Advantage has been taken of these peculiarities of staining for use in identifying bacteria under microscopic examination. Thus in examining sputum for tubercle bacilli or in examining pus for gonococci, dyes are applied to the material spread thinly on a piece of glass. The tubercle bacilli in the one case and the gonococci in the other take up certain dyes, while other bacteria which may be present are not stained by these dyes; the difference in staining allows the bacteria to be differentiated.

Ehrlich, by exercising what he called his "chemical imagination," conceived the idea that it was possible that bacteria and animal parasites might absorb poisons in the same selective way that they absorb dyes. If a poison could be found which would kill the organisms of disease, but at the same time would not kill the tissues of the body, there would then be available an ideal treatment for infectious diseases. The drug quinine behaves in precisely this manner for malaria; it is more poisonous to the malarial parasite than it is to the human body; but it is inactive toward bacteria or the spirochetes of syphilis.

Ehrlich after a long series of experiments developed an organic compound of arsenic which kills the spirochetes of syphilis, but which, in the amount used, can be given human beings safely. In 1911 he announced the discovery of this compound, which he called salvarsan, or 606, this figure representing the number of experiments he had made during his search for the specific. The composition of salvarsan has been modified and improved since its introduction. Used with care, this poison for spirochetes affords a safe medicament for the cure of syphilis.

Salvarsan is most effective in its action during the primary stage of syphilis, but with prolonged administration definite cures can be obtained in the later stages of the disease. After the spirochetes have entered the central nervous system, however, and are causing paresis or locomotor ataxia, they cannot be eradicated with salvarsan.

It is noteworthy that the men who sought for means to

effect the medical control of syphilis ranked among the highest in their profession. This fact is striking in view of the public opinion which still regards syphilis as a disease which is shameful and whose name is not even to be mentioned with propriety. Some moralists and many clergymen still regard syphilis as a fitting punishment for immorality. This standpoint indicates that these moralists and clergymen are actually opposed to the advance of civilization and human welfare. For centuries past the social control of syphilis was in their hands and they failed to effect any improvement in this social and moral scourge. Now modern medicine has taken the control of syphilis out of their hands. In the period of six years, 1905 to 1911, the methods of science applied to the study of syphilis resulted in the isolation of the organism causing the disease and in the development of a reliable prophylaxis, an exact method of diagnosis, and a treatment which failed of perfection in only one respect. This prophylaxis effectively prevents syphilis; but only for those who know how to apply it. Unfortunately, public opinion is still largely controlled by the moralists opposed to the spread of knowledge concerning this prophylaxis. It is therefore largely due to the moralists that many cases of syphilis still occur.

Salvarsan does not cure syphilis when the last stages are reached and paresis and locomotor ataxia appear. In this one respect the medical control of syphilis was incomplete. Therefore the search for means of complete control continued. It led into the most difficult and least developed field of medicine, that which deals with insanity.

The treatment of mental disease is not so well developed as the treatment of other diseases because insanity has only recently been recognized as a medical problem. Even today the diagnosis of insanity, unlike the diagnosis of any other disease, involves the decision of a court of law. Presumably this ancient custom is retained because insanity deprives a man of his freedom and property. But a man may also be deprived of his freedom on account of leprosy or some other infectious disease of shorter duration. The courts are not asked to pass upon each case of smallpox or measles; medical decision is final in such cases, and the patient is quarantined. The insane were formerly treated as criminals and were accordingly locked up in prisons; this attitude has survived in the court decision for insanity. The reason that it has persisted lies in the fact that the medical diagnosis for insanity is not as positive as is the diagnosis for other diseases. The medical diagnosis for insanity is not yet regarded with complete confidence because psychology and its medical aspect, psychiatry, have as yet made very little progress. The uncertainty of diagnosis in cases of suspected insanity is seen clearly in trials for murder involving a plea of insanity. Eminent psychiatrists offer diametrically opposite opinions before the court. If the question were the diagnosis of syphilis or typhoid fever instead of insanity there could be no difference of opinion, for the diagnosis would be positive. Yet thirty years ago the diagnoses of typhoid and syphilis were open to the same uncertainties as is the diagnosis of insanity today.

Throughout all ages the treatment of insanity has been neglected. Only recently have the insane been treated humanely, and even now their condition does not receive as intensive scientific study as is devoted to other diseases. Nor will it receive this consideration until civilization has advanced beyond its present stage and there is developed as great an interest and compassion for men who, because of illness, have lost their mental faculties as for men who, because of illness, have lost their physical faculties.

This distinction between those mentally and those physically ill is of extreme antiquity, but was most marked in Europe during the Middle Ages. The medieval Christians built hospitals and everyone who was physically ill was admitted. But the insane were excluded. If their insanity took the form of religious enthusiasm, as insanity often does, they were as likely as not to be regarded as saints and treated with veneration. If their insanity took on an abusive or maudlin form and did not yield to the exorcisms of the clergy, the insane, and the devils which were supposed to

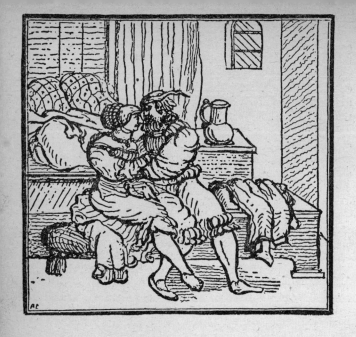

## THE SANGUINE MAN

A woodcut from the medical poem of Salerno. The text characterizes
this type of man as follows:

"Complexions cannot vertue breed or vice,
    Yet may they vnto both giue inclination,
    The *Sanguine* game-fome is, and nothing nice,
    Loue Wine, and Women, and all recreation,
    Likes pleafant tales, and news, playes, cards & dice,
    Fit for all company, and euery fafhion:
    Though bold, not apt to take offence, not irefull,
    But bountifull, and kinde, and looking cheerefull.
    Inclining to be fat, and prone to laughter,
    Loues mirth, & Mufick, cares not what comes after."

In the jargon of the "newer psychology" such a man would be classified as an "extrospect of the sensation, feeling type."

possess them, were chained in madhouses, places even worse than the prisons of those days. There they remained, poorly sheltered, scantily fed, and unclothed, to lie in their own excreta until they died of neglect and exposure. The only treatment they received was an occasional beating when their cries became annoying.

In non-Christian countries during medieval times the care of the insane was much better. In Arabia they were treated kindly and were kept in asylums, where their Oriental love of hearing stories was used to keep them quiet. It was not until 1547 that an insane-asylum was established in London at the hospital of St. Mary of Bethlehem, a name soon abbreviated to "Bedlam." The conditions in it fully justified the significance which the word bedlam acquired. A medical book written at the time Bedlam was opened summarizes the accepted treatment of the insane in these words: "I do advertyse every man which is madde or lunatycke or frantycke or demonyack to be kept in safegarde in some close house or chamber where there is lytell light; and that he have a keeper the which the madde man do fear." The brutality thus implied in regard to the keeper found full expression in the brutalities practiced on the insane.

During the eighteenth century Bedlam was one of the "sights" of London and visitors came to be amused at the antics of the inmates. The insane at some asylums were kept in cages and exposed to view on payment of a small fee. Samuel Johnson and Boswell visited Bedlam and Steele took three school-boys to see "the lions, the tombs, Bedlam, and the other places which are entertainment to raw minds, because they strike forcibly upon the imagination."

The occasional patient who improved at Bedlam in spite of the treatment was allowed to go free and to wander about the country begging. These insane beggars wore a badge and were known as "Tom o' Bedlams." John Aubrey, writing near the close of the seventeenth century, says: "Till the breaking out of the Civil Wars Tom o' Bedlams did travel about the country. They had been poor distracted men, but had been put in Bedlam, where, recovering some soberness,

they were licentiated to go abegging; . . . they had on
their left arm an armilla of tin about four inches long; they
could not get it off. They wore about their necks a great
horn of an ox in a string or baudry, which, when they came
to a house for alms, they did wind, and they did put the
drink given them into the horn whereto they did put the
stopple." Perhaps Edgar in Shakespeare's *King Lear* refers to this custom of drinking from the horn when he says:
"Poor Tom, thy horn is dry." Shakespeare in his treatment
of King Lear showed more knowledge of insanity than is to
be found in any medical book of his time. Shakespeare's
son-in-law was a Dr. Hall, who was noted for his use of
herbs, but he could not have supplied any information about
insanity, nor could any other physician of that time. Shakespeare may well say: "Oh, who can minister to a mind diseased?"

When Shakespeare spoke of insanity as "a mind diseased"
he anticipated physicians in this knowledge by nearly a
century. Thomas Willis, a prominent London practitioner of
the seventeenth century, seems to have been the first physician to consider insanity as a disease. He gave a clear description of paresis, but of course did not recognize that it
is caused by syphilis. Willis, among his many notable contributions to medicine, was the first physician to observe
sugar in the urine of patients with diabetes. The test he used
to detect sugar was the sense of taste; physicians as well as
patients have profited by modern methods of diagnosis.

At the beginning of the nineteenth century the treatment
of the insane was little better than it had been in the Middle
Ages. The Lunatics Tower of Vienna was one of the show
places of that city, and there, as formerly at Bedlam, the
patients were exhibited to the public like animals in a me-
nagerie. The Tower was not closed until 1853. It was only
during the latter part of the nineteenth century that insanity came to be clearly recognized as a disease, but the theories as to its cause were mere speculations. Such symptoms
as egotism, jealousy, laziness, and self-abuse were regarded
as causes of insanity. In fact, even today the study of insan-

ity is concerned largely with the observation of symptoms and attempts to classify the different forms of insanity on the basis of these symptoms. Even after the particular form of insanity is given a name very little is done to treat it; only for cases of paresis is there a specific treatment.

The insane-asylums of today are not hospitals where the mentally ill are treated, but are sanatoria where they are kept. Great improvements have been effected in the care given them during the last century. In the beginning of the nineteenth century the brutalities of earlier times were ameliorated, but the insane were still treated harshly. They were dosed with drugs, bled excessively, locked up in dark damp cellars, and restrained with chains. The idea persisted that the insane were willfully destructive and obstinate, and consequently attempts were made to intimidate and bully or even beat them into submission. This procedure was not followed in malice, but because it was believed that it would help to relieve the insanity; and all this on the supposition that it was good for them.

The first influential champion of more gentle treatment was Philippe Pinel, a physician at the Hôpital Bicetre of Paris. Pinel was led to the study of mental diseases by the fact that one of his friends who had become insane escaped into the forest and was there devoured by wolves. In an effort to improve the condition of the insane he appealed in their behalf to the Common Council of Paris and requested authority to use humane treatment. His act was a bold one, for Paris was still in the turmoil that followed the Revolution, and Pinel was in danger of being killed as an "aristocrat." Couthon, the associate of Robespierre, spoke for the Council in answer to Pinel's plea, and the suspicious attitude of the time is evident in his words: "Citizen, I will visit thee in the Bicetre tomorrow morning, and woe to thee if thou hast deceived us and concealed enemies of the people among thy madmen." Couthon duly visited the hospital and was revolted by the shrieks and blasphemies of the insane patients who were chained to the walls. He said to Pinel: "Ah, citizen, art thou thyself a madman, that thou desirest to turn such cattle loose? I greatly fear thou wilt become thyself a victim of thy preconceived opinions." Nevertheless, Pinel took the chains off his insane patients and put an end

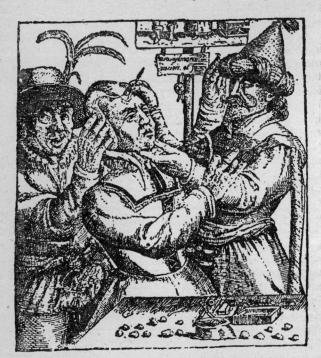

### QUACK REMOVING A STONE FROM THE HEAD OF AN INSANE WOMAN

Prior to the nineteenth century the insane, under the Biblical authority of possession by devils, were treated with outrageous brutality. Even their relatives were sometimes imposed upon; the quack shown here has been employed to remove from the woman's head the stone which was presumed to be the immediate cause of her insanity. He is making a cut in her forehead and next he will palm a stone and exhibit it as coming from the wound. On the table are a collection of stones which he has removed from other patients.

to brutality. He substituted wholesome food and sunlight for the unsanitary and otherwise pitiful conditions under which the patients had previously been kept. The insane patients improved under Pinel's treatment, and the procedures spread gradually to other institutions.

In the United States prior to 1850 there were a few private insane-asylums, but most insane patients were confined in county poorhouses or prisons. Improvement came largely through the efforts of Miss Dorothea Dix. She spread the ideas of Pinel widely in this country and was instrumental in establishing as many as thirty-two state asylums. In such institutions the insane could be better cared for. But even the state institutions are not ideal. In 1894 Dr. Weir Mitchell pointed out the evils of political control and the absolute lack of scientific study in insanity in America. Since then some improvement has been made, but it is slight in comparison with that in other branches of medicine.

The most notable advance in psychiatry has been the discovery that paresis is produced by the spirochetes of syphilis. This fact was demonstrated in 1913 by Noguchi, one of the investigators in the Rockefeller Institute, who recently died while studying yellow fever in Africa. His name is thus added to the long list of medical martyrs who in conquering disease have themselves paid with the last full measure of devotion. Prior to the demonstration that paresis was a form of syphilis the connection between the two diseases was suspected; but since paresis could not be influenced by treatment with mercury or salvarsan, it was assumed that the insanity was in some way the result of syphilis, but not a manifestation of active syphilis. Noguchi, however, demonstrated the living spirochetes in the brain of paretics and thus showed that the functional and anatomical changes in the brain, manifest as paresis, are directly due to their presence and action. He likewise demonstrated that locomotor ataxia is due to the action of spirochetes in the spinal cord. The only difference between this disease and paresis is the part of the nervous system which the spirochetes attack; in the one case the spinal cord, in the other the cerebrum.

Unfortunately, salvarsan does not penetrate into the brain or spinal cord in sufficient amounts to kill the spirochetes there. Salvarsan applied to the treatment of syphilis during its primary or secondary stage prevents the development of paresis and locomotor ataxia by killing the spirochetes before they invade the brain. But many people are ignorant of the serious consequences of the disease and ignore it because it causes no discomfort in its early stages; or they hide their disease because of the moral obliquity which is attached to it. Consequently, many people with syphilis do not have proper treatment. The pseudo-moral attitude which often deprives them of treatment extends even to the hospitals, most of which will not accept for treatment uncomplicated cases of venereal disease. They reject no other disease, but the members of hospital boards are influenced by public and religious opinion. This attitude of the hospitals is not of recent origin, for when Louis XIV established the Salpêtrière as a hospital prison for prostitutes, those with syphilis were at first excluded. Later they were admitted, but were whipped on entering and on leaving, in punishment for having acquired syphilis.

Until recently there were only a few places where syphilitics who are unable to afford the services of a specialist could receive early treatment. Now, however, some of the larger cities have established venereal clinics where syphilitics can obtain treatment at a nominal cost or free. The establishment of these clinics in itself serves to illustrate the artificial distinction which is made between venereal disease and other infectious disease; there are no clinics where any other infectious disease is thus separately treated. These clinics were doubtless established with motives which were strictly humanitarian, but an economic motive is also involved. Paretics form about 10 per cent of the inmates of insane asylums. They are an expense to the taxpayers.

The greatest benefit to be expected from the clinics, however, is a decrease of syphilis. Syphilis is ordinarily transmitted for two to four years after it is acquired. If early treatment is given with salvarsan this period of transmission is cut down to a month or less. The possibilities of transmission are lessened proportionately. It will be ten to twenty years before the full benefits from venereal clinics will be seen in a reduction in the number of paretics admitted to asylums, for it takes that length of time for the insanity to develop. Moreover, since syphilis exists in spite of the fact that a prophylaxis has been available to prevent it now for twenty years past, it is improbable that all cases of syphilis will be treated even when venereal clinics are generally established. Before medical control becomes fully effective it will be necessary to overcome both the moral attitude toward syphilis and the ignorance of its consequences. Ignorance may be overcome by education, but moral attitudes are among the most deep-seated of the mores of a civilization and can be changed only slowly. Therefore cases of paresis will continue to occur for many years in spite of the fact that medical science has an entirely effective means of prevention.

Fortunately, another medical discovery has made it possible to arrest the progress of this form of insanity, although it cannot be cured completely any more than a scar can be removed with drugs. So far as the brain of the paretic is permanently damaged from the action of the spirochetes the changes are irremediable, but further scarring can be prevented. It has been found that when paretics are infected with malaria the paresis is largely arrested. The malaria can then be cured with quinine. Accordingly, paretics are now treated by giving them malaria and much improvement in their condition results. Recent researches show that it may be unnecessary to infect them with malaria, and that the same beneficial effect may be obtained with injections of proteins. The striking fact is, however, that paresis has been picked out from all other forms of insanity as the one for which there is an effective treatment.

As pointed out in a previous chapter, there are two means of controlling syphilis—the social and the medical. The social means has failed; it has nothing practical to offer to prevent prostitution and the immorality which maintains syphilis. On the other hand, the medical control of syphilis has reached a high state of development. If this control were fully accepted, syphilis could be eradicated. The results of this eradication, if less striking than the eradication of bubonic plague, would be as valuable to humanity.

Syphilis has been dealt with in this chapter and in a former chapter rather more extensively than other diseases for the reason that it illustrates in particular the fact that the medical sciences are today contributing actively to the advancement of civilization. The civilization toward which they lead is one of normal-bodied and hence normal-minded human beings with a reasonable expectation of life for useful and productive work.

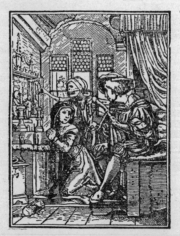

DEATH EXTINGUISHES THE FLAME OF ILLICIT LOVE
After a woodcut of Hans Holbein.

## CHAPTER XVII

### CIVILIZATION AND MEDICINE

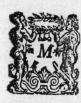 odern science has made the world, and particularly our cities, a far more convenient place in which to live than it was only a generation or two ago. The chemist, the physicist, and the engineer take a proper pride in the fact that their discoveries and inventions have facilitated travel and other forms of human activity and have enormously increased the production of wealth. The extent of the benefits that they have conferred upon civilization may be estimated by considering the difference that it would make to a city like New York or London if it were suddenly deprived of one or more of these inventions and discoveries. For example, suppose that electricity were abolished. The city would be in darkness, electric trains and elevators stopped, telephones and telegraph useless, the machinery in many factories still, and the streets empty of automobiles. If no substitute form of power could be found, civilization would go back half a century to the pre-electric days. Instead of New York and London as they now are these cities would become again the New York and London of 1875, with oil lamps, buildings only a few stories high and horse cars.

Yet, great as would be the inconvenience involved in the loss of electricity or any other product of physical science, the changes in the conditions of life would be small compared with those which would result from the loss of modern medical science.

Let us consider what would happen to New York or London or any other large city if it were deprived of the protection of medical science. Its civilization would go back not merely fifty years, it would go back five hundred years, if indeed the demoralization and panic at first produced did not destroy the city entirely. The result would not be confined to such inconvenience as the loss of electricity or steam or any of the other products of physical science would occasion. It would be a matter of life and death for the greater part of the inhabitants of every city, large and small. The pestilences would return. Epidemics would sweep across the country and within a decade the greater part of the population would have been wiped out. Even those advantages which we owe to the physical sciences and to engineering, instead of assisting in protection, would rather contribute to the spread of disease. Not only would great cities dwindle to a fraction of their present size, but in these disease-ridden towns the people would be sickly and generally short-lived. Large sections of the world which are now prosperous would become uninhabitable. Yellow fever would return to Panama and would block traffic through the canal. Such facilities for travel as the railroad, the steamship, and the airplane would spread disease with far greater rapidity than could the stagecoach or the sailing ship. If the measures of preventive medicine were lost, if drinking-water were no longer protected or purified, if the sanitary disposal of sewage were not practiced, and if vaccination were discontinued, every facility for rapid transportation would be equally effective for the rapid spread of disease. Indeed, the population of the country could continue only in sparse and separate communities connected by slow means of transportation. Diseases now almost forgotten would return to take their place with the existing pestilences. Leprosy would again spread, for the disease has foci in the United States. Surgery would be the rough wound surgery of the ancients. Aseptic obstetrics would be replaced by the medieval midwife or the hospital with an enormous death rate from puerperal fever. Dentistry would be confined to brutal extractions without anesthetics.

It is not mere imagination, but the cold and literal truth, to say that modern civilization and the use of the inventions and discoveries of physical science would be utterly impossible were it not for medical protection. This protection now ranks in importance scarcely behind that of food supply. When any large section of the country suffers from a flood or when a city is destroyed by an earthquake or a hurricane, the first call is for food. But immediately afterward comes the call for medical assistance and for such sanitary control as will prevent epidemic disease.

In spite of the fact that the benefits both of physical science and of medical science are vital to modern civilization, many people take quite different attitudes toward these two essentials. Nearly everyone realizes more or less distinctly the advantages accruing from the telephone, the automobile, the radio, and the airplane. Comparatively few, however, appreciate in equal degree the even greater dependence of civilization upon the service of medical science. The reason why one is appreciated and the other not is probably to be found in the fact that the contribution of the one is positive, and of the other negative. Yet, if a people without automobiles who were scourged with Asiatic cholera could take their choice of having automobiles or being freed from cholera, there can be little doubt which they would choose. On this ground we owe more to science for freeing us from cholera than for giving us automobiles. This is no fanciful comparison. Repeatedly during the nineteenth century Asiatic cholera spread over the United States and took a toll of thousands of lives. Throughout the nineteenth century in the Southern states of this country and in the seaports of the North yellow fever was a continual menace. Both pestilences have been eradicated in this country. But the man of the twentieth century fails to appreciate fully the benefit that he derives. He simply accepts it and forgets that these diseases ever existed here. He is oblivious to the idea that they could return. His appreciation of medical science is to a great extent limited to an ardent desire for the elimination of the diseases which still afflict mankind.

Unfortunately, in many cases the attitude toward medical science is not merely one involving a lack of enthusiasm and an indifference to benefits conferred, but is rather one of active opposition. The anti-vaccinationists, for instance, oppose one of the most essential and best proved measures of preventive medicine; and it is due to them that smallpox persists. The anti-vivisectionists oppose medical investigation both for the winning of new knowledge and for the application of knowledge already won. The adherents of cult-healing advocate the abolition of all medical science. Although they are a minority of the voting population, they are an active minority who take advantage of the indifference of the majority of our people. They continually introduce laws obstructing medical science and at every opportunity create difficulties for the legal maintenance of medical control. Through their activity the compulsory vaccination laws have already been repealed in two states, with the result that most of the smallpox in the United States is now found in these states. Unfortunately, smallpox does not respect state lines or remain where legislation favors it, but is carried into other states. The complete eradication of smallpox in the United States is thus prevented.

Many of the people who are opposed to medical science still cling to the ancient philosophies of primitive medicine which are deeply rooted in human character. They do not refuse all forms of healing; what they object to is the principle or philosophy of modern medicine. Such people accept and adapt themselves to the material conditions of modern life, which are the products of physical science, but they have not kept pace with the changing philosophies of modern life. They are merely savages riding in automobiles.

There are two philosophies of medicine: the primitive or superstitious, and the modern or rational. They are in complete opposition to one another. The former involves the belief that disease is caused by supernatural forces. Such a doctrine associates disease with sin; it is an aspect of religion which conceives diseases as due to certain forms of evil and attempts to control them by ceremonial and superstitious measures or to drive them away by wishful thinking. On the other hand, rational medicine is based on the conception that disease arises from natural causes; it associates sickness with ignorance. Civilized man tries to control the forces causing disease by material, not spiritualistic, means; he does not view disease as supernatural or the outcome of sin against moral laws, but rather as resulting from the violation of sanitary laws. He recognizes that knowledge is the sole means of preventing it. The measures he relies upon both to prevent and to cure disease are those which have resulted from scientific investigation and which have been proved to be effective by experience.

Primitive medicine is still the medicine of the inhabitants of many countries. Millions of people today, in time of illness, look to their priests and gods rather than to the health officer and medical science. To many people, even in civilized countries, there is something mysterious about disease. Rational medicine seeks to remove this element of mystery. But rational medicine is very recent in man's experience; it is a feature of advanced civilization, and civilization is new. Man has lived on the earth two or three million years, whereas even the beginnings of civilization date back only a few thousand years. For example, the Egyptian and Babylonian records show that only five thousand years ago human sacrifices were made by the priest-physicians to placate the angry gods of disease. The man of prehistoric times, only twenty-five thousand years ago, lived by hunting with stone knives and arrowheads. His medicine-man, as shown on page 294 of this book, made rough drawings on the walls of caves to drive away the evil spirits of disease. Now this prehistoric man is the ancestor of modern civilized man. Although we do not know his entire history, we do know his emotions and his reactions to the hazards of life. For, in spite of the fact that civilization has altered man's surroundings, it has not changed his essential nature. Modern man is still largely controlled by instinctive beliefs and impulses developed in primitive man a million years ago, and these instincts and impulses, with their accompanying emotions, are now embodied in the very structure of the human nervous system.

Educated men of today are merely primitive men who by intelligent effort and training have subjugated their instincts and emotions to reason. Children born of civilized peoples do not differ inherently from children born of primitive peoples. If the children of today were not educated and trained in the ways of civilization they would grow up like primitive men. Every child, during its first year or two, even in the most civilized home, is nothing more than an animal, a little beast. From this stage the child develops naturally into the state of a savage. His advancement from that point onward depends upon his training and education.

It is not surprising that rational medicine has opponents. Man's inherent nature is such that he has an almost intuitive belief in primitive medicine, and this intuition can be reformed only by education and reason. Many people, with a merely literary or religious education, have never learned to think logically in matters of health. They do not understand the principles of science, and are, therefore, controlled by sentiment and by opinions which are held tenaciously because they are matters of faith. In the same way savages, when brought into contact with civilization, may adopt some of its conveniences and many of its vices, but they do not adopt its religion or its medicine. They wear conventional clothing, eat canned food, and ride in automobiles, but they remain savages at heart. They hold to the philosophies of their ancestors and in secret are apt to make offerings to the evil spirits and consult the witch doctor.

Thus rational medicine involves the rejection of deeply rooted primitive beliefs. It is a development of civilization which better than any other measures man's intellectual advancement. When civilization progresses rational medicine largely replaces primitive medicine; when civilization deteriorates the opposite is true.

The transition from primitive to rational medicine is seen

in many ancient civilizations. The prophet Moses drew up a rational sanitary code for the Hebrews, but it is typical of the stage of civilization that the Jewish people had then reached that Moses built his sanitary code into their religion. Sanitation became a religious observance and the priests were sanitary police.

The ancient Greeks effected the first complete separation of medicine from religion. Prior to this separation Greek medical treatment was under religious control; Æsculapius was the god of healing. As medicine developed, the temples in which he was worshiped became sanatoria where the sick were cared for. The priests treated disease by such practical measures as rest and diet, but they wisely assumed no responsibility; they held that the will of the gods determined the success or failure of their treatment. In the fifth century before Christ a drastic reform in this temple cult of healing was brought about by Hippocrates, the greatest of all physicians. Under his guidance, medicine for the first time was separated from religion. He relieved the gods of the responsibility for disease and placed it squarely upon the shoulders of man. The will of the gods no longer served to cover man's ignorance; man's condition became man's problem and he must find the solution for himself. The history of medicine from Hippocrates to the present time is the record of the extent of man's acceptance of this responsibility.

Hippocrates did more than separate medicine from religion; he gave rational medicine the general form it holds today. He laid down certain principles of science upon which modern medicine is built. These principles are in substance:

1. There is no authority except facts.
2. Facts are obtained by accurate observation.
3. Deductions are to be made only from facts.

One of the aphorisms of Hippocrates has become part of the literature of all lands. It is opposed to dogma and mere opinion and says: "Life is short and art is long, the occasion fleeting, experience fallacious and judgment difficult." Hippocrates was modest because he recognized man's limitations, but he believed that man is capable of discovering the laws of nature by observation and unbiased reasoning.

Hippocrates was the first physician to differentiate diseases. Prior to his time all sickness was one great disease, and no significance was given to the varying symptoms; they were simply indicative of a single general abnormal condition. Hippocrates, however, recognized that certain symptoms were associated and that in patients with a particular association of symptoms the disease followed a different course from that in patients with another combination of symptoms. He realized, for instance, that a young man who was weak, whose pale and hollow cheeks showed a hectic flush, and whose gaunt frame was shaken by a racking cough was in no immediate danger of dying. Hippocrates saw that such a man would die slowly unless he went to the hills beyond the city and rested in the sunshine. Today physicians call the same condition tuberculosis and recommend the same treatment that Hippocrates prescribed. Again, Hippocrates perceived that a man with high fever, pain in the chest and delirium would not die slowly like the young man whom he had sent to the hills to recuperate, but would in all likelihood die within a few days or else abruptly start to recover. He prescribed, under those circumstances, cooling and nourishing drinks, fresh air, and rest in bed. The descriptions of diseases that Hippocrates has left were based on keen and careful observation; they stand today as models of their kind. After his time such accurate observations were not again made in medicine for eighteen centuries.

Hippocrates attempted to turn medical thought away from speculation and toward accurate observation and common sense. He said: "To know is one thing; merely to believe one knows is another. To know is science, but merely to believe one knows is ignorance." It was a difficult path that he pointed out for medicine to follow, since it involved intellectual honesty. Only the highest types of men have the intelligence, the independence, the honesty, and the courage to admit their errors and to seek without bias after the truth.

Hippocrates recorded his failures for the guidance of future physicians as freely as he did his successes.

Hippocrates lived in the period of the highest achievements of Greek intellect in art, literature, government, and science. He lived in the age of Pericles and but a short time before Plato and Aristotle. After this period civilization deteriorated, and the deterioration is shown most strikingly in the realm of medicine. The impetus given to medicine by Hippocrates carried it on for centuries, but as civilization declined this impetus was lost. Progress was hindered by speculations which displaced observation and clear reasoning. Physicians were divided into groups or schools which held different theories of disease and its treatment. These rival schools were more interested in making converts for their dogmas than they were in seeking honestly for the truth.

Three hundred years after Hippocrates, Corinth was destroyed and Greek medicine migrated to Rome. There in the person of Galen, who lived in the second century A.D., the medicine of Hippocrates was partially revived, but it was the last period of enlightenment for many centuries. Galen did not have the genius of Hippocrates, nor his clarity of thought and intellectual honesty. He was an active physician and an egotistical one. He did not record his medical failures, but only his successes, which were often clever and showy. Galen performed experiments, and therein lies his claim to medical distinction, but his work is overlaid with dogma and with theories derived from mere speculation. If the young man with tuberculosis had come to Galen instead of to Hippocrates, the simple truth would not have been told, nor would the simple treatment of rest in the sunshine have been prescribed. Galen would have made an elaborate diagnosis, and would have explained the disease according to his own speculative theory. He would have said that it belonged to the category of diseases with too much moisture and cold, a maladjustment of the humors. While he would have prescribed rest in the sunshine he would also have prescribed medicines concocted from many herbs. Such medicine was

intended to correct the coldness and moisture and to re-
adjust the humors. If the patient lived, Galen would have
given the credit to his medicaments and not to the rest and
sunshine.

Galen wrote voluminously on medical subjects; he spoke
with an impressive positiveness on matters on which neither
he nor any one else had any real knowledge; he thus disregarded the warning of Hippocrates that "to believe one
knows is ignorance." Sufficient knowledge had not then been
accumulated about the human body or its diseases to support
sound theories. Dissection of the human body was forbidden
among the Greeks and Romans. But Galen refused to admit
deficiency of knowledge and evolved elaborate theories which
gave plausible but usually erroneous explanations for every
phenomenon and specious answers to every question. His
writings obtained great authority and his theories became
dogmas. His extensive use of drugs and his beliefs about
disease became the orthodox medicine of subsequent centuries. They completely obscured the simple principles of
Hippocrates.

After Galen's time the Roman Empire declined. Even before Rome finally fell the deterioration of civilization was
rapid, likewise the deterioration of medicine. Physicians became more and more ignorant, dogmatic, and mercenary,
and the venders of quack remedies increased in number and
prominence. Dealers in magic, professional poisoners, and
courtesans who peddled drugs became familiar figures in
Rome. Medicine ceased altogether to be a science and became an affair of salves and poultices, talismans and spells.

When in the fifth century the Roman Empire fell at the
hands of the barbarians, rational medicine ceased altogether
in Europe. Although the Christian religion survived, the
Christian theology of that time denied liberty of conscience
and taught superstition and dogma. It was bitterly hostile to
the scientific spirit. All knowledge necessary to man's salvation, physical as well as spiritual, was to be found in the
Bible as the Church interpreted the Bible. Since the teachings of the Church were supposed to be sufficient for all

needs, there was no excuse for observations and experimental investigations. The inquisitive spirit was wholly suppressed, the rigorous methods of Greek logic were for many centuries lost from European civilization, and intelligent thought was replaced by revelation, speculation, tradition, and subservience to the written word of the Bible, to the writings of the saints, and later, in medical matters, to the work of Galen. The theological beliefs of the time became the controlling influence in Western civilization.

While men's minds were filled with thoughts of sin, death, judgment, and the after life, the health of the body was of little importance. The salvation of the soul was believed to be jeopardized by the body through so-called "sins of the flesh." The aim of the Christian Church for many centuries was the subordination of the body and perfection of the spirit. Physical health was despised, while disease and other "mortifications of the flesh" were considered to be means of purifying the soul. Like all earthly calamities, disease was the will of God. It was supernatural and its cure was to be effected by the exorcism of some evil spirit or by miracle. The whole responsibility for man's physical state was again placed upon the Deity and men were instructed to accept their lot in resignation. The Middle Ages, which some modern writers profess to admire, were in reality times of low civilization: the proof of this fact is that medicine reverted to its primitive state.

If the young man with tuberculosis, whose treatment at the hands of Hippocrates and of Galen has been already described, had sought treatment during the early Middle Ages, he would not have been told to rest in the sunshine or even to take medicine. He would have been told to fast, pray, repent of his sins, and prepare to die—and he would have died.

While, from a worldly aspect, the theological beliefs of these times were impractical, they nevertheless had elements of idealistic beauty. The idealism led to the founding of orphan asylums and hospitals. But the impracticability and "other-worldliness" of the Middle Ages prevented effective treatment of the diseases of the inmates. Such hospitals were merely dark, crowded, and unsanitary places of refuge for the needy and sick, who received no rational medical attention.

There were intellectual efforts in the Middle Ages, but men "in seeking a heavenly home lost their bearings upon earth." Such men left unsurpassed architectural achievements, the medieval cathedrals, and founded a number of universities. But the subjects taught in these universities were dialectics, moral science, and theology, with very little natural science and no scientific experiments. Never in all history were cities as filthy and the people as disease-ridden as they were in the Middle Ages. Even with a very high birth rate the sparse population found it difficult to maintain its numbers against the inroads of disease. As late as the fifteenth century the population of all Europe was equal only to that of the British Isles today.

The scientific spirit of the Greeks was not, however, entirely dead; from the eighth to the eleventh century the Arabs advanced in civilization, and, as seems always the case in an advancing civilization, they adopted rational medicine. Science flourished among them and reached a dignity and importance which contrasted strongly with its degradation among Europeans. By the commencement of the seventh century Christianity had spread eastward almost to China. By the end of that century the Arabs had swept from Arabia through the eastern Roman Empire and over Egypt, North Africa, and Spain. The fate of western Europe hung in the balance until the Arabs were defeated in the battle of Tours in 732. The Arabs made war in barbarous fashion; they destroyed the great library of Alexandria. But after their conquest they adopted intellectual pursuits. They became interested particularly in the medicine of the Greeks and Romans and translated the manuscripts of Galen into Arabic. Within two centuries Arabic medicine had developed to a high level. Something of the Greek fervor for fact and truth is found in the writings of the Arabic physicians, Rhazes and Avicenna, but the Arabs did not attain to the principles of Hippocrates. They stopped with the theories of Galen. Like the Greeks, they made no dissections of the body.

Arabic medicine was brought back to western Europe by crusaders returning from Palestine in the thirteenth and fourteenth centuries. Europe thus obtained a garbled version of the theories of Galen. These theories were accepted and adhered to with religious veneration, for all knowledge then rested on authority. New facts were, therefore, not sought and any new observation was rejected.

Revival of the principles of Hippocrates began in the sixteenth century during the renaissance of European civilization. At first the efforts were without definite aim; an occasional independent thinker revolted against the ancient authorities and made observations for himself. The keynote of this revolt was struck by Paracelsus, but speculation and obscurantism had so blinded men's eyes that he fell into the same errors that he abused. He was a physician who sought after the truth, but he lived at a time when to stray from the beaten path of authorized knowledge was heresy for which the innovator might be burned at the stake. Nevertheless, he struck out boldly for the right to observe facts for himself and for the right of individual judgment. To show his disregard for the ancient dogmas he burned the works of Galen and Avicenna publicly. But he could not wholly escape the mental habits of his time and his own observations are obscured by fanciful speculations. His writings are now more often quoted in the literature of mysticism than in that of medicine. His bold example, however, started men to thinking independently in regard to medical problems.

Out of this new-found independence of thought came the revival of the scientific spirit, the search for facts and careful observation. Vesalius was the leader of this movement in the sixteenth century. He made the first systematic dissection of the human body and published drawings of great accuracy. The works of Hippocrates were then translated for the first time. The ligature was reintroduced into surgery and podalic version into midwifery by Paré. A book of instructions for midwives was published, the first book of its kind in thirteen centuries.

In the seventeenth century the revival of the scientific spirit was so extended by a few able men that experiments were used to prove facts and their relations. The chief advancement of this period was the demonstration of the circulation of the blood by Harvey, but even his genius for experiment had difficulty in overcoming the persistent belief of the time in the theories of Galen.

By the beginning of the eighteenth century physicians had obtained a knowledge of the general structure of the body and of the action of some of the principal organs. Certain remedies had been discovered by chance, notably quinine for malaria and mercury for syphilis. Medicine, however, had not yet emerged from obscurantism. There was no real knowledge of what disease is or how it is caused. Instead of returning to the simple methods of Hippocrates and making careful observations, most of the physicians still preferred to speculate on the cause of disease and to treat their patients according to theories evolved from their speculations.

In the beginning of the eighteenth century a physician named Morgagni revived in full the Hippocratic principles. Just as Hippocrates by careful observation and reasoning had been able to differentiate the external appearances of the diseases, so Morgagni by careful observation and reasoning was able to show the changes in the internal organs of the body. Hippocrates recognized that tuberculosis and pneumonia were different diseases because a different association of symptoms occurred, but he knew these diseases only through their symptoms. Morgagni, on the other hand, demonstrated the nature of the damage to the body which was the disease itself and which gave rise to the symptoms. He observed and recorded the symptoms of his patients during illness and then made post-mortem examinations to find the derangements in the organs which had occasioned the symptoms. He thus showed that a certain pathological state results in certain symptoms. He was then able by merely observing symptoms to visualize the derangement inside the body and to estimate its extent. The principle established is the basis of all clinical medicine.

In the eighteenth century modern medicine was beginning to take shape under the revival of the scientific spirit. Morgagni's work was the first general advance; soon afterward came one of the greatest single discoveries—vaccination against smallpox. There is no briefer or better statement of the principles of Hippocrates than that of John Hunter. When Jenner came to him and said that he thought he could prevent smallpox by vaccination, Hunter replied: "Don't think; try; be patient, be accurate."

Except in respect to smallpox, medicine had really made little *practical* progress in the treatment or prevention of diseases up to the beginning of the nineteenth century. During the first four decades of the nineteenth century scientific facts were accumulated, methods were developed and the spirit of investigation and observation widely extended. In these forty years Laënnec discovered auscultation, the method of listening with a stethoscope and determining abnormalities in the lungs and heart by the nature of the sounds elicited; John Bright described the disease of the kidneys, nephritis, which is often called Bright's disease; Pinel introduced humane treatment of the insane. Scarpa described arteriosclerosis, the hardening of the arteries usually associated with high blood pressure; Louis founded medical statistics, the only really final test of treatment; and Claude Bernard showed the immense possibilities of experimental medicine and created modern physiology. Although medicine advanced greatly as a science during this period, the advances were of no immediate benefit to the patient. Practical results did not appear until the last sixty years of the nineteenth century. The greatest benefits that medical science has given to mankind have come within the lifetime of men still living.

The first of these benefits was anesthesia, which made surgical operations painless. It was one of the most humane discoveries of mankind.

Next, in 1847, the greatest hazard of childbirth was brought under control. Semmelweis, after years of painstaking observation, demonstrated the contagious nature of puerperal fever. The number of mothers saved and the amount of invalidism prevented since that time reach an enormous total.

Soon afterward the teaching of nurses began; it has given us the modern trained nurse. No practical advance ever made in medicine has brought greater comfort to the sick person than this innovation of Florence Nightingale.

In 1867 the antiseptic principle was introduced into surgery. Modern surgery thus started with the work of Lister. His results were obtained by observation and reason; he perceived that simple fractures of bones healed without the formation of pus, whereas in all other wounds pus was regularly present. He then reasoned that since the only difference between the injuries was that one was exposed to the air and the other not, something from the air caused the formation of pus. Pasteur at about this time had demonstrated that putrefaction in wine resulted from contamination with bacteria from the air. Lister concluded that infection in wounds was analogous to putrefaction in wine, and he applied to the wounds substances—antiseptics—to destroy the infection. Later it was recognized that the infection came not from the air, but from the dirty hands and instruments of the surgeon, and antiseptic surgery was largely replaced by aseptic surgery.

A few years after Lister's work the bacterial cause of infectious diseases was established. Pasteur, by the painstaking application of principles of science, laid the foundation for the preventive medicine and sanitation which are now part of civilization and which, if developed to the fullest extent, will result in the eventual eradication of all infectious diseases.

The medical sciences are today giving the world the healthiest period it has ever known, but they are not yet mature. What has already been accomplished in scientific medicine is small in comparison with future possibilities of preventing disease, alleviating suffering, and prolonging human life. But there is no assurance that these possibilities will ever be realized. In this matter man literally controls his own destiny. Medical science can exist and advance only so long as the scientific spirit survives. The survival of the scientific spirit is dependent upon advancing civilization. Civilization, in turn, is, in the light of history, a very uncertain process, prone to regress as well as to advance. No doubt

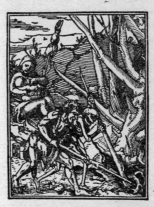

THE CONSEQUENCES OF MAN'S FALL
A woodcut by Hans Holbein.

the Romans of the "golden age" thought that their civilization was stable; yet within a few centuries it passed into the degradation of the Middle Ages.

Recognition of facts and honest deductions are not natural to the human mind. The primitive instincts are for emotion and loose imaginings. The danger to the scientific spirit, to the advance of medicine, and to the integrity of civilization does not come from the masses of unthinking people. This danger comes from intelligent people who play a part in shaping civilization but who have not been educated to think rationally; it comes from sentimental and idle people in whom the primitive instinct escapes from repression and rises to prevent thought. They revive the religious healing cults of the primitive peoples, but with modernized form and terminology; or they join forces with the anti-vivisectionists and revel in the contemplation of cruelties which exist only in their imaginations.

Medicine and civilization advance and regress together. The conditions essential to advance are intellectual courage and a true love for humanity. It is as true today as always in the past that further advance or even the holding of what has already been won depends upon the extent to which intellectual courage and humanity prevail against bigotry and obscurantism.

# INDEX

Abortion, among primitive peoples, 26
  in Middle Ages, 26-27
  to avoid difficult childbirth, 64
Accoucheurs, 45
Adams, John, 239
Adam's missing rib, 134
Æsclepieia, 15
Æsculapius, 15, 405
Agattin, Saint, 225
Agrippina, 22
Albertus Magnus, 27
Alexander VI, 254
Alexander the Great, 372
Anatomical dissection, approved by Church, 153
  edicts against, 147
  in Middle Ages, 147
  opposition to, 159
Anatomical knowledge of Babylonians, 133
  of Egyptians, 132-133
  of Greeks, 134
  of Jews, 134
Anatomical material, scarcity of, 155-156
Anatomical teaching in Colonial America, 156-161
Anatomy, founded by Vesalius, 149-154
  laws, 159, 161
  murders of Scotland, 161 et seq.
Anemia, pernicious, 374-375
Anesthesia, benefits described by Hayden, 101-104
  demonstration of, 97, 103-104
  dentistry, 103
  for childbirth, 96 et seq.
    situation today, 126. See also Twilight sleep

Anesthesia—(Continued)
  nature of, 97
  origin of name, 105
  spinal, 128-129
Anesthetics, first used, 101
  origin of name, 105
  See also, Chloroform, Ether, Narcotics, Nitrous oxide, Soporific potions
Animal magnetism, 321
  malicious, 326-327
Anne, Queen, and royal touch, 307
  as favoring quacks, 52-53
  death of, 141
Anne de Beaupré, Saint, 314
Anthrax, 379-380
Antimony, controversy over, 366-367
  introduction of, 366
  popularization of by Louis XIV, 123
Antiseptics, introduced by Lister, 176 et seq.
Antivaccinationists, 241, 402
Antivivisectionists, 416
Antoninus Pius, Emperor, 16
Aphrodisiacs, 98
Apollo, 15-16
Apollonia, Saint, 225
Apothecaries, in medical practice, 360
  in Middle Ages, 357-358
Apothecary shops, founding of, 357
Appliance cures, 334-335
Aquinas, Thomas, 204
Arabian medicine, 411
Arabian surgery, 168
Aseptic surgery, 181
Asafetida bag, 195

# POCKET BOOK BEST SELLERS

*Are there any you have missed? Of the more than 300 Pocket Book titles that have been published to date, these are the outstanding favorites:*